Clinical Orthopaedic Examination

Ronald McRae FRCS (Eng, Glas) AIMBI

With original drawings by the author

FOURTH EDITION

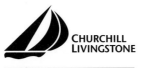

CHURCHILL
LIVINGSTONE

NEW YORK EDINBURGH LONDON MADRID MELBOURNE SAN FRANCISCO
TOKYO 1997

CHURCHILL LIVINGSTONE
Medical Division of Pearson Professional Ltd

Distributed in the United States of America by
Churchill Livingstone Inc., 650 Avenue of the
Americas, New York, N.Y. 10011, and by associated
companies, branches and representatives throughout
the world.

First edition 1976
Second edition 1983
Third edition 1990
Fourth edition 1997

ISBN 0 443 056021
International edition ISBN 0 443 058121

British Library Cataloguing in Publication Data
A catalogue record for this book is available
from the British Library.

Library of Congress Cataloging in Publication Data
A catalog record for this book is available from the
Library of Congress.

Medical knowledge is constantly changing. As new
information becomes available, changes in treatment,
procedures, equipment and the use of drugs become
necessary. The author and the publishers have, as far
as it is possible, taken care to ensure that the
information given in this text is accurate and up to
date. However, readers are strongly advised to
confirm that the information, especially with regard
to drug usage, complies with current legislation and
standards of practice.

Produced by Longman Singapore Publishers (Pte) Ltd
Printed in Singapore

Preface

The ability to make a good clinical examination can only be mastered by practice, and I have no doubt that the basic techniques are best learned by performance under supervision. Unfortunately the size of student classes in relation to teaching staff and the not infrequent dearth of an adequate range of suitable clinical cases make this ideal difficult to achieve in practice. Many students may acquire only a sketchy knowledge of the techniques of examination which are fundamental to diagnosis and treatment. It is hoped that this book may help to fill some of these inevitable gaps until sound practice based on experience is achieved.

The text

It is assumed that the value of good history-taking is appreciated and practised.

Patients parade their complaints on an anatomical basis, and the text has been arranged accordingly. The emphasis in each section is on the common rather than the rare conditions to be found in the region. Although this approach is open to criticism, it is nevertheless true to say that while the obscure will tax the most experienced, the most frequent mistake is a failure to diagnose the common. An encyclopaedic text, commendable on the ground of completeness, may nevertheless often confuse, especially where no indication is given of the incidence of the conditions observed. I have purposely avoided detail, and where this is required a fuller orthopaedic textbook must be consulted. In some areas too I have made deliberate simplifications where a blight of terminology suggests the independence of a number of conditions which cannot be distinguished by symptomatology or investigation.

The illustrations

The illustrations dealing with the practical aspects of clinical examination have been arranged in an essentially linear sequence following the traditional lines of inspection, palpation, and the examination of movements and pertinent anatomical structures. In practice, this logical order is often altered by the experienced examiner to avoid undue movement of the patient. It must be stressed that not all the tests described need be carried out routinely. Many are performed only when a specific condition is suspected, and it is assumed that this will be obvious to the reader. In particular, in any joint assessment, it is necessary to discover if there is any restriction of movement. In many cases simple screening tests will suffice, and these are highlighted in most sections.

The more detailed examination and recording of movement are generally reserved for cases under lengthy continuous observation and for medico-legal work.

Radiographic examination plays an essential part in the investigation of most orthopaedic cases, and to aid the inexperienced I have made some observations regarding the views normally taken and how they may be interpreted. Only a fraction of the possible pathology can be illustrated in a small work, but I have concentrated on the common or informative.

The spatial requirements of the captions have set some restriction on their content; this discipline has resulted in brevity at the expense in places of completeness. Nevertheless, wherever possible I have tried to show not only how each test should be carried out, but also its significance.

An appreciable number of changes have been made in this fourth edition: these include a number of additional tests and the inclusion of more anatomical detail to aid interpretation. The text has been updated and re-organised throughout, and there are a number of additions. I have also included a readily accessible summary of joint movements. I hope that these new features will contribute to the usefulness of this work.

Conventions and references

Where two limbs are illustrated, the pathology is shown on the patient's right side.

Where several conditions are described, and one representative illustration only is given, it refers to the first condition mentioned.

Cross references refer to the illustration number in the appropriate section. They are given thus: (chapter number, illustration number).

When joint movements are being considered, the patient's normal side should if possible be used for comparison. Angular measurement is an approximation, and the figures quoted are in most cases values rounded to the nearest five degrees from figures published by the American Academy of Orthopedic Surgeons[1], Kapandji[2], Lusted & Keats[3] or Boone & Azen[4].

Abbreviations

L & R = left and right.
L & M = lateral and medial.
A & P = anterior and posterior.
N   = normal.

References

1. American Academy of Orthopedic Surgeons 1965. Joint motion: method of measuring and recording. Churchill Livingstone, Edinburgh
2. Kapandji A 1974 The physiology of the joints. Churchill Livingstone, Edinburgh
3. Lusted L B, Keats T E 1972 Atlas of roentgenographic measurement. Year Book Medical Publishers, London
4 Boone C D, Azen P S 1979 Normal range of motion of joints in male subjects. Journal of Bone and Joint Surgery 61A/5: 756–759

Gourock, 1997   R. McR.

Contents

1. General principles in the examination of a patient with an orthopaedic problem

In practice, the primary area of interest of the orthopaedic surgeon is in the joints of the limbs and spine, and how well they function. The major part of most orthopaedic examinations is therefore centred on the joint that troubles the patient, but the examination must often be extended to include the nerves and muscles which are responsible for movements in the joint; and some of the patient's other joints may also have to be checked to see if they are affected as well.

Joints possess a remarkable degree of individuality, and it follows that the techniques for examining one joint may have to be varied when it comes to looking at another. However, a common sequence is followed and it may be helpful to keep it in mind. (It is assumed that a full, relevant history has been obtained, and any general physical examination has been carried out.) The examination of the joint itself may be broken down into six distinct steps:

1. Inspection.
2. Palpation.
3. Examination of movements.
4. Conduction of special tests.
5. Examination of radiographs.
6. Arrangement of further investigations.

It is not always necessary to keep strictly to this order or indeed to carry out all of these procedures.

The contents of each section of this book are generally ordered in this sequence unless special circumstances dictate otherwise.

Step 1 Inspection

Look carefully at the joint, paying particular attention to the following points:

1. Is there swelling? If so, is the swelling *diffuse* or *localised*? If the swelling is diffuse, does it seem confined to the joint or does it extend beyond the joint? *Swelling confined to the joint* suggests distension of the joint with (a) excess synovial fluid (effusion), e.g. from trauma or a non-pyogenic inflammatory process (such as rheumatoid arthritis or osteoarthritis) or (b) blood (haemarthrosis), e.g. from recent acute injury or a blood coagulation defect, or (c) pus (pyarthrosis), e.g. from an acute pyogenic infection. *Swelling extending beyond the confines of the joint* may occur with major infections in a limb, tumours, and problems of lymphatic and venous drainage.

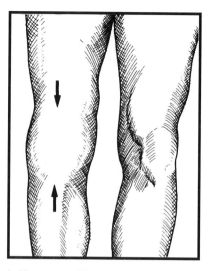

1. Note any swelling confined to the joint.

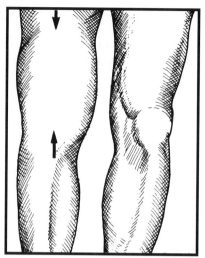

2. Note any swelling extending beyond the joint.

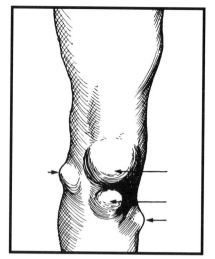

3. Note any localised swelling.

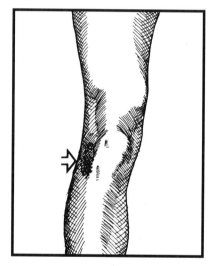

4. Note any bruising or oedema.

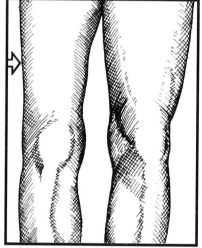

5. Note any muscle wasting.

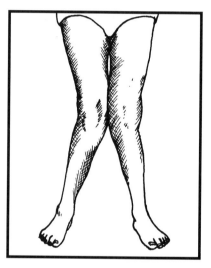

6. Note any alteration of posture or shape.

If there is a localised swelling, note its position in relation to the underlying anatomical structures, as this may give a clue to its possible nature or identity.

2. Is there bruising? This might suggest trauma, with a point of impact or gravitational or other spread.

3. Is there any other discoloration, or oedema? This might occur as a localised response to trauma or infection.

4. Is there muscle wasting? This usually occurs as a result of disuse from pain or incapacity, or from denervation of the muscles affected.

5. Is there any alteration in shape or posture, or is there evidence

of shortening? There are many possible causes for each of these abnormalities (including congenital abnormalities, past trauma, disturbances of bone mineralisation and destructive joint disease); their presence should be noted, and explored in further detail during the course of the examination.

Step 2 Palpation

Some of the points which you should note include the following:

1. Is the joint warm? If so, note whether the temperature increase is diffuse or localised, always bearing in mind the false impression which may be caused by the effects of local bandaging. A *diffuse* increase in heat occurs when a substantial tissue mass is involved, and is seen most commonly in joints involved in pyogenic and non-pyogenic inflammatory processes, and anastomotic dilatation proximal to an arterial block. Away from the joints themselves, infection and tumour should be kept in mind. A *localised* increase in temperature generally pinpoints an inflammatory process in the underlying anatomical structure. Asymmetrical *coldness* of a limb commonly occurs where the limb circulation is impaired, e.g. from atherosclerosis.

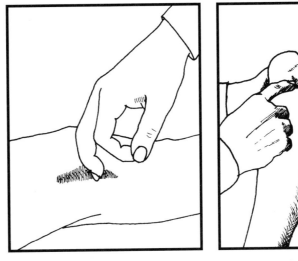

7. Note any increased local heat.

8. Note any tenderness, and whether localised or diffuse.

2. Is there tenderness? If so, note if it is diffuse or localised. Where tenderness is *diffuse*, the cause is likely to be the same as for an increase in local heat. When there is *localised* tenderness, the site of maximal tenderness should be assiduously sought, as this may clearly identify the underlying anatomical structure which is involved.

Step 3 Examination of movements

Most, but not all, orthopaedic conditions are associated with some

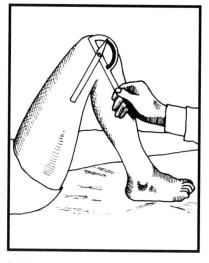

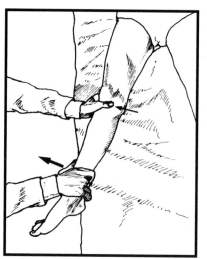

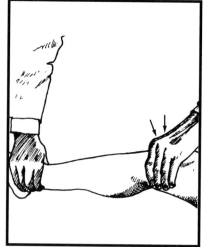

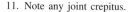

9. Measure the range of movements, and record any fixed deformities.

10. Test for movements in abnormal planes.

11. Note any joint crepitus.

restriction of movements in the related joint(s). Complete loss of movements follows surgical ablation of a joint (arthrodesis), or may occur in the course of some pathological process (such as infection) where fibrous or bony tissue binds the articular surfaces together (fibrous or bony ankylosis); the joint then cannot be moved either actively or passively. In many conditions there is loss of that part of the range of movements which allows the joint to be brought into its neutral position. The commonest loss of this type prevents the joint from being fully extended; this is known as a fixed flexion deformity. *Fixed deformities* may be caused, for example, by the contraction of joint capsules, muscles and tendons, or by the interposition of soft tissues or bone between the articular surfaces (e.g. torn menisci, loose bodies). Estimation of *the range of movements in the joint* is an essential part of any orthopaedic examination. To assess any deviation from normal the good side may be compared with the bad. Where this is not suitable (e.g. when both sides are involved) resort must be made to published figures of calculated average ranges. *Restriction of the range of movements in a joint* is nearly always due to mechanical causes and is consequently a sure indicator of pathology. If the muscles controlling a joint are paralysed, then the *passive range of movements* must be assessed; occasionally pain or other factors may restrict the *active range of movements* to a range less than the passive. Sometimes a partly or totally paralysed joint can be persuaded to move by invoking gravity or movement elsewhere (*trick movements*), and the confirmation of paralysis generally begs the determination of its cause.

In many joints it is also mandatory to look for evidence of *movements in an abnormal plane*. To do this the joint is generally stressed in a particular plane and excessive movements assessed by inspection or by the examination of radiographs. Other accompaniments of movement may require assessment. Rough articular surfaces will produce grating sensations (*crepitus*) when the joint is moved, and this may be detected by palpation or auscultation. *Clicks coming from the joint on movement* may be produced through soft tissues moving over bony prominences (generally of little importance), from soft tissues within the joint (e.g. displaced menisci), or from disturbances in bony contours (e.g. from irregularities in a joint surface following a fracture involving the joint).

The strength of muscle contraction (and hence the strength of each joint movement) must be carefully assessed, and especially if found reduced, recorded on the Medical Research Council (MRC) scale:

M0 — No active contraction can be detected.

M1 — A flicker of muscle contraction can be seen or found by palpation over the muscle, but the activity is insufficient to cause any joint movement.

M2 — Contraction is very weak, but can just produce movement so long as the weight of the part can be countered by careful positioning of the limb.

M3 — Contraction is still very weak, but can produce movement against gravitational resistance (e.g. the quadriceps being able to extend the knee with the patient in a sitting position).

M4 — Strength is not full, but can produce movement against gravity and added resistance.

M5 — Normal power is present.

Muscle strength may be impaired by pain or wasting from disuse, disease or denervation. Finally, attention should be paid to any impairment of overall function in the affected limb as a result of disturbance of movement or muscle power. In the case of the legs, this implies an assessment of *the gait*. Many tests are available to detect disturbance of separate aspects of upper limb function.

Step 4 Conduction of special tests

For most joints there are a number of specific tests developed especially to test some particular aspect of that joint's function. These include tests for the integrity of certain joint ligaments, and for the examination of structures associated with the joint (e.g. the menisci in the knee). Of particular importance is an appropriate neurological examination (e.g. the testing of specific muscle groups and the determination of any sensory loss). When applicable, the MRC gradings of motor and sensory recovery should be recorded. The latter is as follows:

S0 — Absence of all modalities of sensation in the area exclusively supplied by the affected nerve.

S1 — Recovery of deep pain sensation.

S2 — Recovery of protective sensation (skin touch, pain and thermal sensation).

S3 — Recovery of protective sensation with accurate localisation. Sensitivity, and hypersensitivity, to cold are usual.

S3+ — Recovery of ability to recognise objects and texture; any residual cold sensitivity and hypersensitivity should now be minimal. In

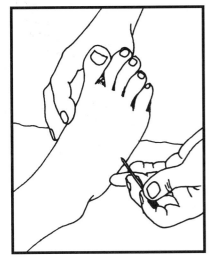

12. Test for sensory loss and any other neurological defect.

the case of the hand, recovery of two-point discrimination to less than 8 mm.

S4   — Normal sensation.

Step 5 Examination of radiographs

Someone experienced in looking at radiographs will recognise the main pathology at a glance without following any analytical procedure, just as a familiar face is identified without apparently paying conscious attention to the relative position and size of its main features. Until such skills are developed, it may be helpful for the student to have some simple scheme to follow. One such is to look at each radiograph as though in the cinematic sequence of long shot, medium shot and close-up. In the long (wide angle) shot a scene is established, and the overall relationship of the important features is made clear. Start by looking at the radiograph in a general, unfocused way, as though you were standing well back from it. Ask yourself the following questions:

1. Are the bones of normal shape, size and contour, or are they thicker or thinner than normal, shorter or longer than usual or abnormally curved or angled?
2. At the joints themselves, are the bony components in correct alignment, or are they displaced or angled?

Looking a little more closely, note if the bone texture appears normal or disturbed, such as in osteoporosis, Paget's disease, avascular necrosis, osteopetrosis etc. Note if there are any areas of new bone formation, such as exostoses, subperiosteal new bone formation etc. Note if there are any areas of bone destruction such as may be found in the presence of many tumours.

Examination of the bone in close-up may be done in two ways: either methodically trace round the contours of the bone noting any abnormality en route, or go through a check list of your own making. Check lists can have different bases, and can be used in combination. A list may be based on *pathology*: you might then look for evidence of congenital abnormality, infection (or an inflammatory process), trauma, neoplasm, metabolic disturbance, degeneration. Alternatively, a list may have an *anatomical* base: you might then assess ligament attachments, joint margins, the joint space and the cortical and cancellous bone elements.

Step 6 Arranging further investigations

This last stage is not always required, but the indications are usually quite clear. The clinical and radiological examination may have resulted in a differential diagnosis which requires additional tests to allow a firm diagnosis to be made; in many cases the additional tests serve to confirm a strong impression. Occasionally clinical examination fails to clarify the problem, and one remains baffled by the cause of the complaint. Further investigation may hopefully throw some light on the situation, perhaps indicating an area which should be concentrated upon, or suggesting that temporisation and observation may be embarked upon with safety, or occasionally suggesting that some at least of the complaint may have a functional basis.

The commonest screening tests include the following:

1. Erythrocyte sedimentation rate (ESR).
2. Full blood count with differential.
3. Latex fixation test.
4. Serum calcium, phosphate and alkaline phosphatase.
5. Serum uric acid.
6. X-ray of chest.

Equipment requirements

The special tools required for examining the patient with an orthopaedic complaint are of a modest character. Four are desirable:

1. A tape measure (preferable of the type used by tailors), for measuring such things as limb lengths and girths (for evidence of inequality in length or evidence of muscle wasting), and sometimes for assessing movement (e.g. in the spine, knee and rib cage).
2. A goniometer, preferably with an easily read scale with reciprocals, for measuring the range of movements in a joint.
3. A tendon hammer, for eliciting limb reflexes.
4. A disposable sharp point (by default a hypodermic needle), fresh for each case, for assessing any disturbance of sensation to pinprick.

2. Segmental and peripheral nerves of the upper limb

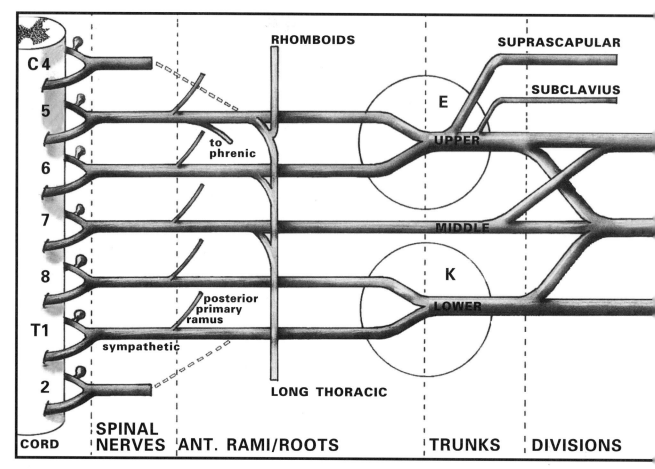

Fig. 2.A

The brachial plexus: cervical part

The *roots* of the brachial plexus are formed by the anterior primary rami of C5–T1 inclusive, with occasional contributions from C4 and T2. The roots lie between the scalene muscles in the neck. (Do not confuse the roots of the *plexus* with the roots of the *segmental spinal nerves*, which are intra-thecal.) C5 and C6 form the *upper trunk*; C7 forms the *middle trunk*; and C8 and T1 form the *lower trunk*. (Pre-ganglionic sympathetic nerve fibres to the upper limb arise from T2–T6, ascend in the sympathetic trunk, synapse in cervico-thoracic ganglia, and pass to the upper limb mainly through the lower trunk of the plexus. An important localising point to note is that pre-ganglionic fibres en route to the eye via the stellate ganglion arise from T1.) The trunks are found in the posterior triangle of the neck. The subclavian artery lies in front of the lower trunk.

Each trunk forms an anterior and posterior division. The *divisions* lie behind the clavicle. The three posterior divisions form the *posterior cord*; the anterior divisions of the upper and middle trunks form the *lateral cord*; and the anterior division of the lower trunk continues as the *medial cord*. The divisions and commencement of the cords lie in the posterior triangle of the neck.

The brachial plexus has a most extensive distribution, and the order in which the nerves come off is of value in determining the site of any lesion. This is of particular importance in traumatic lesions where the prognosis and treatment are closely related to the level of injury.

Branches from nerve roots. *The first branches* of the plexus to be given off arise from the nerve roots themselves. Two important branches in this category are:

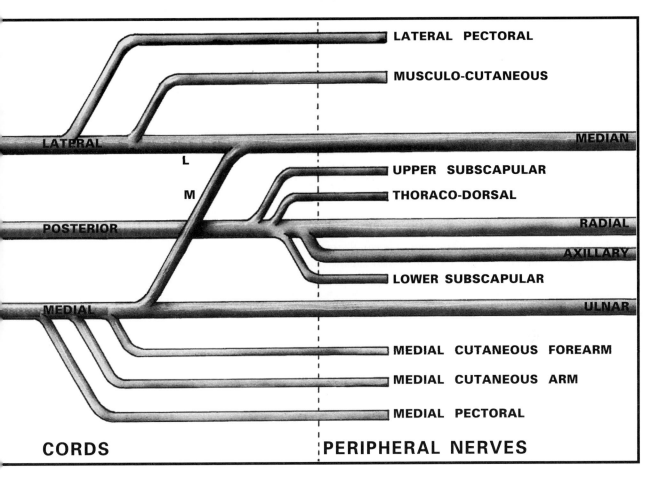

1. The nerve to the rhomboids (dorsal scapular nerve). It arises from the C5 root alone.
2. The nerve to serratus anterior (long thoracic nerve). It has contributions from C5, 6 and 7. Its most proximal part arises in conjunction with the nerve to rhomboids.

C5 also contributes to the phrenic nerve, and C5, 6, 7 and 8 supply the scalenes and longus colli. Although not strictly branches of the brachial plexus, these segmental branches are of some importance; paralysis of the hemidiaphragm, when found after a brachial plexus injury, indicates a proximal lesion.

Branches from the trunks. There are two branches only at this level:

1. The suprascapular nerve is important, supplying the supraspinatus and infraspinatus.
2. The nerve to subclavius: this is of little clinical significance.

Both these nerves arise from the upper trunk. All the branches from the nerve roots and trunks arise above the clavicle (the supraclavicular branches).

Note: 1. In Erb's (upper obstetrical) palsy (E) the C5–6 roots are affected, but the nerve to rhomboids and the long thoracic nerve are spared. 2. In Klumpke's (lower obstetrical) palsy (K) the C8–T1 roots are involved. The sympathetic nerve supply to the eye (arising from T1) is often also affected, leading to a Horner's syndrome. It was said that 80% of birth injuries to the plexus make a full recovery by 13 months, and persisting severe sensory or motor deficits in the hand are rare; recent work suggests that this view is somewhat optimistic. Note that a number of obstetrical injuries to the plexus are accompanied by facial nerve palsy and posterior dislocation of the shoulder. 3. In traumatic plexus lesions in adults, the commonest patterns of injury are (a) C5–6 (Erb type); (b) C5, 6, 7; (c) C5–T1 inclusive.

The brachial plexus: axillary part

The cords for the most part lie in the axilla, and are closely related to the axillary artery. (The axillary artery commences at the outer border of the first rib, and ends at the lower border of teres major. The second part of the axillary artery lies behind the pectoralis minor, with the first and third parts of the artery lying above and below it. The three cords enter the axilla above the first part, embrace the second part in the position indicated by their names, and give off their branches around the third part.)

Branches from the cords.

The lateral cord (C5, 6, 7). This gives off the following branches:

1. The lateral pectoral (which supplies pectoralis major).
2. The musculo-cutaneous (which supplies coraco-brachialis and biceps).
3. The lateral root of the median nerve.

The medial cord (C8, T1). This gives off:

1. The medial pectoral nerve (which supplies pectoralis major).
2. The medial cutaneous nerve of the arm (which supplies the skin over the front and the medial side of the arm).
3. The medial cutaneous nerve of the forearm (which supplies the skin over the lower part of the arm and the medial side of the forearm).
4. The medial root of the median nerve.
5. The ulnar nerve. (In 90% of cases the ulnar nerve receives a branch (C6, 7) from the lateral cord.)

The posterior cord (C5, 6, 7, 8, T1). This gives off:

1. The upper subscapular nerve (C5, 6) (which partly supplies subscapularis).
2. The lower subscapular nerve (C5, 6) (which supplies subscapularis and teres major).
3. The thoraco-dorsal nerve (C6, 7, 8) (which supplies latissimus dorsi).
4. The radial nerve (C5, 6, 7, 8, T1).
5. The axillary nerve (C5, 6).

Details of the most important branches (median, ulnar, radial, axillary) are given later.

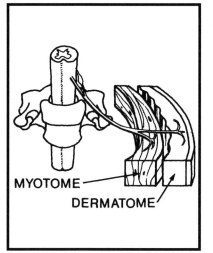

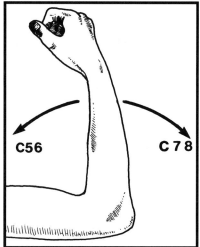

1. *Segmental distribution:* Where you suspect involvement of spinal nerves rather than peripheral nerves (e.g. injuries to the spine or brachial plexus, cervical spondylosis etc.) you must examine myotomes and dermatomes. These are the muscle masses and areas of skin supplied by single spinal nerves (no matter how the nerve fibres within these spinal nerves are finally distributed via the limb plexuses and peripheral nerves).

2. *Myotomes* (1): Normally two roots produce movement of a joint in one direction, and two in another. This is true at the elbow where weakness of elbow flexion and an absent biceps tendon jerk indicate C5, 6 involvement; and where weakness of extension and an absent triceps jerk suggest a C7, 8 lesion. This general rule is followed throughout the lower limb, but is modified in the highly specialised upper limb.

3. *Myotomes* (2): In a distal or proximal joint, the four spinal segments involved differ by plus or minus one so that theoretically the shoulder should be controlled by C4, 5, 6, 7. However, C4 has been suppressed, with the result that abduction is mediated through C5 alone (deltoid, supraspinatus etc.). Adduction (involving pectoralis major principally) is controlled by C6, 7.

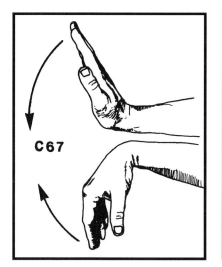

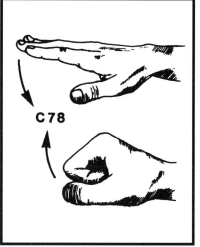

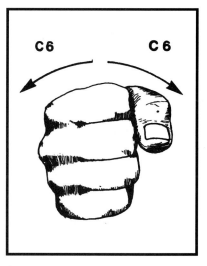

4. *Myotomes* (3): At the wrist, where C6, 7 would have been expected to control palmar flexion only, it is the case that these two segments control dorsiflexion as well.

5. *Myotomes* (4): Both flexion and extension of the fingers are controlled by C7, 8.

6. *Myotomes* (5): In the case of pronation and supination, a single spinal segment is involved, namely C6.

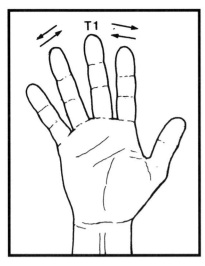

7. *Myotomes* (6): A single segment again, namely T1, is involved in producing abduction and adduction of the fingers — these movements are carried out by the small muscles (intrinsics) of the hand. *Note:* In testing for myotomes, the ability to perform the above movements (2–7) should be assessed (MRC grading) and note made of the segments affected. It is often the case that the defect can be localised to a single segment.

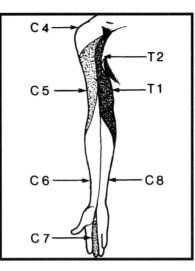

8. *Dermatomes:* Note that the middle finger is supplied by C7, and that there is a regular, easily remembered sequence of sensory distribution round the pre-axial line of the limb.

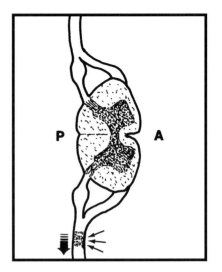

9. *Types of brachial plexus injury: lesions in continuity:* More than half of plexus injuries are of this pattern. Traction is the commonest cause, and the nerve roots are affected between the intervertebral foramina and the clavipectoral fascia. The lesions may be transient (neuropraxia); if the axons degenerate (axonotmesis), regeneration occurs at the rate of 1 mm per day, provided the axons can penetrate the intra-neural scar.

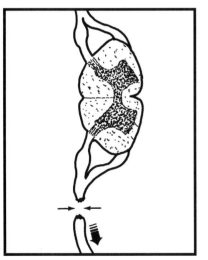

10. *Lesions with ruptured nerve roots:* In more severe injuries the nerves are disrupted at the same level. Only surgical intervention can offer any hope of recovery, but repair, even with nerve grafting, may be impossible because of extensive *intra-neural* damage. It is important to differentiate between lesions of this type, lesions in continuity (where the treatment is expectant) and cord avulsion lesions (where the prognosis is hopeless).

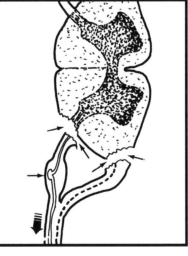

11. *Complete avulsion lesions:* The nerve is avulsed from the cord, and surgical repair is impossible. Motor axons degenerate, and the paralysed muscles show denervation fibrillation potentials on the electro-myograph (EMG). The cells of the sensory nerves in the dorsal root ganglion remain intact; although sensation is lost, conduction within the distal nerve remains, and may be detected through externally applied electrodes.

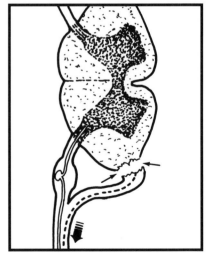

12. *Partial avulsion lesions:* Rarely, the posterior roots are spared so that there may be the paradox of muscle paralysis accompanied by preservation of sensation. The prognosis for the motor loss is in these circumstances also hopeless. While the exact nature of the lesion may seem fairly clear after clinical examination and further investigation, in many cases the picture is complex due to the fact that one or more of these injuries may be combined.

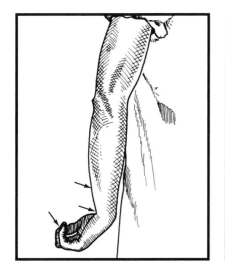

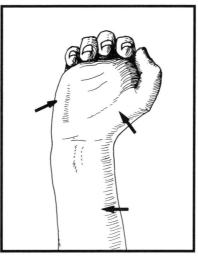

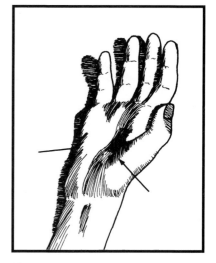

13. *Long-standing plexus lesions* (1): In *Erb's palsy* (upper obstetrical palsy), which affects the upper trunk of the brachial plexus and hence C5, 6, there is deformity of the limb which is held in a characteristic position: the wrist is flexed and pronated, and the fingers flexed. The elbow is extended and the shoulder internally rotated (waiter's tip deformity). The nerve to rhomboids and the long thoracic nerve are usually spared.

14. *Long-standing plexus lesions* (2): In *Klumpke's paralysis* the small (intrinsic) muscles including the hypothenar and thenar groups are wasted and there is a claw hand deformity. There is sensory loss on the medial side of the forearm and wrist. In many cases there is an associated Horner's syndrome. (Note also that 38% of patients who receive radiotherapy for breast carcinoma develop a brachial neuropathy.)

15. *Long-standing plexus lesions* (3): The T1 root alone may be involved, the sole signs being wasting of the small muscles of the hand including the thenar group, along with sensory loss on the medial side of the hand only. Lesions of this type are seen in incomplete lower obstetrical palsy, cervical spondylosis, cervical rib syndrome, neurofibromatosis, and apical and metastatic carcinoma.

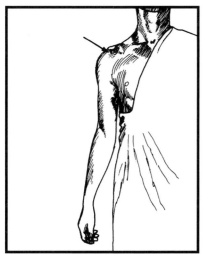

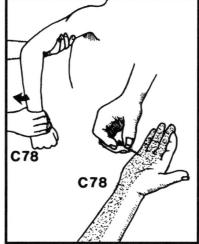

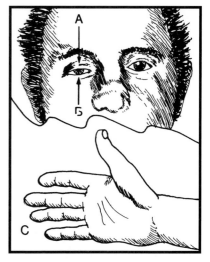

16. *Acute traumatic lesions of the brachial plexus:* The commonest mechanisms of injury involve depression of the shoulder combined with lateral flexion of the neck to the opposite side; or traction on the arm. Motor cycle accidents are the commonest cause. On inspection, look for the presence of tell-tale bruising over the shoulder or at the root of the neck. In the more severe cases the arm hangs flaily at the side.

17. *Assessment* (1): Begin by determining the *extent* of the lesion — i.e. which segments are involved, and whether the involvement is partial or complete. Start by testing for active movements in the shoulder, elbow, wrist and fingers, relating your findings to the myotomes responsible for these movements. Then check for sensation to pinprick and light touch, again noting the dermatomes involved (which normally correspond with the previously determined myotomes).

18. *Assessment* (2): After determining which segments are affected, you should try to form an opinion as to the *type* of injury. This may be difficult to clarify, but the more evidence there is of *proximal* damage, the greater the chance of cord avulsion and a poor prognosis. *Horner's syndrome*, characterised by (A) pseudo-ptosis, (B) smallness of the pupil on the affected side, and (C) dryness of the hand from absence of sweating, occurs when the T1 root is involved close to the canal.

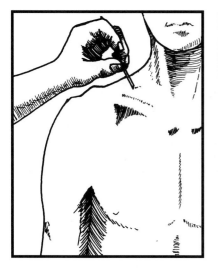

19. *Assessment* (3): Look for sensory loss above the clavicle. This area is normally supplied by C3, 4 and if this is affected, it generally indicates that the injury has been so severe that it has not only involved the plexus but the roots above; it is usually indicative of a proximal injury with a poor prognosis. Deep bruising in the posterior triangle is also strongly suggestive of a pre-ganglionic lesion.

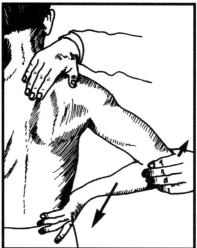

20. *Assessment* (4): Now test the first nerves which come off the plexus. *Nerve to rhomboids* (C5): Ask the patient to place the hand on the hip and to resist the elbow being pushed forwards; feel for contraction in the rhomboid muscles. *Absence* of activity is indicative of a lesion proximal to the formation of the upper trunk of the plexus (and suggestive of cord avulsion). *Presence* of activity means a lesion distal to the intervertebral foramen.

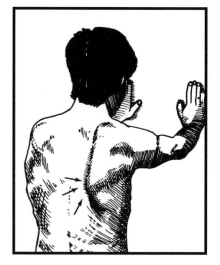

21. *Assessment* (5): *nerve to serratus anterior* (C5, 6, 7): Damage to this nerve produces winging of the scapula, which is normally demonstrated by asking the patient to lean with both hands against a wall, but this test may have to be abandoned in the presence of an extensive plexus lesion. Note that the nerve to serratus anterior may be damaged *in isolation* through lifting very heavy weights.

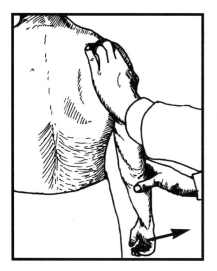

22. *Assessment* (6): *suprascapular nerve* (C5, 6): This nerve arises from the *upper trunk* of the plexus and supplies the supraspinatus and infraspinatus. To test for activity in the supraspinatus, ask the patient to try to abduct the arm against resistance; feel for muscle contraction above the spine of the scapula. (The *infraspinatus* may be tested by feeling for muscle contraction *below* the spine of the scapula while the patient attempts to externally rotate the shoulder.)

23. *Assessment* (7): Other tests, observations and investigations:
(1) *Tinel's sign:* Tap vigorously with a finger at the side of the neck, working from above downwards in the line of the nerve roots as they emerge from the spine. The test is positive if there is marked, painful paraesthesia in the corresponding dermatomes: for example, if tapping over the C6 root produces severe pain and tingling in the thumb. *A positive test* generally indicates a ruptured nerve root and a post-ganglionic lesion. (It is said, however, that the test may also be positive in the presence of an avulsed posterior root ganglion.)
(2) *X-ray:* (a) Plain films of the cervical spine should be obtained. Although these are of principal value in eliminating other pathology, they may occasionally reveal a transverse process fracture. Such a fracture is indicative of the severity of an injury and the probability of an irrecoverable lesion. (b) A plain PA radiograph of the chest may reveal paralysis of a hemidiaphragm, indicative of a proximally sited lesion.
(c) Myelography may give valuable information regarding the presence or absence of signs of avulsion of roots from the cord. Signs indicative of a poor prognosis include traumatic meningocoele; loss, diminution or exaggeration of root pouches; and cystic accumulations of cerebro-spinal fluid (CSF) within the spinal canal. (d) An MRI scan may clarify the site of nerve disruption, particularly in the case of pre-ganglionic lesions.
(3) *Electro-myography:* It has been recommended that at least two muscles supplied by each root should be examined by the insertion of needle electrodes: the presence of any action potentials will indicate some continuity in that root.

(4) *Sensory conduction:* Sensory conduction may be assessed in two ways: (a) by electrically stimulating (say) the median nerve at the wrist and by means of separate electrodes attempting to pick up resultant potentials over the plexus or in the neck (evoked potentials); or (b) stimulating (say) the median nerve at the wrist, and attempting to pick up potentials *distally* by means of ring electrodes round the index finger (sensory action (antidromic) potentials). The latter method appears preferable. One side is compared with the other. If the sides are the same, this suggests a severe or complete pre-ganglionic lesion (avulsion of nerve roots from the cord). If no sensory action potentials are obtained on the injured side, this suggests a post-ganglionic lesion; and if diminished action potentials are present, a mixed lesion is likely.

(5) *Histamine test:* A drop of 1% histamine is placed over the centre of each affected dermatome, and the skin pricked through it; the normal side is used as a control. On the normal side there should be the usual triple response with the flare fully developed within 10 minutes. Absence of a flare on the injured side suggests post-ganglionic damage.

24. *Summary of signs indicative of a poor prognosis in traumatic lesions of the plexus:*

1. A complete lesion involving all five roots.
2. Severe pain in an anaesthetic arm.
3. Sensory loss above the clavicle and bruising in the posterior triangle.
4. Fracture of a transverse process.
5. Horner's syndrome.
6. Paralysis of rhomboids and serratus anterior.
7. Retention of sensory conduction in the presence of sensory loss.

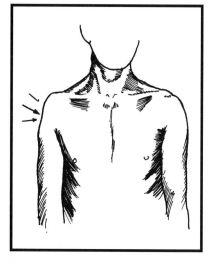

25. *Examination of the peripheral nerves of the upper limb: the axillary (circumflex) nerve (posterior cord) C5, 6 (1):* This nerve is most commonly damaged during shoulder dislocations and displaced fractures of the proximal humerus (humeral neck). Spontaneous recovery usually occurs. Flattening over the lateral aspect of the shoulder develops when muscle wasting is at its height.

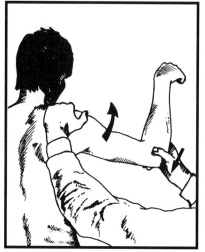

26. *Axillary nerve (2):* Ask the patient to attempt to move the arm from the side (pain permitting) while you resist any movement. Look and feel for deltoid contraction. Sometimes this is difficult to assess, and the two sides should be carefully compared if there is any doubt.

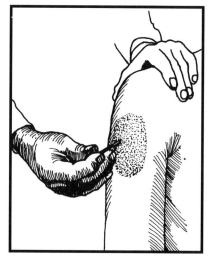

27. *Axillary nerve (3):* Look for loss of sensation over the 'regimental badge' area of the shoulder: this is the area exclusively supplied by the axillary nerve. Where the shoulder is too painful to move (e.g. if dislocated), loss of sensation is sufficient evidence of axillary nerve involvement without testing muscle power.

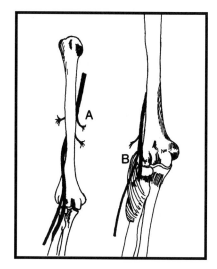

28. *Radial nerve (posterior cord) C5, 6, 7, 8 (T1): motor distribution:* (A) In the upper arm the radial nerve supplies triceps. (B) In front of the elbow, it supplies brachioradialis, extensor carpi radialis longus and brachialis. Its posterior interosseous branch, before it enters the supinator tunnel, supplies extensor carpi radialis brevis and part of supinator.

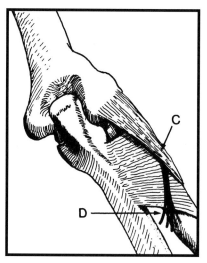

29. *Radial nerve (motor) ctd:* (C) In the supinator tunnel the posterior interosseous branch of the radial supplies the rest of supinator. (D) On leaving supinator below the elbow it supplies extensor digitorum communis, extensors digiti minimi and indicis, extensor carpi ulnaris, abductor pollicis longus, and extensors pollicis longus and brevis.

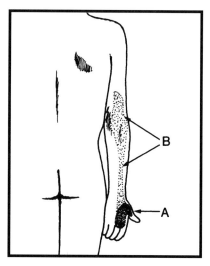

30. *Radial nerve: sensory distribution:* (A) The terminal part (superficial radial) supplies the radial side of the back of the hand. (B) The posterior cutaneous branch of the radial, given off in the upper part of the arm, supplies a variable area on the back of the arm and forearm.

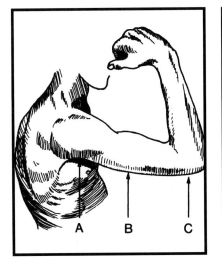

31. *Radial nerve: common sites affected:*
(A) In the axilla (e.g. from crutches, or the back of a chair in the so-called 'Saturday night' palsy); (B) mid-humerus (from fractures and tourniquet palsies); (C) at and below the elbow (e.g. after dislocations of the elbow, Monteggia fractures, ganglions and sometimes surgical trauma following exposures in this region).

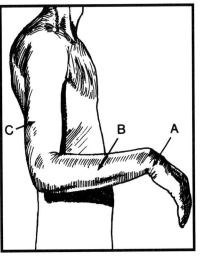

32. *Examination of the radial nerve* (1): Note in particular the following: (A) Is there an obvious wrist drop? (B) Is there wasting of the forearm muscles? (C) Is there wasting of the triceps, suggesting a high (proximal) lesion?

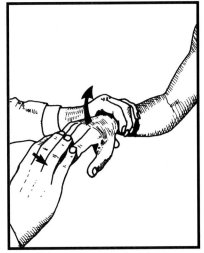

33. *Examination of the radial nerve* (2): Test the extensors of the wrist and fingers. The elbow should be flexed and the hand placed in pronation. Support the wrist, and ask the patient first to try to straighten the fingers, and then to pull back the wrist: if there is any activity, judge the strength by applying counter-pressure on the fingers or hand.

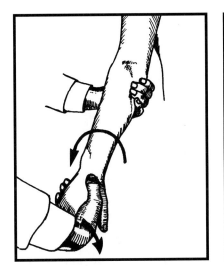

34. *Examination of the radial nerve* (3): Now test the supinator muscle. The elbow must be extended to eliminate the supinating action of biceps. Ask the patient to turn his hand while you apply counter-force. Loss of supination suggests a lesion *proximal to the exit of the supinator tunnel.*

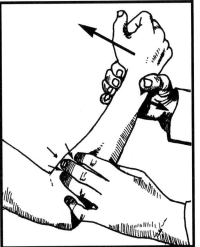

35. *Examination of the radial nerve* (4): Test the brachio-radialis. Ask the patient to flex the elbow in the mid-prone position against resistance. Feel and look for contraction in the muscle. Loss of power suggests a lesion *above* (proximal to) the supinator tunnel.

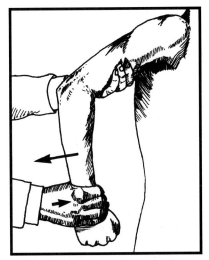

36. *Examination of the radial nerve* (5): Now test the triceps. Extend the shoulder, and ask the patient to extend the elbow against gravity and then resistance. Weakness of triceps suggests a lesion at mid-humeral level, or an incomplete high lesion; loss of all triceps activity suggests a high (plexus) lesion.

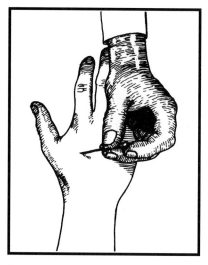

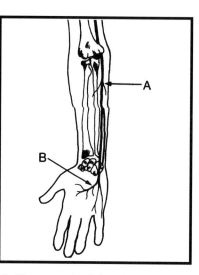

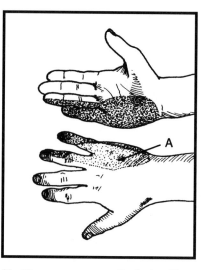

37. *Examination of the radial nerve* (6): Test for sensory loss in the areas supplied by the nerve (see 2, 30). Loss confined to the hand indicates that the lesion is unlikely to be much proximal to the elbow. Careful analysis of both the motor and sensory deficits should allow accurate localisation of the lesion.

38. *Ulnar nerve (medial cord) C8, T1: motor distribution:* (A) In the forearm, it supplies flexor carpi ulnaris and half of flexor digitorum profundus. (B) In the hand, it supplies the hypothenar muscles, the interossei, the two medial lumbricals and adductor pollicis.

39. *Ulnar nerve: sensory distribution:* Note that there are variations in the areas supplied by the median and ulnar nerves in the hand: the commonest pattern is illustrated. The branch supplying the dorsum (A) arises in the forearm; loss here indicates a lesion *proximal to the wrist.*

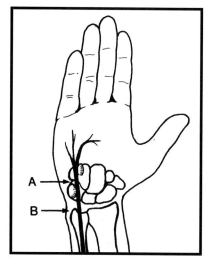

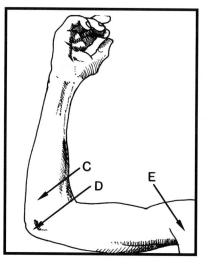

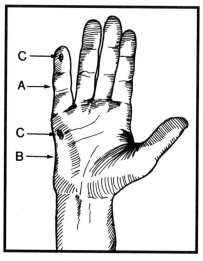

40. *Ulnar nerve: common sites affected* (1): (A) In the ulnar tunnel syndrome, where the nerve passes between the pisiform and the hook of the hamate (e.g. from the pressure of a ganglion, or a hook of hamate fracture). The most distal lesions affect the deep palmar nerve and are entirely motor; (B) at the wrist, especially from lacerations, occupational trauma, and ganglions.

41. *Ulnar nerve: common sites affected* (2): (C) Distal to the elbow, by compression as it passes between the two heads of flexor carpi ulnaris; (D) at the level of the medial epicondyle (e.g. in ulnar neuritis secondary to local friction, pressure or stretching as may occur in cubitus valgus and osteo-arthritis); (E) in the brachial plexus, as a result of trauma, or from other lesions in this area.

42. *Ulnar nerve examination* (1): Note the presence of (A) involuntary abduction of the little finger; (B) hypothenar wasting; (C) ulceration of the skin, brittleness of the nails and any other evidence of trophic change.

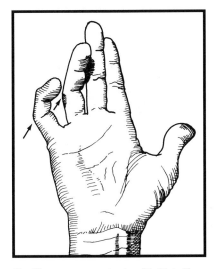

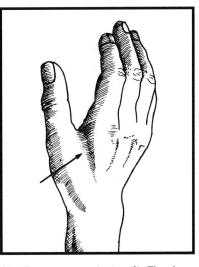

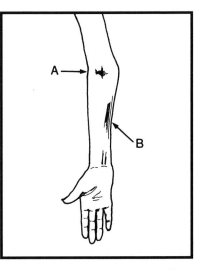

43. *Ulnar nerve examination* (2): Note if there is an ulnar claw hand, with flexion of the ring and little fingers at the proximal IP joints. If the distal interphalangeal (DIP) joints are flexed as well, this suggests that the flexor digitorum profundus is intact, and the lesion is distally placed: i.e. paradoxically, the deformity of the hand is *less* marked in lesions proximal to the wrist where there is *more* motor involvement.

44. *Ulnar nerve examination* (3): The ulnar nerve supplies all the interossei, so look for the presence of any interosseous muscle wasting. The first dorsal interosseous muscle is almost always the first to become noticeably affected, and the hollowing of the skin on the dorsal aspect of the first web space is often most striking.

45. *Ulnar nerve examination* (4): Note if there is (A) any cubitus valgus or varus deformity suggesting an old injury such as a supracondylar fracture (of significance in tardy ulnar nerve palsy); (B) muscle wasting on the medial side of the forearm, confirming a lesion proximal to the wrist. Compare one forearm with the other.

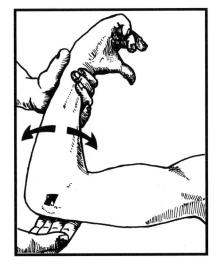

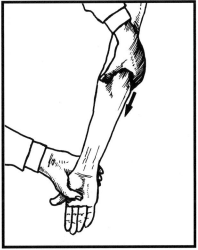

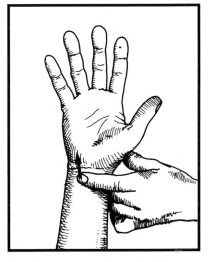

46. *Ulnar nerve examination* (5): Flex and extend the elbow, looking for abnormal mobility in the nerve where it passes behind the medial epicondyle. If the nerve is seen to snap over the medial epicondyle, a traumatic ulnar neuritis (secondary to a deficiency in the tissues which normally anchor it in position) may be diagnosed with reasonable confidence.

47. *Ulnar nerve examination* (6): Roll the nerve under the fingers above the medial epicondyle and follow it distally until it disappears under cover of flexor carpi ulnaris — about 4 cm distal to the medial epicondyle. Note the presence of any tenderness, thickening or the production of an unusual degree of paraesthesia.

48. *Ulnar nerve examination* (7): Palpate the nerve as it lies just lateral to the tendon of flexor carpi ulnaris at the wrist. Follow it down to the region of the ulnar tunnel, again looking for undue tenderness and paraesthesia.

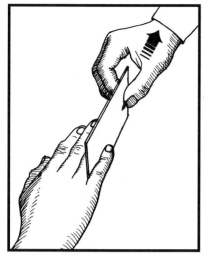

49. *Ulnar nerve examination* (8): Testing the interossei. Ask the patient to hold a sheet of paper between the ring and little fingers. The fingers *must* be fully extended. Withdraw the paper, and note the resistance offered. In a complete palsy, the patient will be unable to grip the paper at all.

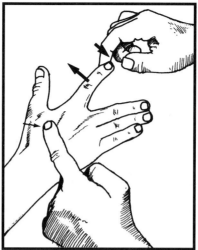

50. *Ulnar nerve examination* (9): Testing the first dorsal interosseous muscle. Place the patient's hand in a palm downwards position, and ask him to resist while you attempt to adduct the index. Look and feel for contraction in the first dorsal interosseous.

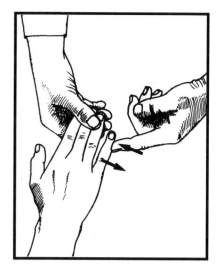

51. *Ulnar nerve examination* (10): Testing abductor digiti minimi. Ask the patient to resist as you adduct the extended little finger with your index. Note the resistance offered, and compare one hand with the other.

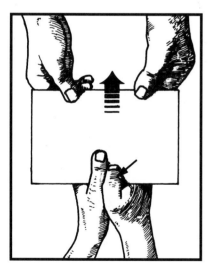

52. *Ulnar nerve examination* (11): *testing adductor pollicis* (1): Ask the patient to grasp a sheet of paper between the thumbs and sides of the index fingers while you attempt to withdraw it. If the adductor of the thumb is paralysed, the thumb will flex at the interphalangeal joint (Froment's test).

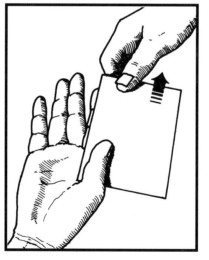

53. *Ulnar nerve examination* (12): *testing adductor pollicis* (2): Alternatively, test the patient's ability to grasp a sheet of paper held between the thumb and the *anterior* aspect of the index metacarpal.

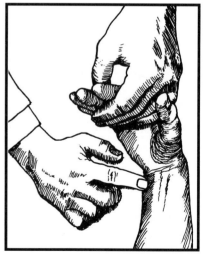

54. *Ulnar nerve examination* (13): *testing flexor carpi ulnaris* (1): Ask the patient to resist while you attempt to extend the flexed wrist. Feel for the tendon tightening at the wrist while you note the resistance offered.

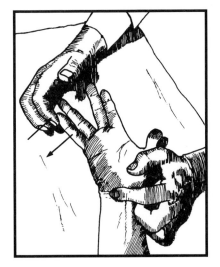

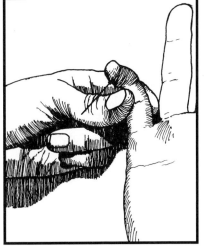

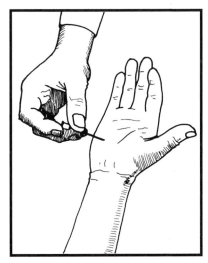

55. *Ulnar nerve examination (14): testing flexor carpi ulnaris (2):* Place the hand on a flat surface and ask the patient to resist while you attempt to adduct the little finger. Again feel for contraction in the tendon. Loss of activity indicates a lesion proximal to the wrist.

56. *Ulnar nerve examination (15): testing flexor digitorum profundus:* The ulnar half only of this muscle is supplied by the ulnar nerve. Support the middle phalanx of the little finger, and ask the patient to try to flex the distal joint. Apply counter-pressure to the finger tip, and note the resistance. Loss of power indicates a lesion near, or above the elbow.

57. *Ulnar nerve examination (16): testing for sensation:* Test for any disturbance of pinprick sensation in the area supplied by the nerve. Note that sensory loss *on the dorsum* is indicative of a lesion proximal to the wrist.

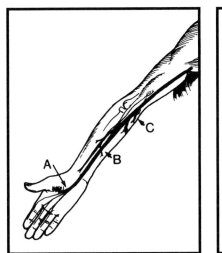

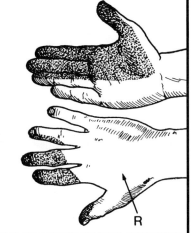

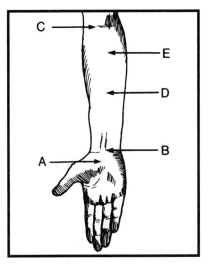

58. *The median nerve (lateral and medial cords) C(5) 6, 7, 8, T1: motor distribution:* (A) Hand: the thenar muscles and the lateral two lumbricals; (B) forearm (through its anterior interosseous branch): flexor pollicis longus, half of flexor digitorum profundus, pronator quadratus; (C) near elbow: flexor digitorum superficialis, flexor carpi radialis, palmaris longus and pronator teres.

59. *Median nerve: sensory distribution:* Note that there is considerable variation in the relative areas supplied by the median and ulnar nerves. Note also that the lateral side of the posterior aspect of the hand is supplied by the terminal part of the radial nerve (superficial radial nerve) (R). The commonest pattern of sensory distribution is shown.

60. *Median nerve: common sites affected:* (A) In the carpal tunnel (e.g. carpal tunnel syndrome, and sometimes after fractures and dislocations about the wrist); (B) at the wrist (e.g. from lacerations here); (C) at the elbow (e.g. after elbow dislocations in children); (D) in the forearm (anterior interosseous nerve) from forearm bone fractures; (E) just distal to the elbow, in the pronator teres nerve entrapment syndrome.

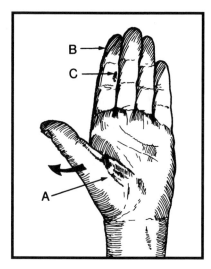

61. *Median nerve examination* (1): Note (A) thenar wasting. In long-standing cases the thumb may come to lie in the plane of the palm (simian thumb); (B) atrophy of the pulp of the index, cracking of the nails and other trophic changes; (C) cigarette burns and other signs of skin trauma secondary to local sensory deprivation.

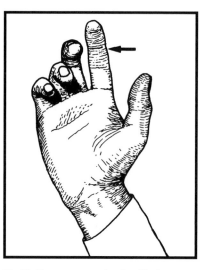

62. *Median nerve examination* (2): In lesions of the anterior interosseous branch or of the median nerve itself at or above the elbow, there may be wasting of the lateral aspect of the forearm, and the index is held in a position of extension (benediction attitude).

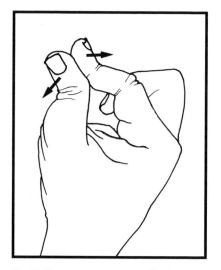

63. *Median nerve examination* (3): Isolated anterior interosseous nerve palsy may be caused by an anomalous band at the origins of sublimis, and if suspected, ask the patient to pinch his index and thumb together. In anterior interosseous nerve palsy, the terminal phalanges of the thumb and index will hyperextend (due to paralysis of flexor pollicis longus and the lateral half of flexor digitorum profundus), but the thenar muscles will remain intact.

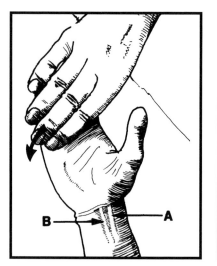

64. *Median nerve examination* (4): First locate the position of the nerve at the wrist. Ask the patient to flex his wrist, then attempt to extend it while he resists. Look for the tendons which are prominent at the front, near the midline, palpating the area if necessary. The nerve lies between (A) flexor carpi radialis longus and (B) palmaris longus (or medial to flexor carpi radialis longus if the latter is absent).

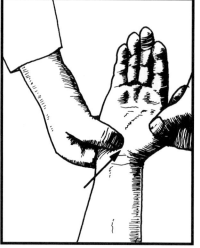

65. *Median nerve examination* (5): Apply firm pressure over the area of the nerve at the wrist and distally in the line of the carpal tunnel, looking for tenderness. (If the carpal tunnel syndrome is suspected, apply pressure with both thumbs, timing the onset of paraesthesia, and carry out the other tests detailed later in Chapter 6.)

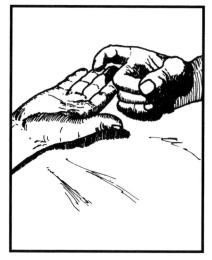

66. *Median nerve examination* (6): *testing abductor pollicis brevis* (1): This muscle is invariably and exclusively supplied by the median nerve. To test it, begin by placing the patient's hand, palm upwards, on a flat surface. Hold your index finger above the palm.

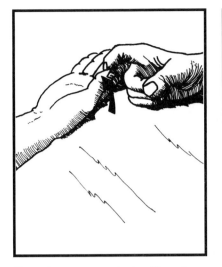

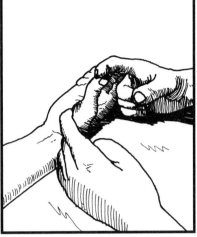

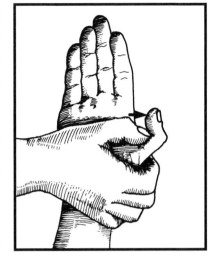

67. *Median nerve examination* (7): *testing abductor pollicis brevis* (2): Now ask the patient to raise his thumb and try to touch your finger. If he tends to move his hand while doing so, steady it with your other hand. Assess his ability to carry out the movement (he may not be able to do it), and look for contraction in the muscle.

68. *Median nerve examination* (8): *testing abductor pollicis brevis* (3): Ask the patient to resist while you attempt to force the thumb back into the starting position. Note the resistance offered; palpate the muscle to confirm its tone and bulk; and compare the power on the affected side with that of the other.

69. *Median nerve examination* (9): Test the power of flexor pollicis longus in the thumb, and flexor digitorum profundus in the index. Do so by asking the patient to try to flex the appropriate distal joint while you support the phalanx proximal to it. Loss of power indicates a lesion proximal to the wrist, either of the median nerve itself, or of its anterior interosseous branch.

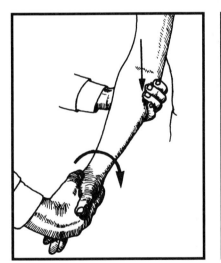

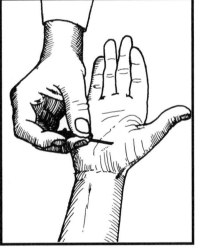

70. *Median nerve examination* (10): *testing pronator teres:* Extend the patient's elbow, and feel for contraction in the muscle as he attempts to pronate the arm against resistance. Loss indicates a lesion at or above the elbow. Accompanying pain and tenderness over pronator teres is found in the pronator teres entrapment syndrome.

71. *Median nerve examination* (11): *testing for sensation:* Look for impairment of sensation to pinprick in the area of distribution of the nerve.

3. The cervical spine

Postural neck pain

In this common condition, pain in the neck and shoulders occurs in association with some abnormality of neck posture. It is commonest in females under the age of 40, many of whom have sedentary jobs (such as typists or computer operators) in which the head may be maintained for long periods in a position which may be short of ideal. In some cases there may be a history of minor trauma which exacerbates or precipitates the complaint. Clinically the head and neck may be held in a somewhat protracted position, but there is usually a full range of neck movements with normal radiographs. Analgesics and physiotherapy are usually helpful in the acute case, but in the long term change of work practices and in the patient's working environment are likely to be of the greatest benefit.

Acute neck pain in the young adult

In the 20–35 age group, often before there is any radiological evidence of arthritic change in the spine, a sudden movement of the neck may produce severe neck and arm pain accompanied by striking protective muscle spasm and limitation of cervical movements. In some cases these symptoms are produced by an acute disc prolapse similar to those occurring more familiarly in the lumbar region. In others, with identical symptoms, investigation by magnetic resonance imaging (MRI scan), or myelography followed by computed axial tomography (CAT) scanning may be quite negative, and some disturbance of the facet joints or related structures is often thought responsible. Most cases respond to a period of rest in a cervical collar, or physiotherapy in the form of traction. In a few resistant cases manipulation may be helpful.

Cervical spondylosis (cervical osteoarthrosis; osteoarthritis of the cervical spine)

Cervical spondylosis is easily the most common condition affecting the neck. Degenerative changes appear early in life in the cervical spine, often during the third decade. The disc space between the 5th and 6th cervical vertebrae is most frequently involved. The earliest changes are confined to the disc, but the facet joints and the unco-vertebral joints (joints of Luschka) may soon become involved. There is inevitable restriction of movements at the affected level, but this is often impossible to detect clinically as it is masked by persisting mobility in the joints above and below. The condition may in fact never attract attention, but unfortunately in many cases symptoms do occur, sometimes being triggered off by minor trauma. Pain may be felt centrally in the neck and may radiate to the occiput, giving rise to severe occipital headache which may be confused with migraine; pain may also radiate in a downward direction further than might be expected on anatomical grounds, to the region of the lower scapulae. Often there is pain at the side of the neck, quite sharply localised, or in the supraclavicular region. With nerve root involvement from arthritic changes in the facet or unco-vertebral joints, there may be radiation of pain into the shoulders, arms and hands, with paraesthesia and on rare occasions demonstrable neurological involvement; this may include absent arm reflexes, muscle weakness and sensory impairment.

In cervical spondylosis the cervical canal may be narrowed by osteophytic lipping of the facet or unco-vertebral joints, by central disc herniations, by thickening of the ligamentum flava, or even from local cervical vertebral subluxations associated with ligamentous laxity. Developmental narrowing of the canal may be an additional factor. The reduction in the size of the canal may lead to cord compression (*cervical spondylotic myelopathy*). The disturbance of cord function which results may cause neck pain, difficulty in walking and unsteadiness on the feet, numbness, paraesthesia, weakness, and loss of upper limb dexterity. There is often co-existing compression of cervical nerve roots leading to radicular symptoms which may complicate the clinical picture. Bladder dysfunction may occur, but is not common, and extensor plantar responses may appear late. Severe progressive myelopathy often requires operative treatment by decompression and stabilisation.

Vertebral artery involvement by osteophytic outgrowths or local spinal instability may cause drop attacks precipitated by extension of the neck. Osteophytes arising from the anterior vertebral margins may sometimes by their size give rise to dysphagia.

The mainstay of treatment in spondylosis is the judicious use of a cervical collar and the prescription of analgesics. If root symptoms are prominent, intermittent or continuous, cervical traction is often employed. Manipulation of the cervical spine, especially in the younger age groups with no neurological involvement, is sometimes advocated. Severe, protracted symptoms may be investigated further by MRI scans, or myelography followed by CAT scanning. If a positive lesion is demonstrated, exploration may be carried out; if not, a local cervical fusion may sometimes be advised.

Cervical rib syndrome

Symptoms in the arm from involvement of the brachial plexus and axillary artery by a cervical rib are a definite but rare occurrence. Slightly more commonly, the same structures may be kinked by fibrous bands or abnormalities in the scalene attachments at the root of the neck. Paraesthesia in the hand is severe, and there may be hypothenar and less commonly thenar wasting. There is sometimes sympathetic disturbance with increased sweating of the hand. The radial pulse may be absent, and other signs of vascular impairment may be present. Complete vascular occlusion, sometimes accompanied by thrombosis and emboli, may lead to gangrene of the fingertips. In some cases symptoms may be precipitated by loss of tone in the shoulder girdle, with drooping of the shoulders; in such cases, physiotherapy is often successful in restoring tone to the affected muscles and relieving symptoms. When vascular involvement predominates, arteriography and exploration may be required.

Whiplash and extension injuries of the neck

Whiplash injuries are now a common cause of persistent cervical symptoms. A true whiplash injury occurs classically when, as a result of a rear impact, an initially stationary or slowly moving vehicle strikes another vehicle or object in front. Because of the inertial mass of the head of the car occupant, there is rapid extension of the cervical spine followed by flexion. In the partial whiplash injury, the main element is extension of the neck; this also commonly occurs as a result of a rear impact, but in this case the vehicle in which the occupant is travelling comes to rest more gradually without striking anything ahead. Unfortunately the attractive nature of the term has led to its misuse, and some recommend that because of its present imprecision it should be avoided altogether. If, however, it is going to be used, then it should be reserved for soft tissue injuries of the neck where extension is the main element. In the majority of cases the radiographs show normal alignment of the cervical vertebrae but occasionally small avulsion fractures of the anterior margins of the vertebral bodies give evidence of the forcible extension of the spine. In some cases there are minor fractures involving the unco-vertebral joints. Where there are spondylotic changes which interfere with the dissipation of the forces involved (because of localised areas of rigidity in the spine), there may be avulsion of anterior osteophytes. The flexion element may sometimes produce wedge compression fractures of the vertebral bodies or avulsion fractures of the spinous processes. These injuries produce symptoms of all degrees of severity. There is always pain and stiffness in the neck, sometimes with neurological disturbance involving the upper and occasionally the lower limbs. Even minor symptoms may be most protracted, often lasting 18 months or longer. In some cases, disability is permanent. Cervical collar supports, local heat and analgesics are usually advised.

Severe extension injuries may occur in falls (often downstairs) when the neck is forcibly extended as the head strikes the ground. There is often tell-tale bruising of the forehead. In a car accident an unbelted occupant may also suffer severe extension of the neck in the early phases of deceleration when the forehead strikes the roof and ricochets backwards. In both sets of circumstances the head injury may attract prior attention, but the possibility of these injuries must not be overlooked. Cervical spondylosis again has a deleterious localising effect on the forces involved, and the neurological disturbance may be profound. In some cases thrombosis extends from the area of local cord involvement, so that there may be a deteriorating and sometimes fatal neurological outcome.

Rheumatoid arthritis in the cervical spine

Rheumatoid arthritis frequently involves the neck, often in a patchy fashion, so that additional stresses are thrown on the remaining mobile elements. With the ligamentous stretching that often accompanies rheumatoid arthritis there may be progressive subluxation of the cervical spine, particularly at the atlanto-axial and mid-cervical levels. As this progresses, pain and stiffness in the neck become accompanied by root and cord symptoms. In the case of atlanto-axial subluxations, there may be severe occipital headache. The gait tends to become ataxic and there is progressive paralysis, often with bladder involvement. These lesions are usually treated by local cervical fusion if the patient's general condition will allow.

Klippel-Feil syndrome

In this condition there is restriction of movements in the cervical spine due to a congenital abnormality characterised by a failure of the cervical vertebrae to differentiate. One or more groups of vertebrae are fused together, and the condition may be associated with congenital elevation of the shoulder (Sprengel's shoulder). The condition gives rise to an increased susceptibility to injury and often neurological compromise.

Neoplasms in the cervical region

Tumours of the cervical spine are rare, secondary deposits however being the most common. They may cause vertebral body erosion or collapse, affect issuing nerve roots, or give rise to cord involvement. Of the primary tumours in this region sarcoma and multiple myeloma are the most common. Primary involvement of the cord may arise with meningiomas and intra-dural neurofibromata, which may also affect isolated nerve roots.

Osteitis of the cervical spine

Osteitis affecting the cervical vertebrae is a rare occurrence in the UK. Tuberculosis, when it occurs, is seen most frequently in children, and may produce widespread bone destruction, vertebral collapse and cord involvement.

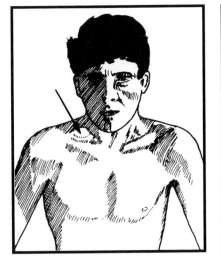

1. *Inspection* (1): (A) Note any *asymmetry in the supraclavicular fossae:* this will require separate investigation (e.g. Pancoast tumour). (B) Note the presence of *torticollis*, where the head is pulled to the affected side, and the chin often tilted to the opposite. In *congenital torticollis*, there may be in the infant a small tumour in the sternomastoid muscle, and in the untreated case, some facial asymmetry. *NB:* in about a third of cases the abnormal head posture is due to *ocular muscle weakness*, and a specialist ocular assessment is mandatory in *every* case.

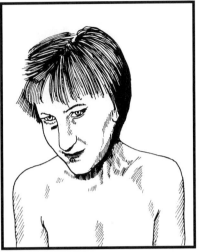

2. *Inspection* (2): (B ctd) In *acquired torticollis*, affecting the older child or adult, protective spasm of the sternomastoid muscle may result from tonsillar infection or vertebral body disease. It is sometimes seen accompanying the Klippel-Feil syndrome. It may also be due to a vertebral malalignment (especially at the C1/C2 level) from trauma or upper respiratory infection. In advanced infections and tumours, the head may be supported by the hands.

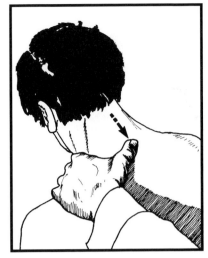

3. *Palpation* (1): Begin by looking for tenderness in the midline from the occiput downwards. Tenderness localised to one space is common in cervical spondylosis and in the very much rarer infections of the cervical spine.

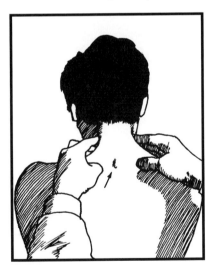

4. *Palpation* (2): Now palpate the lateral aspects of the vertebrae looking for masses and tenderness. Note that the most prominent spinous process is that of T1, and *not* the vertebra prominens, C7.

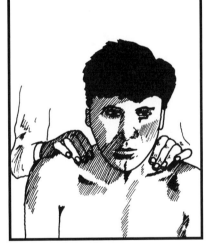

5. *Palpation* (3): Continue palpation into the supraclavicular fossae, looking particularly for the prominence of a cervical rib with local tenderness; look also for tumour masses and enlarged cervical lymph nodes.

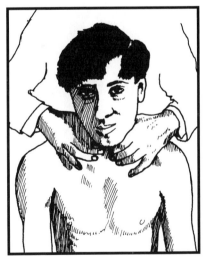

6. *Palpation* (4): Complete palpation of the neck by examining the anterior structures including the thyroid gland.

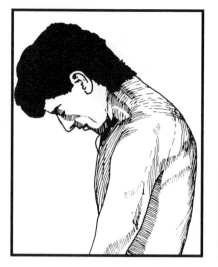

7. *Movements* (1): *flexion:* Ask the patient to bend the head forwards. Normally the chin can be brought down to touch the region of the sterno-clavicular joints. The chin–chest distance may be measured for record purposes.

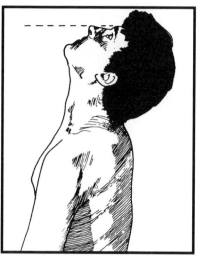

8. *Movements* (2): *extension:* Ask the patient to tilt the head backwards. The patient should be seated and erect. The plane of nose and forehead should normally be nearly horizontal but guard against contributory thoracic and lumbar spine movements.

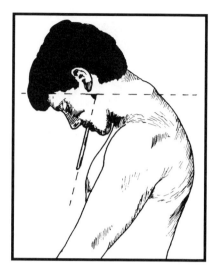

9. *Movements* (3): Recording motion in the cervical spine with any accuracy is difficult, but may be attempted using a spatula in the clenched teeth as a pointer. Stand back, and ask the patient to flex the head forwards. Line up the legs of a goniometer with the spatula and the horizontal respectively. Read off the included angle. *Normal: 80°.*

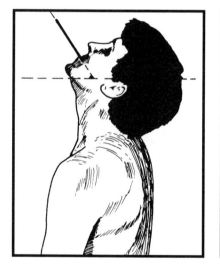

10. *Movements* (4): Now ask the patient to extend the head to measure the range of extension from the neutral position. *Normal range: 50°.* The *total* range in the flexion and extension plane should be assessed, either by a single measurement, or by the summation of flexion and extension. *Normal range: 130°.* Of this total about a fifth occurs in the atlanto-axial and atlanto-occipital joints.

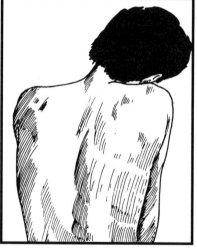

11. *Movements* (5): *lateral flexion* (1): Ask the patient to tilt his head on to his right shoulder. Lateral flexion with slight shoulder shrugging will allow the ear to touch the shoulder. Repeat on the other side and note any difference.

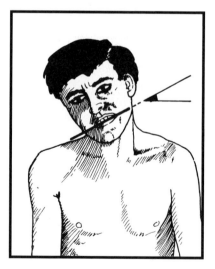

12. *Movements* (6): *lateral flexion* (2): For greater accuracy, a spatula clenched in the teeth may again be used as a pointer. *Normal range: 45°.* About a fifth of this movement occurs at the atlanto-axial and atlanto-occipital joints. Loss is common in cervical spondylosis.

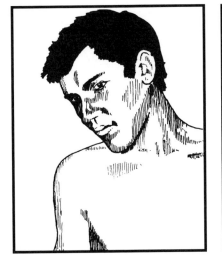

13. *Movements* (7): If lateral flexion cannnot be carried out without forward flexion, this is indicative of involvement of the atlanto-axial and atlanto-occipital joints.

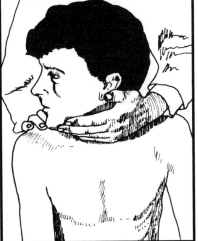

14. *Movements* (8): *rotation* (1): Ask the patient to look over the shoulder. The movement may be encouraged with one hand, and movement of the shoulder restrained with the other. Normally the chin just falls short of the plane of the shoulders.

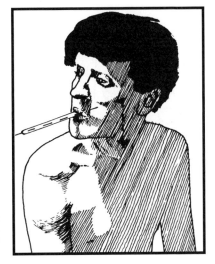

15. *Movements* (9): *rotation* (2): Again a spatula may be used as a pointer for measurement. *Normal range: 80° to either side.* About a third of this occurs in the first two cervical joints. Rotation is usually restricted and painful in cervical spondylosis.

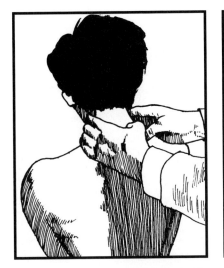

16. *Crepitus:* Spread the hands on each side of the neck and ask the patient to flex and extend the spine. Facet joint crepitus is normally detectable in this fashion, and is a common finding in cervical spondylosis. If in doubt, auscultate on either side of the spine while the patient flexes and extends.

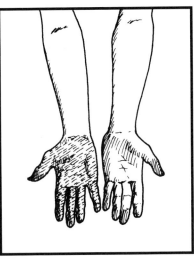

17. *Cervical rib* (1): Look for evidence of ischaemia in one hand (e.g. coldness, discoloration, trophic changes). Bilateral changes are more in favour of Raynaud's disease.

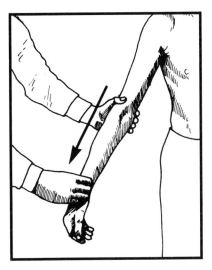

18. *Cervical rib* (2): Palpate the radial pulse and apply traction to the arm. Obliteration of the pulse is not diagnostic, but when the test reveals no change when repeated on the other side it is suggestive.

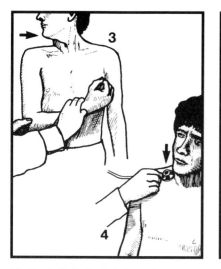

19. *Cervical rib (3):* Ask the patient to turn his head towards the affected side and to take a deep breath (and hold it). If the radial pulse is obliterated (from scalenus anterior obstruction) this is suggestive of the syndrome. (4) Auscultate over the subclavian artery. A murmur is suggestive of a mechanical obstruction, but repeat on the other side.

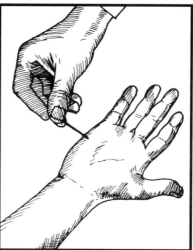

20. *Neurological examination:* (A) *Suspected nerve root involvement:* Pay particular attention to myotomes and dermatomes. (B) *Suspected cord compression* (1): In cervical myelopathy, *lower* motor signs occur in the *upper* limbs at the level of the compression, while *upper* motor signs appear distally, mainly in the *lower* limbs. Flexor plantar responses are late in onset, and the sensory deficit is **not** dermatomal: there is often hypoalgesia or analgesia of the whole hand, wrist and forearm.

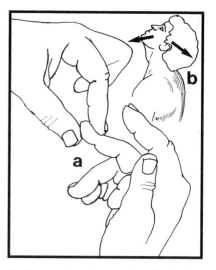

21. *Suspected cord compression* (2): Look for other evidence of cervical myelopathy. (a) *Hoffmann's test:* Rapidly extend the distal phalanx of the middle finger by flicking its anterior surface (pulp). The test is positive (indicating cortico-thalamic dysfunction) if it results in flexion of the interphalangeal (IP) joints of the thumb and index. (b) *Dynamic Hoffmann test:* Repeat while the patient flexes and extends the neck, which often facilitates the response.

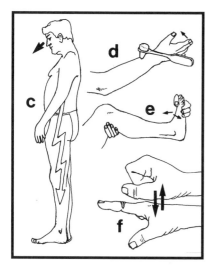

22. *Suspected cord compression* (3): (c) *Lhermitte's test:* Flexion or extension of the neck produces electric shock-like sensations, particularly in the legs. (d) *Inverted radial reflex:* This highly specific test is positive if the fingers flex when the radial reflex is elicited. (e) *Clonus.* (f) *Myelopathy hand* (indicative of pyramidal tract damage): This has two elements: (i) *Kinetic:* there is inability to flex and extend the fingers rapidly. Time the patient over 10 seconds. *The normal is in excess of 20 cycles.*

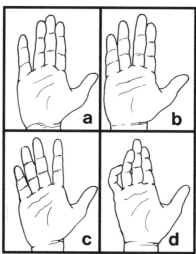

23. *Suspected cord compression* (4): *Myelopathy hand (ctd):* (ii) *Postural:* There is deficient adduction, and often extension, of the ulnar 1–3 fingers. In the mildest cases, when the fingers are extended, the little finger lies in slightly *abduction* (a); if it can adduct, this position cannot be held for long. *Abduction power* is normal. In severe cases, the little, ring (b) and sometimes the middle finger (c) may abduct, and/or the same fingers may *flex* (d) and lose their power of extension.

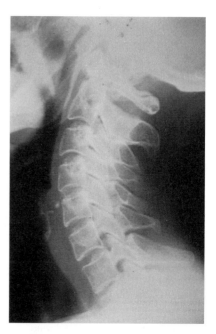

24. *Radiographs* (1) *lateral:* The standard projections are the lateral and antero-posterior views of lower and upper cervical vertebrae.

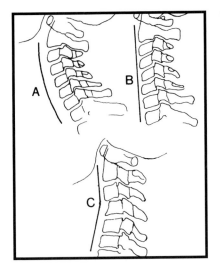

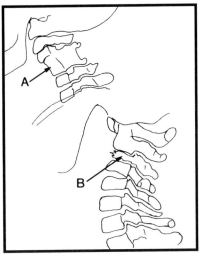

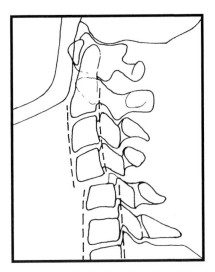

25. *Radiographs* (2): Begin your study of the lateral projection by noting the cervical curve which is normally slightly convex anteriorly: (A) normal, regular curve; (B) loss of curvature: this can be a positional error, but in those with chronic neck pain it may be due to protective muscle spasm. This is, however; a rather unreliable sign; (C) kinking (from a local lesion such as a subluxation, or from intense local muscle spasm).

26. *Radiographs* (3): Now look at the general shape of the bodies of the vertebrae, comparing one with another. Note for example, (A) congenital vertebral fusion, such as occurs in the Klippel-Feil syndrome; (B) vertebral collapse, from tuberculosis, tumour or fracture.

27. *Radiographs* (4): Note the relationship of each verterbra to the one above and below. It is helpful to trace the posterior margins of the bodies. Displacement occurs in dislocations, and may be small when the facet joints on one side only are involved.

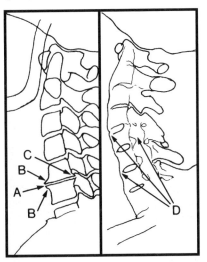

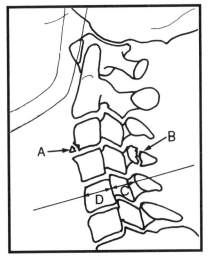

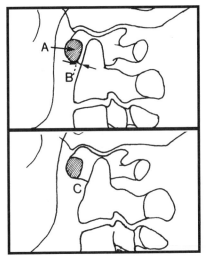

28. *Radiographs* (5): Look at the disc spaces and the related margins of the vertebrae. Note (A) disc space narrowing; (B) anterior lipping; (C) posterior lipping (all typical of cervical spondylosis). Note any evidence of fusion (D) typical of ankylosing spondylitis.

29. *Radiographs* (6): Note the presence (A) of an osteophyte or marginal fracture, suggestive of an extension injury of the neck; (B) fracture of a spinous process, suggestive of a flexion injury of the cervical spine. Syringomyelia (which can produce pain in the head, neck and limbs) may cause vertebral body erosions and dilatation of the canal. The diameter of the canal at C5 (C) should not exceed the vertebral body diameter (D) by more than 6 mm.

30. *Radiographs* (7): (A) Note that the anterior arch of the atlas lies in front of the lower cervical vertebrae. (B) The distance between the arch and the axis is normally 1–4 mm. A greater distance (C) suggests rupture or laxity of the transverse ligament (e.g. from trauma, rheumatoid arthritis or infection).

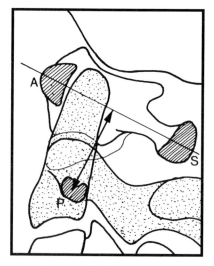

31. *Radiographs* (8): Upward (cranial) migration of the odontoid process is also commonly seen in rheumatoid arthritis. In the adult this may be assessed by noting the distance between the pedicle (P) of C2 (shown stippled) and a line connecting the spinous process (S) with the arch (A) of C1. If this is less than 11.5 mm, upward migration is considered to be present.

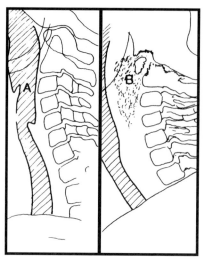

32. *Radiographs* (9): Note the pharyngeal shadow which normally lies fairly close to the bodies of the vertebrae as at (A). Displacement suggests a retro-pharyngeal mass, e.g. (B) suboccipital tuberculosis with abscess. Other causes include haematoma and tumour.

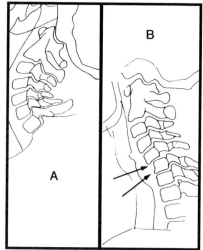

33. *Radiographs* (10): Where instability is suspected, the lateral projection should be supervised with the neck (A) in extension, and (B) in flexion. Any latent instability should be discernible by comparing these views. If doubt remains, intensifier screening of movement may help.

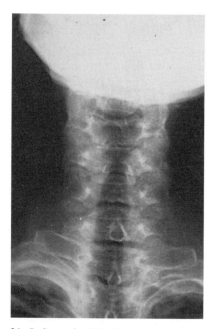

34. *Radiographs* (11): Normal antero-posterior view of the lower cervical vertebrae.

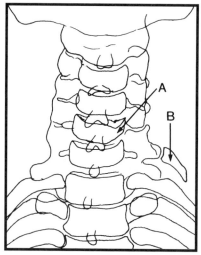

35. *Radiographs* (12): In the anterio-posterior view, interpretation is difficult due to the complexity of the superimposed structures. Note the shape of the vertebral bodies, observing (A) any lateral wedging, e.g. from fracture, tumour or infection. Note (B) the presence of any cervical rib.

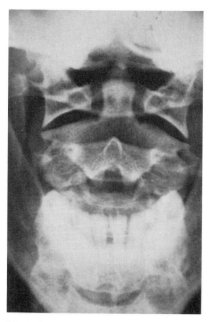

36. *Radiographs* (13): Normal antero-posterior (through-the-mouth) view of C1–3.

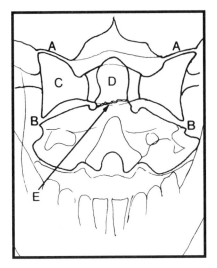

37. *Radiographs* (14): In the antero-posterior view of C1–3, note (A) the atlanto-occipital joints; (B) the atlanto-axial joints; (C) the lateral masses of the atlas. Note any lack of symmetry in the alignment of the odontoid process (D) with the atlas, and look for any evidence of fracture (E). Occasionally congenital abnormalities of the odontoid process (such as hypoplasia or failure of fusion between its ossification centre and the main mass of the axis) may cause difficulties in interpretation.

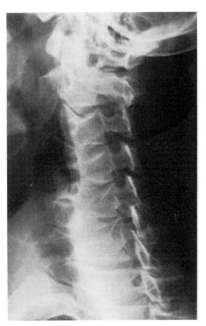

38. *Radiographs* (15): Normal oblique projection of the cervical spine (one of two).

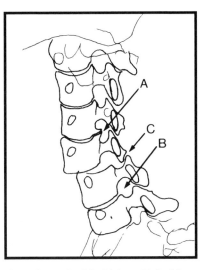

39. *Radiographs* (16): Right and left oblique projections are invaluable in demonstrating (A) localised lipping in the unco-vertebral joints (joints of Luschka) which may be encroaching on the neural foramina (B). They may also show overlapping (locked) facet joints (C) in cervical subluxations.

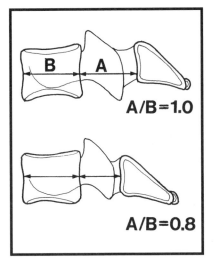

40. *Radiographs* (17): *suspected cervical myelopathy* (1): *the Pavlov ratio:* Normally, the depth (A) of the cervical canal, as seen in the lateral projection, is as great as that of its related vertebral body (B), giving a Pavlov ratio (A/B) of 1.0, and more than adequate room for the spinal cord. A Pavlov ratio of 0.8 or less indicates a developmentally narrow cervical canal, with risk of cord compression. If the ratio is reduced, check the lumbar spine, as there may well be an associated lumbar spinal stenosis.

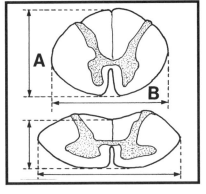

41. *Radiographs* (18): *suspected cervical myelopathy* (2): If there are axial MRI scans (or post-myelographic CAT scans) which show the cord at the suspect levels, the presence and degree of cord compression may be assessed by working out the *cord compression ratio.* This is calculated by dividing the (sagittal) diameter (thickness) (A) of the cord by its width (B). (As this is a ratio, the reduction effects of the scans are immaterial.) Note also that the cord may be considerably distorted, so use its *minimal* sagittal diameter for the calculation. A value of 0.4 is indicative of a serious degree of compression, and if decompression surgery is planned it is best done before a figure as low as this is reached.

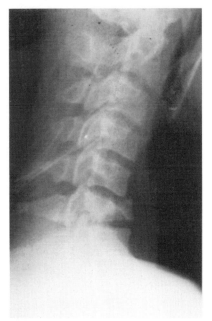

42. *Cervical spine radiographs: examples of pathology* (1): The cervical curvature is reversed; there is wedging of the body of C6. Diagnosis: fracture of C6.

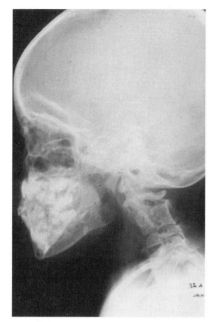

43. *Pathology* (2): C3, 4 and 5 are represented by a solid bony mass. Diagnosis: congenital fusion of cervical spine.

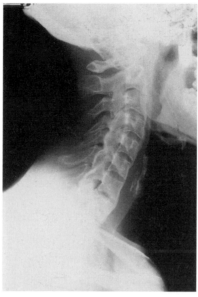

44. *Pathology* (3): There is widespread fusion of the intervertebral facet joints, and the anterior longitudinal ligament is calcified. Diagnosis: ankylosing spondylitis.

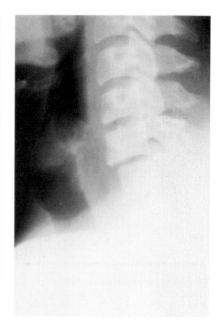

45. *Pathology* (4): There is slight forward shift of the body of C6 relative to that of C7. Diagnosis: unilateral facet dislocation of C6 on C7.

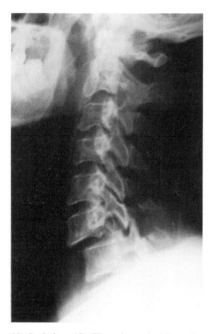

46. *Pathology* (5): There is marked loss of vertebral alignment, and the inferior articular processes of C6 are lying in front of the superior articular processes of C7. The spinous processes of C5 and C6 are fractured. Diagnosis: dislocation of cervical spine (C6 on C7) with locked facets.

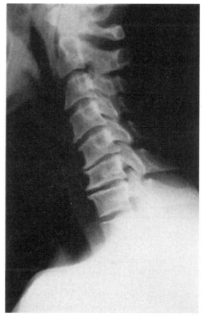

47. *Pathology* (6): There is narrowing of the C5–6 disc space, and to a lesser extent that of C6–7. There is anterior lipping of C4, 5, 6, 7. There is posterior lipping of C5. Diagnosis: moderate degree of cervical spondylosis.

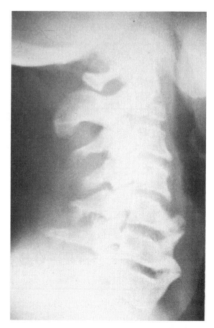

48. *Pathology* (7): There is gross anterior lipping of C5, 6 and 7, with near anterior interbody fusion. The pharyngeal shadow is distorted. Diagnosis: severe cervical spondylosis, associated in this case with dysphagia. Similar appearances are found in Forestier's disease, a condition in which there is excessive, widespread osteophyte formation and abnormal ligamentous calcification (especially of the anterior longitudinal ligament).

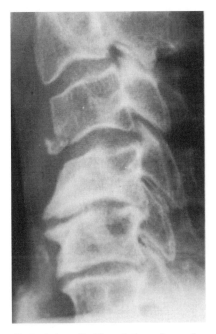

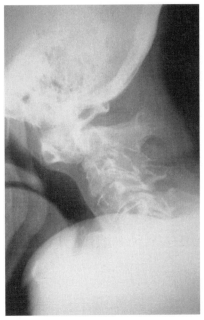

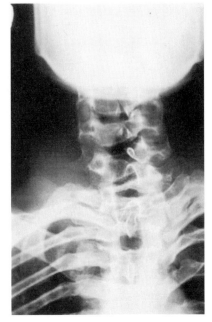

49. *Pathology* (8): There is loss of normal cervical curvature, narrowing of the C5–6 space and anterior lipping. There is an avulsion fracture of the anterior inferior margin of C4. Diagnosis: extension injury of the spine with a marginal fracture and cervical muscle spasm in a patient susceptible to injury because of pre-existing cervical spondylosis.

50. *Pathology* (9): The radiograph has been taken in flexion (one part of a flexion and extension pair) and shows an excessive gap between the anterior arch of the atlas and the odontoid process. There is generalised vertebral demineralisation. Diagnosis: rheumatoid arthritis with an atlanto-axial subluxation.

51. *Pathology* (10): There is deformity of the cervical spine with the presence of only half of a vertebral body at the C6 level. Diagnosis: congenital deformity of the cervical spine (hemivertebra cervicalis).

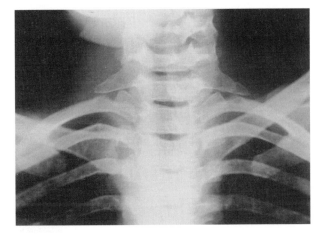

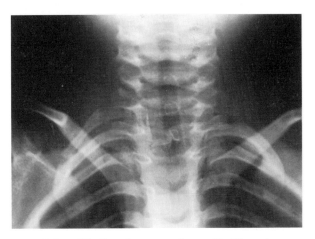

52. *Pathology* (11): The transverse processes of the 7th cervical vertebra are enlarged on both sides. Diagnosis: congenital deformity of the cervical spine related to cervical rib.

53. *Pathology* (12): There is an extra rib one side. Diagnosis: unilateral cervical rib.

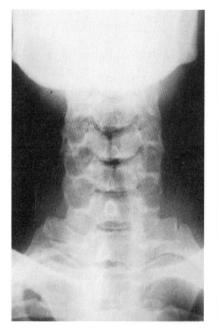

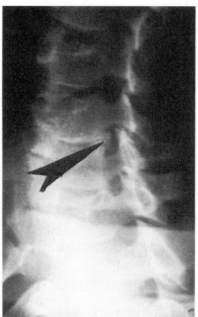

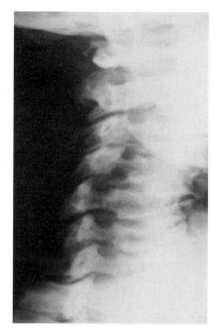

54. *Pathology* (13): There is a vertical fissure in the body of C5 and, less obviously, in C6. Diagnosis: fracture of C5 and C6.

55. *Pathology* (14): This oblique projection shows osteophytes arising from the unco-vertebral joint. Diagnosis: cervical spondylosis, associated in this case with unilateral compression of the C6 nerve root.

56. *Pathology* (15): The inferior articular process of C4 is displaced anteriorly over the upper articular process of C5. (The corresponding oblique projection of the other side is normal.) Diagnosis: unilateral facet joint dislocation, with in this case entrapment of C5.

4. The shoulder

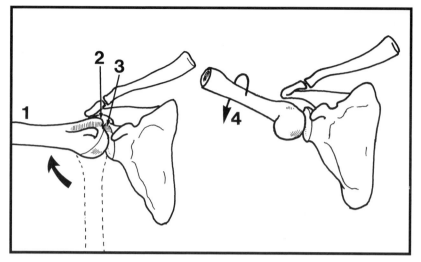

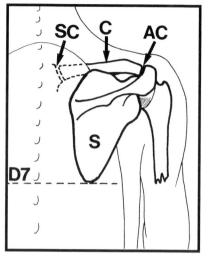

Anatomical features

Fig. 4.A The shoulder is complex, and it is important to note that it has two main components, namely the gleno-humeral joint (between the head of the humerus and the glenoid), and the scapulo-thoracic joint (between the scapula and the chest wall). The latter is a physiological rather than an anatomical joint as it has no synovial cavity.

The *gleno-humeral joint* accounts for about half of shoulder abduction (1), and this comes to an end when the greater tuberosity (2) impinges on the glenoid rim (3); the range of gleno-humeral movement (about 90°) can be increased if the arm is externally rotated (4), thereby delaying the impingement of the greater tuberosity. Note that shoulder *rotation* occurs mainly in the gleno-humeral joint.

Fig. 4.B In the *scapulo-thoracic joint*, the scapula (S), moves over the rib cage and serratus anterior. It is supported by the *clavicle* (C) (which articulates with the scapula at the acromio-clavicular joint (AC), and with the sternum at the sterno-clavicular joint (SC)), and by *trapezius, rhomboids, levator scapulae* and *serratus anterior*. The inferior angle of the scapula normally lies at the level of D7.

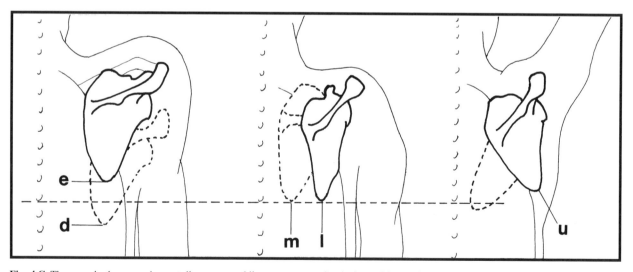

Fig. 4.C The scapula, however, is normally a very mobile structure, varying in its position, and permitting a wide range of *scapulo-thoracic movements*. The scapula may be *elevated* (e) or *depressed* (d) with a maximal total excursion in the order of 12 cm. (Note that *elevation of the shoulder* is a pure scapulo-thoracic movement, and must be distinguished from *elevation of the arm*. The latter term enjoys some popularity as a replacement for abduction or flexion, but because it is somewhat confusing, it is probably best avoided.) The scapula may be *rotated* medially, or laterally and forwards (m, l) round the chest wall. It may also be *tilted* upwards (u) or downwards, with the glenoid angling in a corresponding fashion. When the glenoid is directed upwards, the angle between the vertebral border of the scapula and the vertical may reach 60°. Scapular movement is only possible if there is freedom at the acromio-clavicular and sterno-clavicular joints, and between the scapula and the chest wall.

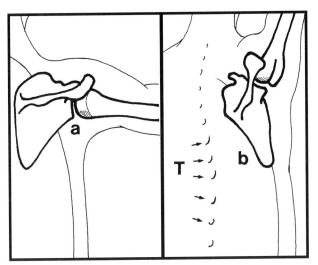

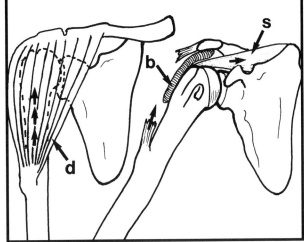

Fig. 4.D *Abduction of the shoulder* (1): During the first 90° of abduction, the gleno-humeral joint is involved more than the scapula (a), while beyond 90°, abduction is continued mainly by scapular movement (b). During the last 30° of abduction, when the gleno-humeral joint is locked and the scapular attachments are tightening, movements *of the spine* may make a contribution: e.g. abduction of the right shoulder may lead to some *lateral flexion* of the thoracic spine (T). The cervical spine may also laterally flex to the other side, to preserve the posture of the head. When both arms are abducted, neither the thoracic nor cervical spine laterally flex, but there may be an increase in lumbar lordosis.

Fig. 4.E *Abduction* (2): The deltoid muscle (d) arises from the lateral end of the clavicle, the acromion, and the spine of the scapula; it is attached to the deltoid tubercle of the humerus. When the arm is at the side, the deltoid acting alone is incapable of *initiating* abduction; its contraction tends to raise the head of the humerus relative to the glenoid. On the other hand, when the arm is at the side, the supraspinatus (s) is in its position of greatest mechanical advantage; with deltoid it forms a couple, and *initiates* abduction (which is then taken over by deltoid). A tear of the supraspinatus (or relevant part of the shoulder cuff) will prevent the normal initiation of abduction which will then only be possible by trick movements. (b = subdeltoid bursa)

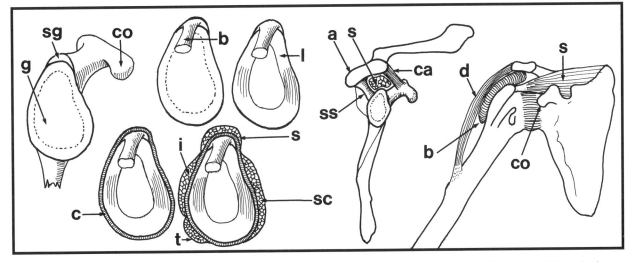

Fig. 4.F *Abduction* (3): In spite of the tendency for gleno-humeral and scapular movements to dominate specific portions of the abduction arc, it should be noted that there is no abrupt transition from one to the other, and indeed all the shoulder girdle joints make a contribution to nearly every movement that takes place in this region. The exceptions are shrugging movements, which do not involve the gleno-humeral joint, and external rotation, which does not involve scapular movement.

The shoulder cuff: The glenoid (g) is widest inferiorly. Anteriorly lies the coracoid (co), and above is the supraglenoid tubercle (sg) from which the long head of biceps (b) arises. The fibro-cartilaginous labrum (l) deepens the glenoid concavity, and is attached to its peripheral margin, along with the joint capsule (c). The capsule is reinforced with the musculo-tendinous insertions of supraspinatus (s), subscapularis (sc), infraspinatus (i) and teres minor (t), which fuse with the capsule laterally, forming a complete tissue annulus (the shoulder cuff). The supraspinatus is its most important part. This in effect runs through a tunnel formed by the spine of the scapula (ss), the acromion (a) and the coraco-acromial ligament (ca). It is partly separated from the acromion by the subdeltoid bursa (b).

Common pathology round the shoulder

The commonest cause of shoulder pain is cervical spondylosis. Pain from irritation of nerve roots in the neck is referred to the shoulder in the same way as pain originating in the lumbar spine may be referred to the hip. There may on occasion be simultaneous pathology in both shoulder and neck, but differentiation is usually straightforward; in particular, restriction of movements of the shoulder with pain at the extremes points to the shoulder as the site of the principal pathology.

Impingement syndromes

The rotator cuff may be compressed during gleno-humeral movement, giving rise to pain and disturbance of scapulo-thoracic rhythm. The commonest site is *subacromial*, causing a painful arc of movement between 70° and 120° abduction. Compression may also occur beneath the *subacromial joint* itself, when there may be a painful arc of movement during the last 30° of abduction, or deep to the *coraco-acromial ligament*. Symptoms may occur acutely (e.g. in young sportsmen and sportswomen) or be chronic, particularly in the older patient, with degenerative changes in the acromio-clavicular (AC) joint which lead to a reduction in size of the supraspinatus tunnel. (Severe shoulder pain in those on haemodialysis is often due to subacromial impingement on amyloid deposits.)

In the acute type, symptoms generally respond to rest or modification of activities. In the chronic case, physiotherapy, analgesics, and the targeted injection of local anaesthetic and steroids may be helpful. If symptoms become persistent and remain disabling, surgery may be required. The commonest procedure is a decompression of the subacromial space; this may involve excision of osteophytes, an AC joint arthroplasty, and excision of the coraco-acromial ligament.

Rotator cuff tears

In the young, athletic patient the shoulder cuff may be torn as the result of a violent traumatic incident. In the older patient, tears may occur spontaneously (e.g. in a cuff weakened as a result of chronic impingement and attrition) or follow more minor trauma, such as sudden arm traction. Most commonly, the supraspinatus region is involved, and the patient has difficulty in initiating abduction of the arm. In other cases, the torn shoulder cuff impinges on the acromion during abduction, giving rise to a painful arc of movement. Although the range of passive movements is not initially disturbed, limitation of rotation may supervene, so that many of these cases, particularly in the older patient, become ultimately indistinguishable from those suffering from frozen shoulder (see later). In the young patient, surgical repair of acute tears is generally advised. In the older patient the indications for surgery are less clear, but operative repair, often combined with a decompression procedure, is becoming increasingly recommended. Prolonged post-operative physiotherapy is usually required.

Rotator cuff arthropathy

If complete rotator cuff tears are neglected, the loss of soft tissue above the head of the humerus may lead to its proximal migration. Friction between the humeral head and the acromion may result in bony collapse and gross degenerative changes in the gleno-humeral joint. In severe cases joint replacement may have to be considered.

'Frozen shoulder'

'Frozen shoulder' is a clinical syndrome which can probably be produced by a variety of pathological processes in the shoulder joint. These can seldom be differentiated and treatment is somewhat empirical. It is a condition affecting the middle-aged, in whose shoulder cuffs degenerative changes are occurring. The outstanding feature is limitation of movements in the shoulder. This restriction is often severe, with virtually no gleno-humeral movements possible, but in the milder cases rotation, especially internal rotation, is primarily affected. Restriction of movements is accompanied in most cases by pain, which is often severe and may disturb sleep. There is frequently (but not always) a history of a minor trauma, which is usually presumed to produce some tearing of the degenerating shoulder cuff, thereby initiating the low-grade prolonged inflammatory changes and contraction of the shoulder cuff responsible for the symptoms. In a number of cases there are fibrotic changes in the coraco-humeral ligament which resemble those found in Dupuytren's disease. Radiographs of the shoulder are almost always normal. In some cases the condition is initiated by a period of immobilisation of the arm, not uncommonly as the result of the inadvised prolonged use of a sling after a Colles' fracture. It is commoner on the left side, and in an appreciable number of cases there is a preceding episode of a silent or overt cardiac infarct. It is commoner in diabetics. If frozen shoulder is untreated, pain subsides after many months, but there may be permanent restriction of movements. The main aim of treatment is to improve the final range of movements in the shoulder, and graduated shoulder exercises are the mainstay of treatment. In some cases where pain is a particular problem, hydrocortisone injections into the shoulder cuff may be helpful. In a few cases, once the acute stage is well past, manipulation of the shoulder under general anaesthesia may be helpful in restoring movements in a stiff joint.

Calcifying supraspinatus tendinitis

Degenerative changes in the shoulder cuff may be accompanied by the local deposition of calcium salts. This process may continue without symptoms, although radiographic changes are obvious. Sometimes, however, the calcified material may give rise to inflammatory changes in the subdeltoid bursa. Sudden, severe, incapacitating pain results; the shoulder becomes acutely tender, and is often swollen and warm to the touch. It is important to differentiate the condition from an acute infection or an acute attack of gout. Symptoms are relieved by the removal of the material by aspiration or curettage, but often local injections of hydrocortisone suffice. The joint is frequently so acutely tender that general anaesthesia is necessary for any attempted aspiration and injection of hydrocortisone.

Osteoarthritis of the acromio-clavicular joint

Arthritic changes in the acromio-clavicular joint may give rise to prolonged pain associated with shoulder movements (with or without shoulder cuff involvement). There is usually an obvious prominence of the joint from arthritic lipping, with well-localised tenderness. Conservative treatment with local heat and exercises may be helpful, but occasionally, in severe persistent cases, acromionectomy may be considered.

Osteoarthritis of the gleno-humeral joint

Osteoarthritis of the gleno-humeral joint is rare, and when it occurs is most frequently secondary to aseptic necrosis of the humeral head. This may be of idiopathic origin, or follow a fracture of the proximal humerus which interferes with the blood supply of its head. It may result from faulty decompression regimes in deep-sea divers, caisson workers and pilots, and it may follow radiotherapy (radionecrosis), particularly treatment for carcinoma of the breast. If empirical treatment fails, joint replacement may have to be considered.

Rheumatoid arthritis of the shoulder

Rheumatoid arthritis is more common than osteoarthritis, and the features are similar to those of the condition in other joints. It is necessary to localise the site of the main pathology so that treatment may be effectively directed, and diagnostic sequential injections may be of help in this respect. Medical treatment and intra-articular injection therapy are tried first. In more advanced cases, where the symptoms are the result of impingement, decompression procedures may be highly effective. Where the gleno-humeral joint is severely diseased, joint replacement will generally produce pain relief and and improved function.

Recurrent dislocation of the shoulder

This condition is seen in the 20–40 age group. There is a history of previous frank dislocations of the shoulder in which the causal trauma has usually become progressively less severe. The shoulder is generally symptom-free between incidents. Surgical repair is generally advised if there have been four or more dislocations.

Recurrent dislocation of the shoulder should be differentiated from habitual dislocation. In the latter the patient is often psychotic or suffering from a joint laxity syndrome. The shoulder repeatedly dislocates without much in the way of pain; the patient is often able to dislocate and reduce the shoulder voluntarily and with ease; and the radiological changes which are found in recurrent dislocation are not present in habitual dislocation. When habitual dislocation is found in children the prognosis is good, and surgery is never indicated. In the adult, surgery is usually best avoided (as the results are often poor), with however good results being claimed for bio-feedback re-education of the shoulder muscles.

Infections round the shoulder

Staphylococcal osteitis of the proximal humerus. This is the commonest infection occurring near the shoulder in the UK at present; nevertheless it is comparatively uncommon.

Tuberculosis of the shoulder. This is now rare. In the moist form, commonest in the first two decades of life, the shoulder is swollen, there is abundant pus production, and sinuses may form; the progress is comparatively rapid and destructive. In the dry form, *caries sicca*, an older age group is affected and the progress is slow with little destruction or pus formation. (It is thought that many of the cases of caries sicca described in the past were in fact suffering from frozen shoulder.)

Gonococcal arthritis of the shoulder. This infection is uncommon, but when it occurs there is moderate swelling of the joint and great pain which often seems out of keeping with the physical signs.

Miscellaneous conditions round the shoulder

Acromio-clavicular dislocation. The acromio-clavicular joint may be disturbed as a result of a fall on the outstretched hand or on the point of the shoulder. If care is taken during examination a lesion of this joint will not be confused with one of the gleno-humeral joint. In major injuries, the conoid and trapezoid ligaments are torn and the clavicle is very unstable; surgical fixation of the clavicle to the coronoid is sometimes advised. In less severe cases, the acromio-clavicular capsular ligaments only are torn; although the outer end of the clavicle becomes prominent, it follows the movement of the acromion and conservative treatment with a sling for several weeks is all that is required. These injuries are frequently missed, as they often do not show in the routine recumbent radiographs of the shoulder.

Clavicle. Primary pathology in the clavicle is uncommon, but a cause of confusion is pathological fracture due to radionecrosis years after treatment for breast carcinoma. The fracture may be preceded by pain for many months, and be mistaken for metastatic spread.

Snapping scapula. A patient may complain of a grinding sensation arising from beneath the scapula. This is often due to a rib prominence, but in some cases it may be caused by an exostosis arising from the deep surface of the scapula. When symptoms are persistent, excision of such an exostosis may give relief.

High scapula. There are several related congenital malformations affecting the neck and shoulder girdle. In the most minor cases one scapula may be a little smaller than the other and be more highly placed; in more severe cases one or both shoulders are highly situated, the scapulae are small, and there may be webs of skin running from the shoulder to the neck (Sprengel's shoulder). In the Klippel-Feil syndrome the neck is short and there are multiple anomalies of the cervical vertebrae which may include vertebral body fusions and spina bifida. Apart from highly placed scapulae, other congenital lesions may be found in association with the Klippel-Feil syndrome; these include diastomatomyelia resulting in tethering of the spinal cord and neurological involvement, lumbo-sacral lipomata and renal abnormalities.

Winged scapula. The patient complains of prominence of the scapula, which is raised along its vertebral border from the chest wall. This is due to weakness of the serratus anterior. The cause may be primarily muscular (as in progressive muscular dystrophy) or follow traumatic paralysis of the long thoracic nerve. Active treatment is seldom necessary.

Ruptured biceps tendon. Rupture of the long head of biceps may occur spontaneously or as a result of a sudden muscular effort, usually in an elderly or middle-aged person in whom degenerative tendon changes are present. No treatment is usually required.

Sterno-clavicular joint. Dislocation of the sterno-clavicular joint is comparatively uncommon; there is always a history of trauma, and the joint asymmetry is obvious if looked for. Good radiographs are often hard to obtain and their interpretation is difficult. The diagnosis should be made primarily on clinical grounds. Symptoms of pain on movement normally settle spontaneously, and only rarely is surgical repair required.

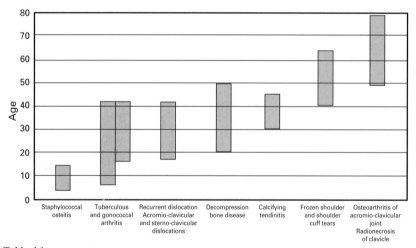

Table 4.1

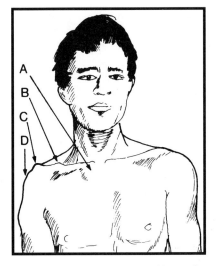

1. *Inspection* (1): *the front:* Note if any of the following are present: (A) prominent sterno-clavicular joint (subluxation); (B) deformity of clavicle (old fracture); (C) prominent acromio-clavicular joint (subluxation or osteoarthritis); (D) deltoid wasting (disuse or axillary nerve palsy).

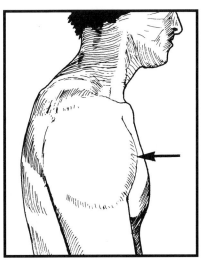

2. *Inspection* (2): *the side:* Note if there is any swelling of the joint, suggesting infection or inflammatory reaction, from, for example, calcifying supraspinatus tendinitis, or from trauma.

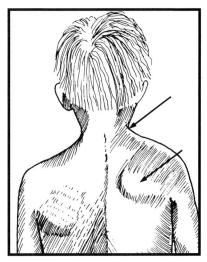

3. *Inspection* (3): *from behind:* Are the scapulae normally shaped and situated, or small and high as in Sprengel's shoulder and the Klippel-Feil syndrome? Is there webbing of the skin at the root of the neck, also typical of the latter? Is there winging of the scapula due to paralysis of serratus anterior (see 4, 38)?

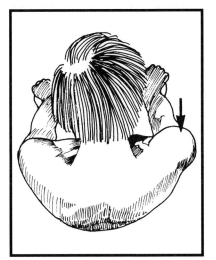

4. *Inspection* (4): *from above:* Again look for swelling of the shoulder, deformity of the clavicle, asymmetry of the supraclavicular fossae.

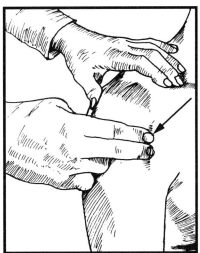

5. *Palpation* (1): Palpate the anterior and lateral aspects of the gleno-humeral joint. *Diffuse* tenderness is suggestive of infection or calcifying supraspinatus tendinitis.

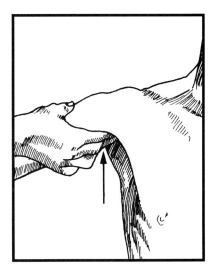

6. *Palpation* (2): Continue the examination by palpating the upper humeral shaft and head via the axilla. Exostoses of the proximal humeral shaft are often readily palpable by this route.

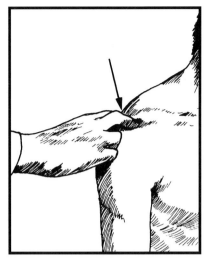

7. *Palpation* (3): Tenderness over the acromio-clavicular joint is found after recent dislocations, and in osteoarthritis of the joint. In the latter, lipping is usually palpable, and crepitus may be detectable when the arm is abducted.

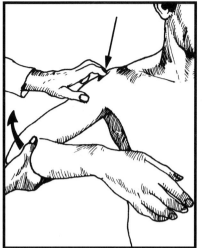

8. *Palpation* (4): Press below the acromion and abduct the arm. Sudden tenderness occurring during a portion of the arc of movement is found in tears and inflammatory lesions involving the shoulder cuff and/or the subdeltoid bursa.

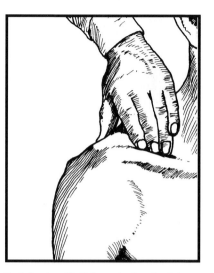

9. *Palpation* (5): Palpate the length of the clavicle. Tenderness is found in sterno-clavicular dislocations and infections (particularly tuberculosis), tumours (rare) and radionecrosis (usually after treatment for breast cancer). Radiological examination of the clavicle is essential if local tenderness is found.

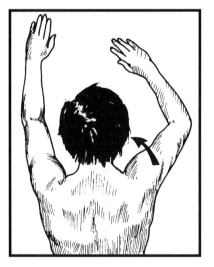

10. *Movements: abduction* (1): Ask the patient to abduct both arms; observe the smoothness of the movement and the range achieved. A full, free and painless range is rare in the presence of any significant pathology in the shoulder region.

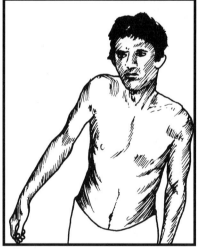

11. *Movements: abduction* (2): Note any difficulty in initiating abduction. Difficulty in doing so is suggestive of a major shoulder cuff tear. A history of violent injury may be obtained in the young adult. In the middle-aged or elderly patient, a tear may follow comparatively minor trauma, or occur spontaneously in a shoulder cuff weakened by attrition from chronic impingement.

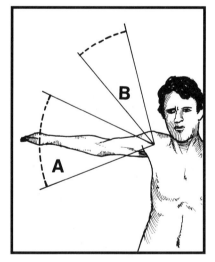

12. *Movements: abduction* (3): Note pain during abduction (which may have to be assisted): (A) during the arc 70–120°, suggestive of shoulder cuff impingement in the region of the acromion; (B) during the latter phase of abduction, suggestive of shoulder cuff impingement in the region of the acromio-clavicular joint or coraco-acromial ligament, or from osteoarthritis of the acromio-clavicular joint.

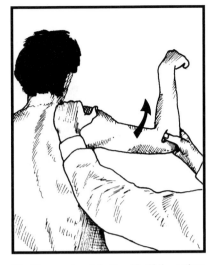

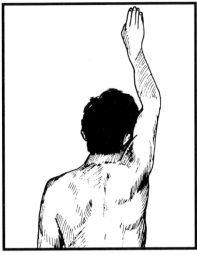

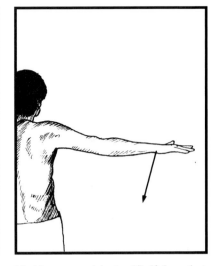

13. *Movements: abduction* (4): If the patient cannot abduct the arm actively, attempt to do this passively, remembering to rotate the arm externally while doing so. A full range indicates an intact gleno-humeral joint.

14. *Movements: abduction* (5): Ask the patient to hold the arm himself in the vertical position. If he can do so, deltoid and the axillary nerve are likely to be intact.

15. *Movements: abduction* (6): If the patient has passed the last test, ask him to lower the arm to the side. Again note the presence of any painful arc of movement.

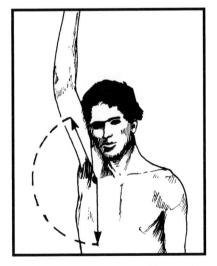

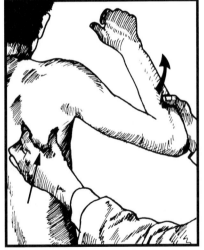

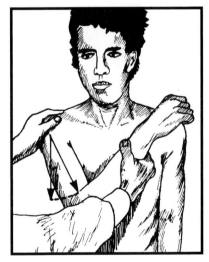

16. *Movements: abduction* (7): Measure the range of abduction. In the normal shoulder, the arm can touch the ear with only slight tilting of the head. The shoulders have already been compared (4, 10). *Normal range: 0–170°.*

17. *Movements: abduction* (8): If both active and passive movements are restricted, fix the angle of the scapula with one hand, and try to abduct the arm with the other. Absence of movement indicates a fixed gleno-humeral joint, the previously noted movements having been entirely scapular.

18. *Movements: adduction in extension:* Place one hand on the shoulder and swing the arm, flexed at the elbow, across the chest. *Normal range: 0–50°.*

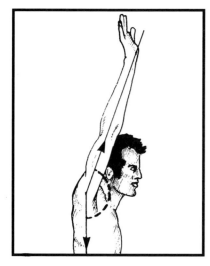

19. *Movements: forward flexion:* Ask the patient to swing the arm forwards and lift it above his head. View the patient from the side. *Normal range: 0–165°.*

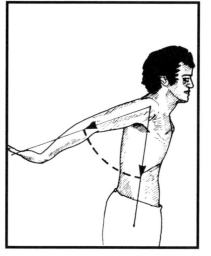

20. *Movements: backwards extension:* Ask the patient to swing the arm directly backwards, again viewing and measuring from the side. *Normal range: 0–60°.*

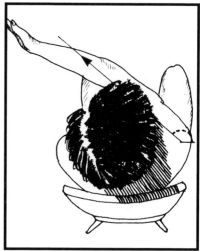

21. *Movements: horizontal flexion and adduction:* Occasionally measurement of this angle may be helpful, but it need not be routine. View the patient from above. The arm is moved forwards from a position of 90° abduction. *Normal range: 0–140°.*

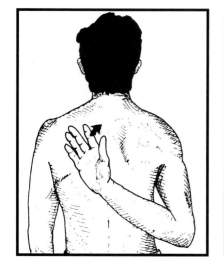

22. *Movements: rotation screening tests* (1): Ask the patient to place the hand behind the opposite shoulder blade. This is a useful test of *internal rotation in extension.*

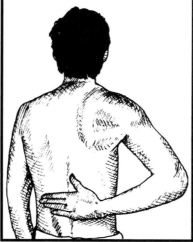

23. *Movements: rotation screening* (2): With slight restriction, he will not be able to get the hand far up the back, and with severe restriction, he will not be able to get it behind the back at all. This movement is commonly affected in frozen shoulder. *To test subscapularis* (which may be torn by violent external rotation, hyperextension or anterior dislocation of the shoulder), ask the patient if he can draw the hand away from contact with the back, when in the position shown.

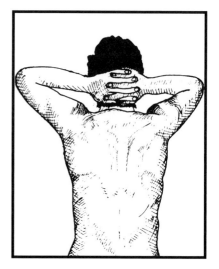

24. *Movements: rotation screening* (3): Ask the patient to place both hands behind the head to screen *external rotation at 90° abduction.* Compare the two sides. Lack of success or restriction is common in frozen shoulder.

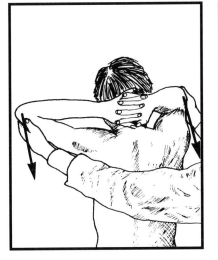

25. *Movements: rotation screening* (4): Sometimes in the last test the patient gets the hand on the affected side behind the head, but in horizontal flexion. If so, gently pull both elbows backwards, noting any difference. (Pain and restriction common in frozen shoulder.)

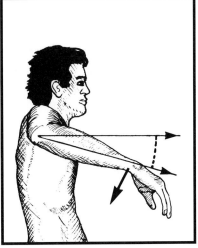

26. *Movements: internal rotation in abduction:* Abduct the shoulder to 90°, and flex the elbow to a right angle. Ask the patient to lower the forearm from the horizontal plane. *Normal range: 70°.*

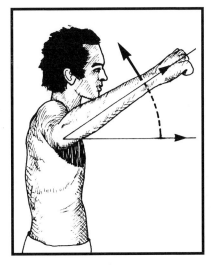

27. *Movements: external rotation in abduction:* From the same starting position with the forearm parallel to the ground, ask the patient to raise the hand, keeping the shoulder in 90° abduction. *Normal range: 100°.*

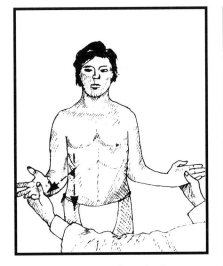

28. *Movements: external rotation in extension:* Place the elbows into the sides, and flex to 90°, with the hands facing forwards. Move the hands laterally, comparing one side with the other. *Normal range: 70°.* An *increase* in external rotation in extension is a feature of tears of the subscapularis muscle (see also 4, 23).

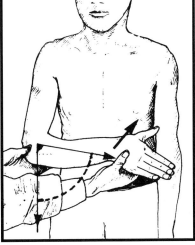

29. *Movements: internal rotation in extension:* Move the hand to the chest from the facing forward position. *Normal range: 70°. For clinical work, assessment of abduction and screening rotation should suffice (but record angular range of movements in all planes for monitoring progress and for medico-legal reports).*

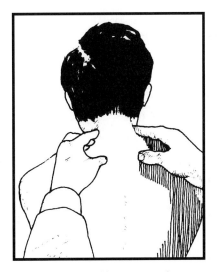

30. *Cervical spine:* Always screen the cervical spine in examining a case of shoulder pain; this is doubly important if shoulder movements are found to be normal.

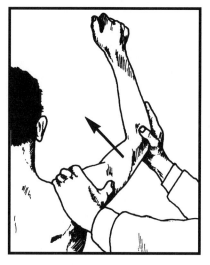

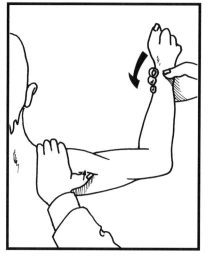

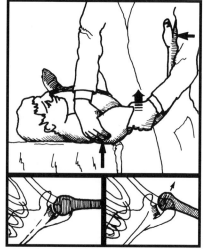

31. *Crepitus:* Place one hand over the shoulder, with the middle finger lying along the acromio-clavicular joint. Abduct the arm with the other hand. Detect any crepitus coming from the shoulder, and locate its source (gleno-humeral or acromio-clavicular). Repeat while the arm is actively abducted, and if in doubt, auscultate. *Clicking* may arise from a number of sources, including scapular exostoses and coracoid impingement. (The latter may cause shoulder pain and coracoid tenderness.)

32. *Suspected gleno-humeral instability* (1): *the apprehension test:* Stand behind the patient (who is preferably seated), and abduct the shoulder to 90°. Externally rotate the shoulder slowly with one hand, while at the same time pushing the head of the humerus forwards with the thumb of your other hand. Apprehension, fear or refusal to continue is evidence of chronic anterior instability of the shoulder.

33. *Suspected gleno-humeral instability* (2): *drawer tests of Gerber and Ganz* (1): Support the (supine) patient's relaxed arm against your side, with his shoulder in 90° abduction, slight flexion and external rotation. Steadying the scapula with the thumb on the coracoid and the fingers behind, try to move the humeral head anteriorly with your other hand. Observe any movement, clicks and patient apprehension, and compare the sides. Axial radiographs may be taken in confirmation during the procedure, which is sometimes performed under anaesthesia.

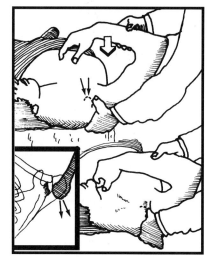

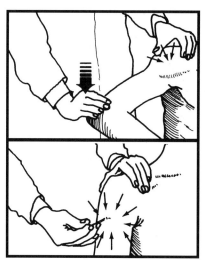

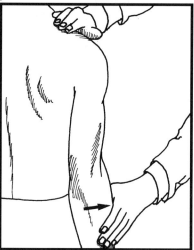

34. *Suspected gleno-humeral instability* (3): *drawer tests* (2): Where recurrent *posterior* dislocation is suspected, hold the relaxed, supine patient's forearm with the elbow flexed and the shoulder in 20° flexion and 90° abduction. Place the thumb just lateral to the coracoid. Now internally rotate the shoulder and flex it to about 80°, pressing the humeral head backwards with the thumb; any backward displacement of the humeral head should be detected with the thumb, but X-ray confirmation may also be made.

35. *Deltoid power:* Ask the patient to try to keep the arm elevated in abduction while you press down on his elbow: look and feel for deltoid contraction. Traction injuries of the axillary nerve resulting in deltoid involvement are seen most frequently after dislocations of the shoulder. If axillary nerve palsy is suspected, test for sensory loss in the 'regimental badge' area on the lateral aspect of the arm.

36. *The suprascapular nerve* (1): *supraspinatus:* Palpate the scapula and identify its spine. Place the fingers of one hand above the spine, over the supraspinatus muscle. Steady the forearm with the other hand, and ask the patient to attempt to abduct the arm against this resistance. If the suprascapular nerve is intact, the contraction of the supraspinatus should be easily felt.

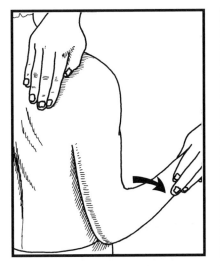

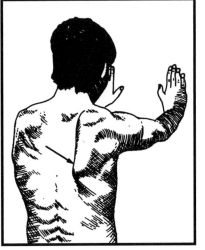

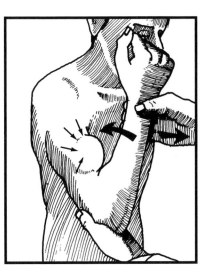

37. *The suprascapular nerve* (2): *infraspinatus:* In a similar manner palpate the infraspinatus, caudal to the spine of the scapula, while asking the patient to externally rotate the shoulder against resistance. Paralysis of the muscle, with pain and weakness of the shoulder, may result from a ganglion in the spino-glenoid (greater scapular) notch. The diagnosis may be confirmed by MRI scan.

38. *Long thoracic nerve:* Where paralysis of serratus anterior is suspected, ask the patient to lean with both hands against a wall. Any tendency to winging of the scapula immediately becomes apparent.

39. *Long head of biceps:* Support the patient's elbow with one hand. Grasp his wrist, and ask him to pull towards his shoulder, while you resist this movement. If the long tendon of biceps is ruptured, the belly of biceps will appear globular in shape. Compare the two sides.

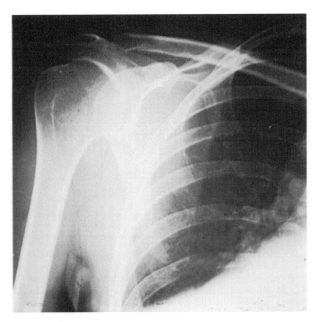

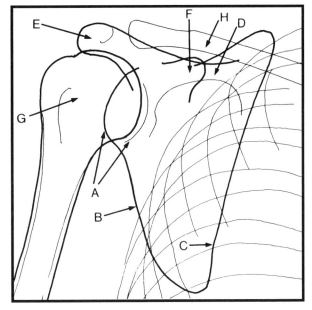

40. *Radiographs* (1): Antero-posterior view of the normal shoulder.

41. *Radiographs* (2): The standard shoulder projection is the antero-posterior taken in recumbency. Examine the radiograph methodically by identifying (A) the glenoid; (B) the lateral border of the scapula; (C) the medial border; (D) its spine; (E) the acromion; (F) the coracoid. Note the relations of the humeral head (G) and the clavicle (H) to the glenoid and the acromion.

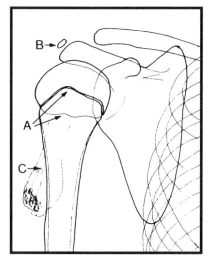

42. *Radiographs* (3): In the child or adolescent, do not mistake (A) the anterior and/or posterior margins of the epiphyseal plate for fracture or (B) the acromial ossification centre for a loose body. Note (C) the typical appearance of a simple exostosis (ossifying chondroma) of epiphyseal plate origin.

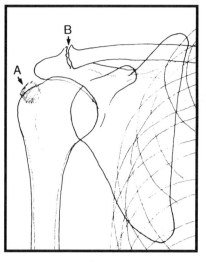

43. *Radiographs* (4): Calcification in the supraspinatus tendon in the upper part of the shoulder cuff has an amorphous appearance (A) and is characteristically situated. It may be symptom-free. Note (B) arthritic changes in the acromio-clavicular joint.

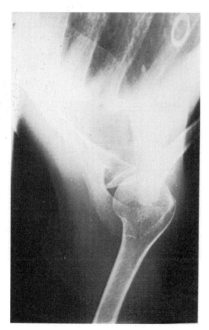

44. *Radiographs* (5): Normal axial (per-axillary or axillary) lateral.

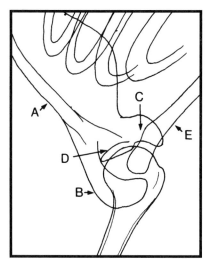

45. *Radiographs* (6): The axial lateral gives the most useful additional information, but is dependent on the patient being able to abduct the arm. It is very helpful in clarifying the relationships of the glenoid and humeral head. (A) lateral border in continuity with scapular spine; (B) acromion; (C) coracoid; (D) glenoid; (E) clavicle.

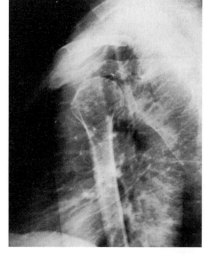

46. *Radiographs* (7): *normal translateral* (1): If the patient is not able to have the arm abducted, a translateral is another view which may be employed to give additional information. Unfortunately detail is often poor, especially in the stout patient. (Some prefer an apical oblique projection, taken with the plate at 45° and the beam angled appropriately; this duplicates and foreshortens the features seen in 41, but helps clarify the gleno-humeral relationship.)

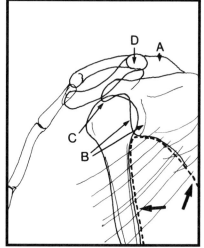

47. *Radiographs* (8): *normal translateral* (2): Note (A) scapular spine, (B) glenoid, (C) coracoid, (D) acromio-clavicular joints and superimposed clavicular shadows. Note the parabolic curve formed by the humeral shaft and the lateral border of the scapula. This is disturbed in most shoulder dislocations and subluxations.

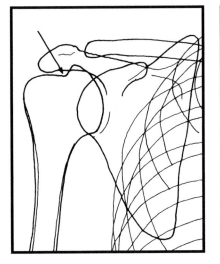

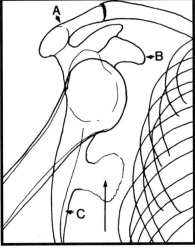

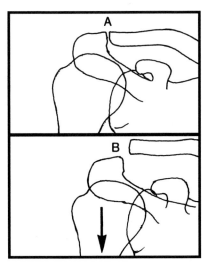

48. *Radiographs* (9): In suspected recurrent dislocation of the shoulder, an additional antero-posterior view should always be taken with the arm internally rotated. This may show a confirmatory defect in the postero-lateral part of the head ('hatchet head'). An axial lateral will help to confirm this.

49. *Radiographs* (10): In cases of clicking or snapping shoulder, tangential views of the blade of the scapula will reveal any causal exostosis, particularly on the costal surface. (A) Acromion; (B) glenoid; (C) blade of scapula.

50. *Radiographs* (11): Where subluxation of the acromio-clavicular joint is suspected, it is *essential* that the antero-posterior view of the shoulder is taken with the patient erect and holding a weight on the affected side. (A) Normal joint; (B) acromio-clavicular dislocation.

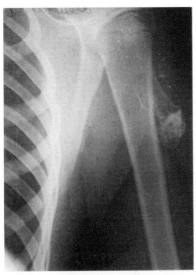

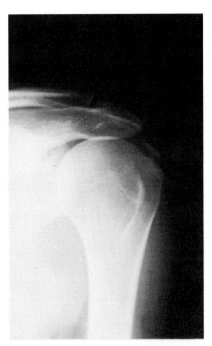

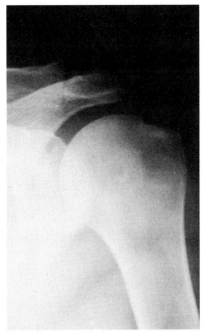

51. *Shoulder radiographs: examples of pathology* (1): There is a calcified mass over the humeral shaft: its pedicle is attached to the metaphysis. The appearances are of a simple exostosis (ossifying chondroma, enchondroma).

52. *Pathology* (2): There is an amorphous mass of calcified material situated over the humeral head. Diagnosis: calcifying supraspinatus tendinitis.

53. *Pathology* (3): There is narrowing of the joint space, some irregularity of the surfaces, and a little lipping in keeping with a diagnosis of osteoarthritis of the acromio-clavicular joint. There is a minimal degree of calcifying supraspinatus tendinitis also present.

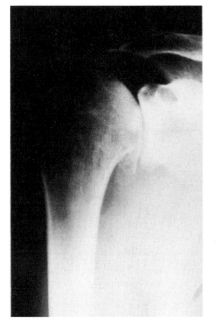

54. *Pathology* (4): There is marked narrowing of the gleno-humeral joint space, with a large exostosis arising from the humeral head. Diagnosis: osteoarthritis of the gleno-humeral joint.

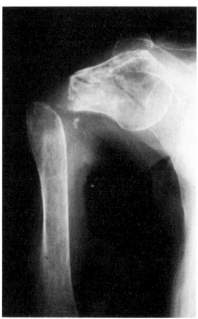

55. *Pathology* (5): There is non-union in a fracture of the proximal humerus. The bone ends are rounded off and rather osteoporotic. This has been a pathological fracture resulting from radionecrosis following therapy for breast carcinoma.

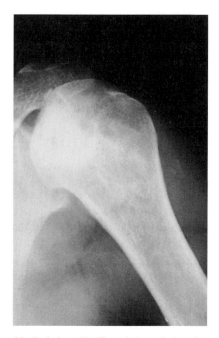

56. *Pathology* (6): There is irregularity of the humeral head, with patches of increased density. The appearances are characteristic of the type of avascular necrosis seen in caisson disease.

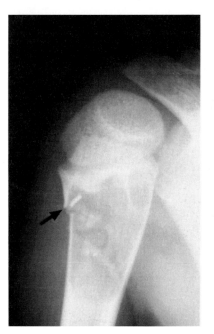

57. *Pathology* (7): The arrow points to a fracture through the proximal humerus of a child. The bone is expanded and there is thinning of the cortex. This is a pathological fracture through a simple (unicameral) bone cyst.

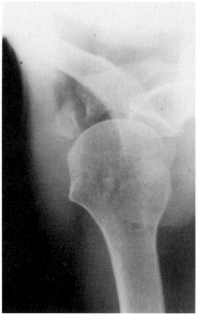

58. *Pathology* (8): This axial projection shows non-union in a fracture of the coracoid.

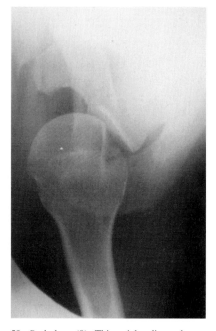

59. *Pathology* (9): This axial radiograph shows an anterior subluxation of the shoulder associated with a defect in the humeral head. The findings confirm a clinical diagnosis of recurrent dislocation of the shoulder.

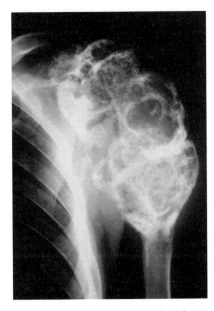

60. *Pathology* (10): The humeral head has been replaced by a huge mass of poorly differentiated bone; the appearances are typical of osteoclastoma (giant cell tumour of bone), a locally malignant condition which may become invasive and metastasise.

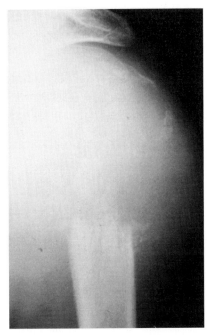

61. *Pathology* (11): The head of the humerus has been destroyed by a (malignant) chondrosarcoma.

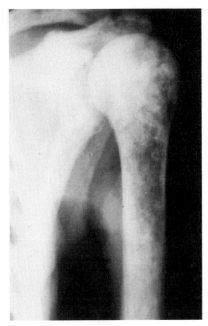

62. *Pathology* (12): The humerus and scapula show widespread sclerotic changes typical of metastatic spread from a carcinoma of the prostate.

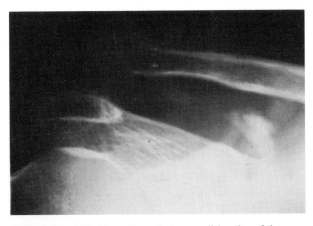

63. *Pathology* (13): The radiograph shows a dislocation of the acromio-clavicular joint. In addition, there is evidence of calcification in the haematoma which has resulted from the tearing of the conoid and trapezoid ligaments.

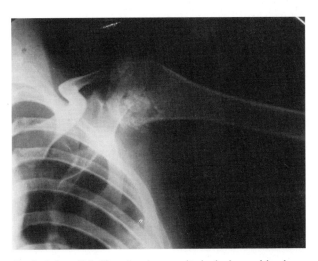

64. *Pathology* (14): There is a large cavity in the humeral head containing a sequestrum; calcified pus is also present. The appearances are typical of tuberculosis of the shoulder joint.

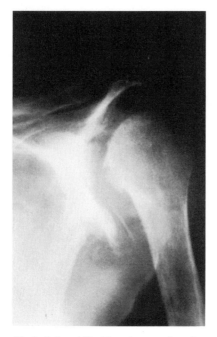

65. *Pathology* (15): There is gross distortion of the humeral head and the glenoid, with alteration of bone texture and destructive changes typical of Charcot's disease.

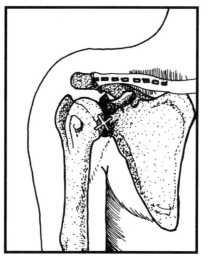

66. *Special investigations* (1): *aspiration:* Consider if pus is suspected. *Method:* with the patient supine, follow the clavicle laterally and find the coracoid, which lies about 5 cm obliquely below the acromio-clavicular joint. Now rotate the arm, when you should be able to feel the head of the humerus. After local infiltration, pass a large-bore needle directly backwards into the joint below and just lateral to the coracoid.

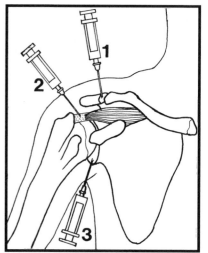

67. *Special investigations* (2): Where there is shoulder pain related to movement, and the source is uncertain, serial injections with local anaesthetic may be tried. Start with the acromio-clavicular joint (1); if pain on movement is not relieved after 5–10 minutes, proceed to the upper part of the shoulder cuff (2); and if this also fails, infiltrate the gleno-humeral joint (3). This may be approached as detailed in the previous figure.

68. *Special investigations* (3): Other investigations can include the following:

(1) *Suspected infections:*
White cell count and differential blood count; blood culture; erythrocyte sedimentation rate (ESR); X-ray of the chest; aspiration of the joint, with the appropriate examinations to exclude pyogenic, gonococcal and tubercular infections.

(2) *Undiagnosed mechanical problems or painful arc syndromes:*
Examination of the joint by CAT scan or MRI scan.
Arthrography, with the use of radio-opaque dye in (a) the gleno-humeral joint, or (b) the subdeltoid bursa.
Examination of the joint under general anaesthesia.
Athroscopy.

5. The elbow

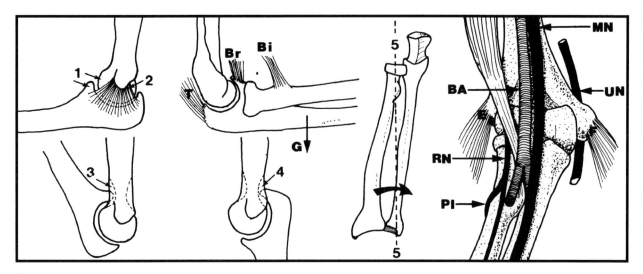

Fig. 5.A

Anatomical features

General points. The calliper-like close fit between the ulna and the trochlea (1) contributes to the impressive stability of the normal elbow; this is aided by the strong collateral ligaments (2). Instability may be seen following certain fractures of the coracoid or olecranon, or when the ligaments become lax in the course of rheumatoid arthritis or joint infection.

At the end of flexion, the coronoid process tucks into the coronoid fossa (3); and at full extension, the olecranon process fits into the olecranon fossa (4). The clearances are small, and only a little local disturbance such as a small loose body in one of the fossae may produce a significant restriction of movement.

The elbow joint is normally extended by gravity (G); forced extension is powered by triceps (T); and triceps acting with the elbow flexors (biceps (Bi) and brachialis (Br)) holds the elbow straight and rigid.

The axis (5) of pronation and supination passes through the radial head and the attachment of the triangular fibro-cartilage. Mechanically, pronation and supination may be restricted by problems involving the elbow, wrist, or forearm bones. Pronation is controlled by pronator teres and pronator quadratus; supination is carried out by biceps and supinator.

Important relations. The median nerve (MN) and brachial artery (BA) lie medial to the biceps tendon, and superficial to the brachialis muscle.

The radial nerve (RN) and its important posterior interosseous nerve branch (PI) lie lateral to the biceps tendon.

The ulnar nerve (UN) at the elbow lies behind the medial epicondyle.

The main extensor muscle origin (E) is from the lateral epicondyle.

The main flexor origin (F) is from the medial epicondyle.

Tennis elbow

This is by far the commonest cause of elbow pain in patients attending orthopaedic clinics. It is generally believed to be due to a strain of the common extensor origin, but fibrosis in extensor carpi radialis brevis or a nerve entrapment syndrome have been suggested as alternative causes. The patient, usually in the 35–50 age group, complains of pain on the lateral side of the elbow and difficulty in holding any heavy object at arm's length. There may be a history of recent excessive activity involving the elbow — e.g. dusting, sweeping, painting or even playing tennis.

In sportsmen and sportswomen, a period of rest or modification of a flawed game-playing technique may allow the condition to settle. In manual workers, relief may follow avoidance of the suspected causal activity, although this may not always be possible. When these basic measures fail, an elbow clamp (employed to redirect the pull of the forearm extensors) can be effective. Symptoms are also usually relieved by 1–3 injections of local anaesthetic and hydrocortisone into the painful area, and local ultrasound may be tried. Excellent results have been claimed from extra-corporeal shock wave therapy. In resistant cases, when all conservative measures have failed, exploration of extensor carpi radialis brevis may be considered (with excision of any fibrous mass or lengthening of the tendon).

In golfer's elbow, there is a similar history, but here pain and tenderness involve the common flexor origin on the medial side of the elbow. This condition is much less common than tennis elbow.

Cubitus varus and cubitus valgus

Decrease or increase in the carrying angle of the elbow generally follows a supracondylar or other elbow fracture in childhood. While the normal child has great powers of spontaneous recovery following injury, there may nevertheless be some epiphyseal damage which fails to correct; where there is evidence of interference with the carrying angle the child should be observed for a number of years. If there is failure of spontaneous correction or even deterioration, and the deformity is very unsightly, correction by osteotomy may be undertaken. In later life either of these deformities may be followed by a tardy ulnar nerve palsy.

Tardy ulnar nerve palsy

This ulnar nerve palsy is of slow onset and progression. It appears usually between the ages of 30 and 50, and the preceding injury to the elbow, considered responsible for the ischaemic and fibrotic changes in the nerve, has usually been in childhood. It is seen most frequently where there is a cubitus valgus deformity. The progress of the palsy may be arrested by transposition of the nerve from its normal position behind the medial epicondyle to the front of the joint.

Ulnar neuritis and the ulnar tunnel syndrome

Ulnar neuritis, with its frequent accompaniment of small muscle wasting and sensory impairment in the hand, may occur as a complication of local trauma at the elbow or at the wrist. At the elbow, it is also seen where the nerve is abnormally mobile. In these circumstances it is exposed to frictional damage as it slips repeatedly in front of and behind the medial epicondyle. In such cases re-anchorage or transposition may prevent further deterioration.

The nerve is also subject to pressure as it passes between the two heads of flexor carpi ulnaris below the elbow, or as it lies in the ulnar tunnel in the hand. Where the local findings are not clear enough to localise the site of involvement, nerve conduction rate studies are often most helpful.

In a number of cases no obvious cause for an ulnar neuritis may be found.

Olecranon bursitis

Swelling of the olecranon bursa is common in carpet-layers and others who repeatedly traumatise the posterior aspect of the elbow joint. Swelling of the bursa is also common in rheumatoid arthritis, and there may be associated nodular masses in the proximal part of the forearm. The condition is usually painless unless there is an associated bacterial infection within the bursa. Excision is sometimes advised for cosmetic reasons.

Pulled elbow

This condition occurs in young children under the age of 5, and is produced by traction on the arm, as for example when a mother snatches the hand of a child wandering towards the edge of a pavement. The radial head slides out from under cover of the orbicular ligament, and the child complains of pain and limitation of supination. The orbicular ligament and radial head may be reduced by forced supination while pushing the radius in a proximal direction (by forced radial deviation of the hand). On the other hand, spontaneous reduction, without manipulation, usually occurs within 48 hours of the incident if the arm is rested in a sling.

Osteoarthritis and osteochondritis dissecans

Primary osteoarthritis of the elbow joint is not uncommon in heavy manual workers. Osteoarthritis is also seen secondary to old fractures involving the articular surfaces of the elbow. It may also follow osteochondritis dissecans.

Both osteoarthritis and osteochondritis dissecans may give rise to the formation of loose bodies which restrict movements or cause locking of the joint. The joint may lock in any position, and the patient often develops the trick of unlocking the joint himself. If loose bodies are found, they should be removed to prevent further incidents of locking and to reduce the risks of their causing more damage to the articular surfaces. Joint replacement surgery in those suffering from osteoarthritis of the elbow is seldom indicated, as the physical demands are likely to exceed the capabilities of any current replacement.

Rheumatoid arthritis

Rheumatoid arthritis may affect either one or both elbows. If both elbows are involved, the functional disability may be particularly great.

Clinically there may be marked synovitis, painful restriction of movements, and a fixed flexion deformity. Pronation and supination may be restricted and painful, although in some cases the distal radio-ulnar joint may be responsible. When there is gross destruction of the elbow, the ulnar nerve may be affected, and the joint may become flail.

Medical treatment and steroid injections may help in the early stages. Later, synovectomy with excision of the radial head may delay progress; and in the advanced case, with gross instability, joint replacement may be considered.

Tuberculosis of the elbow

Tuberculosis of the elbow is now very uncommon; marked swelling of the elbow with profound local muscle wasting is usually so striking that there is unlikely to be delay in further investigation by aspiration and synovial biopsy.

Myositis ossificans

This condition occurs most commonly after supracondylar fractures and dislocations of the elbow. Calcification occurs in the haematoma which forms in the brachialis muscle covering the anterior aspect of the elbow joint. It is particularly common in association with head injuries, and may also follow over-vigorous physiotherapy. It leads to a mechanical block to flexion. If discovered at an early stage, complete rest of the joint is necessary to minimise the mass of material formed. In later cases it may be excised after the lesion has appeared quiescent for many months.

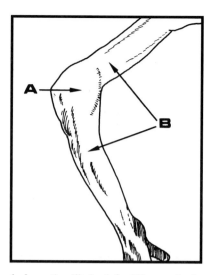

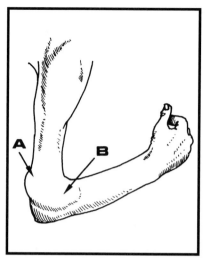

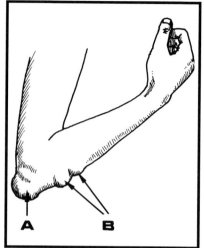

1. *Inspection* (1): Look for (A) generalised swelling of the joint; (B) muscle wasting, both suggestive of infective arthritis (e.g. tuberculosis) or rheumatoid arthritis. The swollen elbow is always held in the semiflexed position.

2. *Inspection* (2): (A) Note that the earliest sign of effusion is the filling out of the hollows seen in the flexed elbow above the olecranon. (B) The next sign is swelling of the radio-humeral joint. Fluid may be squeezed between these two areas.

3. *Inspection* (3): Note if there are any localised swellings round the joint — e.g. (A) olecranon bursitis; (B) rheumatoid nodules.

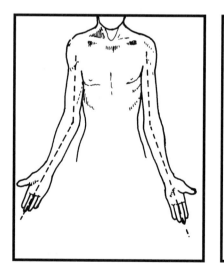

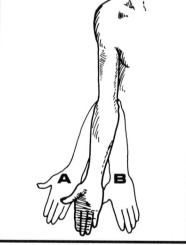

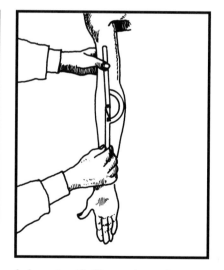

4. *Inspection* (4): Ask the patient to extend both elbows and note the carrying angle on both sides. Any small difference between the sides will then be obvious.

5. *Inspection* (5): (A) In cubitus valgus there is an increase in the carrying angle. (B) In cubitus varus there is a decrease in the carrying angle. The commonest cause of unilateral alteration in the carrying angle is an old supracondylar fracture.

6. *Inspection* (6): The carrying angle may be measured with the goniometer. *Average values: Males: 11° (range 2–26°); Females: 13° (range 2–22°).*

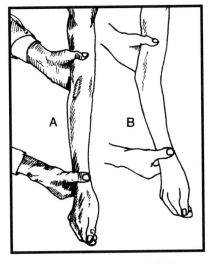

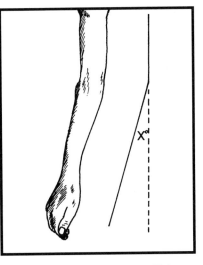

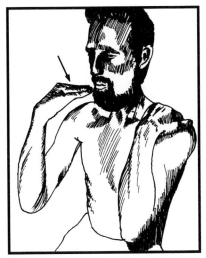

7. *Movements* (1): *extension:* (A) Full extension: 0° is present if the arm and forearm can be made to lie in a straight line. (B) Loss of full extension is especially common in osteoarthritis, rheumatoid arthritis, and old fractures (particularly of the radial head) involving the elbow joint.

8. *Movements* (2): *hyperextension:* If the elbow can be exended beyond the neutral position, record as 'X° hyperextension'. Up to 15° is accepted as normal, especially in women. Beyond this, look for hypermobility in other joints (e.g. Ehlers-Danlos syndrome).

9. *Movements* (3): *flexion* (1): (Screening test) Ask the patient to attempt to touch both shoulders. A slight difference in flexion between the sides is then usually obvious.

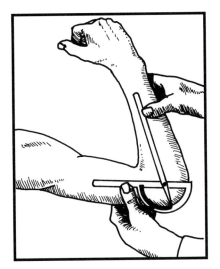

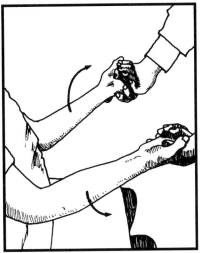

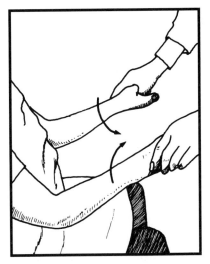

10. *Movements* (4): *flexion* (2): The range of flexion may be measured. *Normal range: 145°.* Restriction of flexion is common after all fractures round the elbow and in all forms of arthritis.

11. *Movements* (5): *pronation/supination screening* (1): Ask the patient to hold the elbows closely to the sides. Turn the palms upwards into supination, comparing the sides.

12. *Movements* (6): *pronation/supination screening* (2): Now turn the palms downwards in pronation, again comparing the sides.

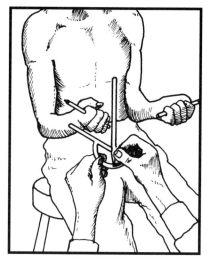

13. *Movements* (7): *supination:* Supination may be recorded. Give the patient a pencil to hold, and note the angle achieved from the vertical. *Normal range: 80°.*

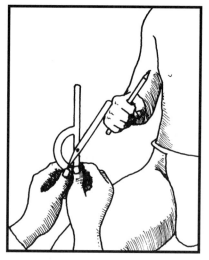

14. *Movements* (8): *pronation:* This may be measured in the same way. *Normal range: 75°.* Pronation/supination movements may be reduced after fractures at the elbow, forearm and wrist (e.g. most commonly after Colles' fracture). Loss may also occur after dislocation of the elbow and rheumatoid and osteoarthritis. Pure supination loss may occur in children with pulled elbow.

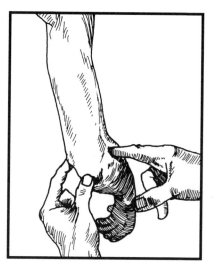

15. *Palpation* (1): Begin by locating the epicondyles and the olecranon. If in doubt, flex the elbow and note the equilateral triangle normally formed by these structures. This relationship is disturbed in elbow subluxations.

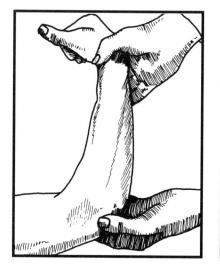

16. *Palpation* (2): Palpate the lateral epicondyle with the thumb. Sharply localised tenderness here or just distal is almost diagnostic of tennis elbow. Carry out confirmatory tests (5, 22). Note that after the injection of hydrocortisone locally (e.g. for tennis elbow) tenderness becomes more diffuse.

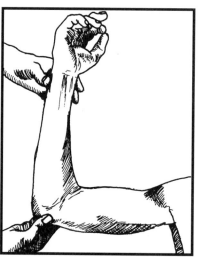

17. *Palpation* (3): Palpate the medial epicondyle. Tenderness occurs here in golfer's elbow, tears of the ulnar collateral ligament, and injuries of the medial epicondyle.

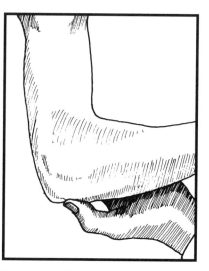

18. *Palpation* (4): Tenderness over the olecranon is uncommon, apart from fracture and infected olecranon bursitis, both of which are usually obvious.

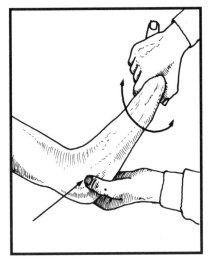

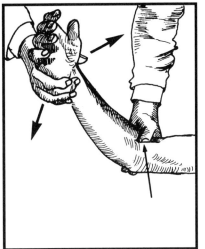

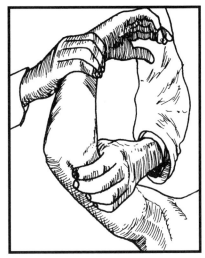

19. *Palpation* (5): Press the thumb firmly into the space on the lateral side of the elbow between the radial head and humerus. Now pronate and supinate the arm. Tenderness here is common after injuries of the radial head, osteoarthritis and osteochondritis dissecans.

20. *Palpation* (6): Palpate the front of the elbow on both sides of the biceps tendon while flexing and extending the elbow through 20°. Note the presence of any abnormal masses (e.g. myositis ossificans, loose bodies).

21. *Palpation* (7): Roll the ulnar nerve under the fingers behind the medial epicondyle. Note if there is any difference between the sides. If indicated, carry out a fuller examination of the nerve (see 2, 39).

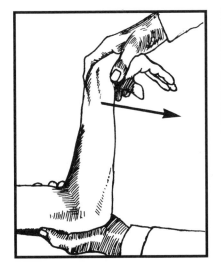

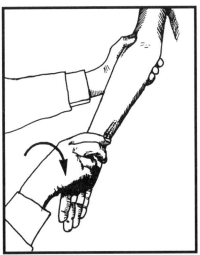

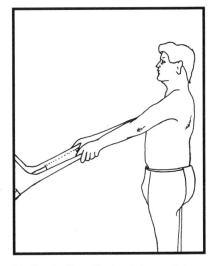

22. *Additional tests: tennis elbow* (1): Flex the elbow and fully pronate the hand. Now extend the elbow. Pain over the lateral epicondyle is almost diagnostic of tennis elbow.

23. *Tennis elbow* (2): As an alternative, pain may be sought by pronating the arm with the elbow fully extended.

24. *Tennis elbow* (3): *the chair test:* Ask the patient to attempt to lift a chair (of about 3.5 kg in weight), with the elbows extended and the shoulders flexed to 60°. Difficulty in performing this manoeuvre, with complaint of pain on the lateral aspect of the affected elbow, is suggestive of tennis elbow.

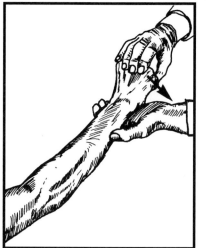

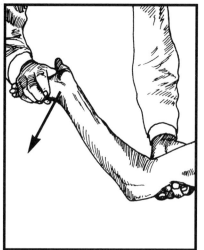

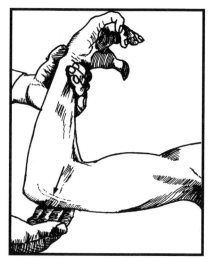

25. *Tennis elbow* (4): *Thomsen's test:* Ask the patient to clench the fist, dorsiflex the wrist, and extend the elbow. Try to force the hand into palmar flexion while the patient resists. Severe pain over the external epicondyle is again most suggestive of tennis elbow. (5) Repeat, only this time attempting to flex the extended middle finger rather than the wrist.

26. *Additional tests: golfer's elbow:* Flex the elbow, supinate the hand, and then extend the elbow. Pain over the medial epicondyle is very suggestive of golfer's elbow.

27. *Additional tests: ulnar nerve* (1): Inspect the medial side of the elbow carefully while the patient flexes and extends the joint. The nerve is visible in the thin patient, and displacement on movement may be obvious.

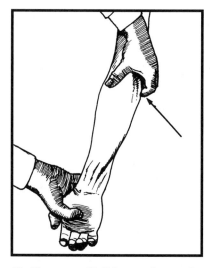

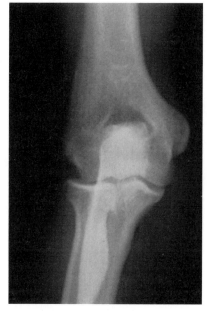

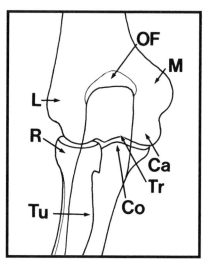

28. *Ulnar nerve* (2): Palpate again; note the extent of any tenderness, and whether the nerve is thickened. Look again for cubitus valgus. Look for evidence of ulnar nerve palsy (see 2, 39).

29. *Radiographs* (1): Normal antero-posterior (AP) radiograph of the elbow.

30. *Radiographs* (2): In examining the standard AP view, trace out the outline of (M) medial epicondyle; (OF) olecranon and coronoid fossae; (L) lateral epicondyle; (Ca) capitulum; (R) radial head; (Tu) tuberosity of the radius; (Co) coronoid process of ulna; (Tr) trochlea.

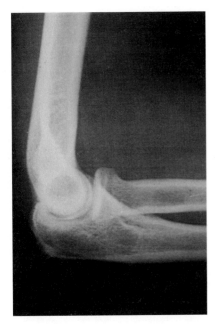

31. *Radiographs* (3): Normal lateral radiograph of the elbow.

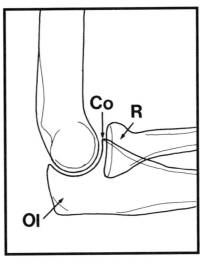

32. *Radiographs* (4): In examining the standard lateral projection, note (R) radial head; (Co) coronoid process of the ulna; (Ol) olecranon.

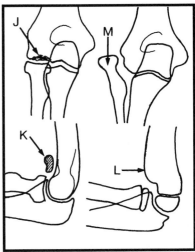

33. *Radiographs* (5): Look for (J) any defects in the capitulum suggesting osteochondritis dissecans; (K) loose bodies (usually secondary to osteoarthritis or osteochondritis); (L) incompletely remodelled supracondylar fracture (usually associated with loss of flexion); (M) old Monteggia fracture (fracture of ulna and dislocation head of radius), usually associated with reduction of pronation and supination.

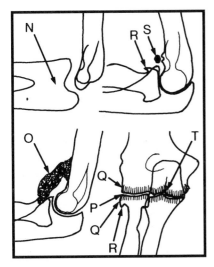

34. *Radiographs* (6): Note the presence of (N) a congenital synostosis (with inevitable loss of pronation and supination); (O) myositis ossificans (with clinical restriction of flexion). Note any osteoarthritic changes, with for example (P) joint space narrowing; (Q) sclerosis; (R) osteophytes; (S) loose body formation, or (T) evidence of previous fracture.

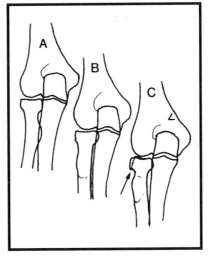

35. *Radiographs* (7): Where the radial head is suspect, radiographs should be taken in the antero-posterior plane (A) in mid-position; (B) in supination; (C) in pronation. These may bring an area of osteochondritis of the radial head or an old fracture into profile.

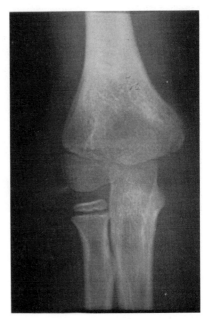

36. *Radiographs* (8): Normal antero-posterior radiograph of the elbow of a child of 8.

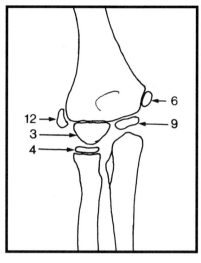

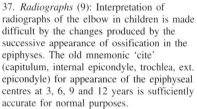

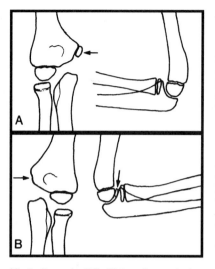

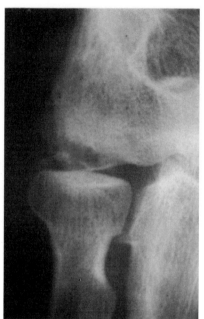

37. *Radiographs* (9): Interpretation of radiographs of the elbow in children is made difficult by the changes produced by the successive appearance of ossification in the epiphyses. The old mnemonic 'cite' (capitulum, internal epicondyle, trochlea, ext. epicondyle) for appearance of the epiphyseal centres at 3, 6, 9 and 12 years is sufficiently accurate for normal purposes.

38. *Radiographs* (10): If there is any doubt, radiographs of both sides should be taken. Note that if a child over 6 has injured the elbow there is every likelihood that the medial epicondyle has become displaced into the joint if it *cannot* be seen in the antero-posterior view or if it *can* be seen in the lateral. (A) Normal; (B) displaced.

39. *Elbow radiographs: examples of pathology* (1): This radiograph shows the typical appearance of osteochondritis of the capitulum. In this case the condition was responsible for aching pain in the joint of several months' duration.

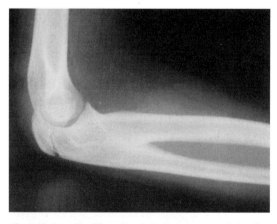

40. *Pathology* (2): The radiograph shows a congenital radio-ulnar synostosis. No pronation/supination movements are possible. The epiphysis of the olecranon has not yet united.

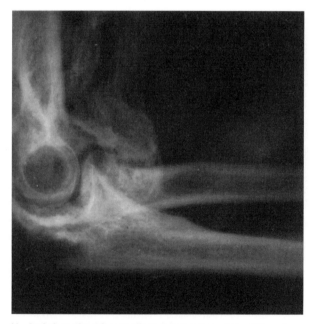

41. *Pathology* (3): After an elbow injury a large mass of bone has formed in the front of the joint, and has virtually obliterated all movements: myositis ossificans.

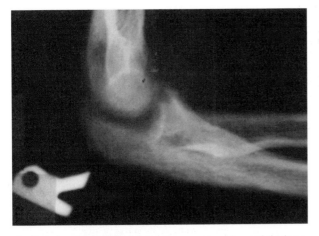

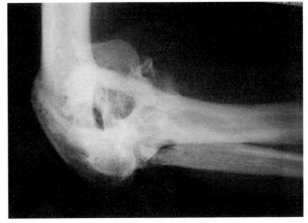

42. *Pathology* (4): All the joint surfaces are irregular, and the bone texture has a moth-eaten appearance. This is a septic arthritis of the elbow.

43. *Pathology* (5): Following a gunshot wound of the elbow with extensive bone damage, bony ankylosis has occurred.

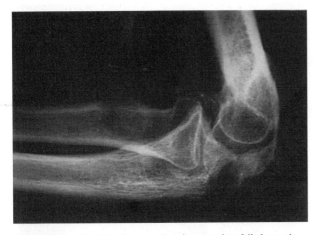

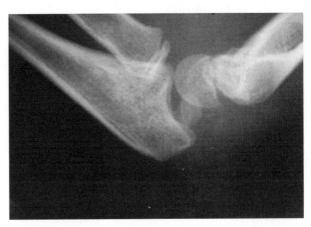

44. *Pathology* (6): After fracture, the olecranon has failed to unite with the rest of the ulna. Injuries of this type may have surprisingly few symptoms, but there is often weakness and restriction of extension.

45. *Pathology* (7): Following a dislocation of the elbow there is marked restriction of movements due to the medial epicondyle having been trapped between the joint surfaces.

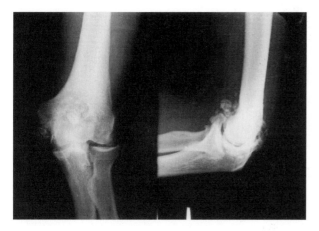

46. *Pathology* (8): There is osteoarthritis of the elbow with the formation of multiple loose bodies in the joint. Synovial chondromatosis may have a similar appearance.

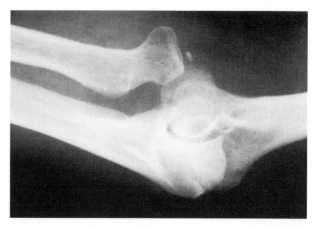

47. *Pathology* (9): There has been an old Monteggia injury of the elbow, with long-standing persistent dislocation of the radial head and a cubitus varus deformity; this was followed by a tardy ulnar nerve palsy.

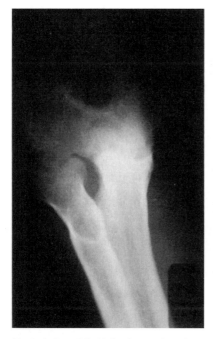

48. *Pathology* (10): Following a tuberculous infection of the joint there has been a fibrous ankylosis, with the articular surfaces of the ulna and trochlea being virtually obliterated.

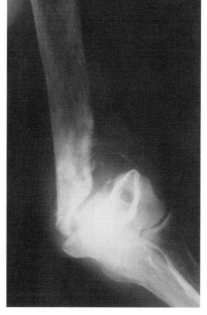

49. *Pathology* (11): An old supracondylar fracture of the humerus has failed to unite, forming a pseudarthrosis. In this case, very little movement remained in the elbow joint, most of the rather unstable range of flexion and extension occurring at the old fracture site.

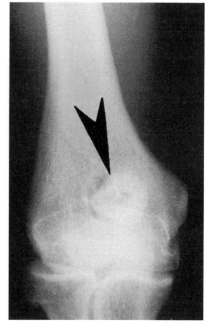

50. *Pathology* (12): The arrow points to a large loose body lying in the coronoid fossa. Such a mass would be responsible for substantial restriction of flexion in the joint.

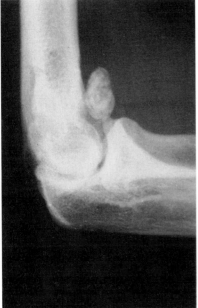

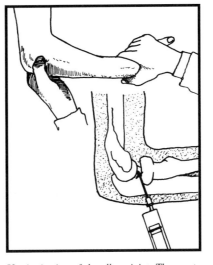

51. *Pathology* (13): This lateral radiograph shows a large loose body lying in the front of the joint; in some cases, loose bodies of this type may be extruded and come to lie in the brachialis muscle where their mechanical effects are less obtrusive.

52. *Aspiration of the elbow joint:* The most direct and safest approach is from the lateral side. Flex the elbow to 90°; to locate the radial head, pronate and supinate the arm, and feel with the thumb for its rotation. After infiltration of the area with local anaesthetic, introduce the aspirating needle in the area of the palpable depression between the proximal part of the radial head and the capitulum.

6. The wrist

Study of the wrist cannot be separated from the hand, and in many cases careful examination of both may be required.

Complications occurring after Colles' fracture

Considering the incidence of Colles' fracture, the commonest of all fractures, it is surprising that complications from this injury are not seen more frequently. Nevertheless they do occur and are of importance. Excluding initial weakness of the wrist, the commonest complaints are of residual deformity, restriction of movements and pain.

The common deformities are radial deviation of the hand and prominence of the ulna. Due to resorption of bone at the fracture site during healing, there is shortening of the radius with radial deviation of the hand. This may be aggravated by a poor reduction. At the back of the wrist, the head of the ulna becomes prominent. (Gross subluxations of the ulna of this pattern are sometimes referred to as Madelung's deformity; this term was used initially to describe a condition occurring in adolescents, where following some disturbance of growth in the distal radial epiphysis, often idiopathic in origin, the ulna becomes relatively prominent.)

In all Colles' fractures there is disturbance of the inferior radio-ulnar joint. In some cases this is responsible for persisting pain and tenderness just lateral to the ulnar styloid.

Again, disruption of the inferior radio-ulnar joint is partly responsible for loss of movements in the wrist. This certainly accounts for the loss of supination which causes patients the greatest concern. Although restriction of palmarflexion occurs after most Colles' fractures, this seldom gives rise to any functional problems.

Two other important complications are seen after Colles' fracture: (a) delayed rupture of extensor pollicis longus tendon may occur some months after injury and is due to ischaemia or attrition of the tendon; and (b) Sudeck's atrophy, which is usually diagnosed some weeks after cast fixation has been discontinued, is characterised by marked swelling of the wrist, hand and fingers, gross stiffness of the fingers, and carpal decalcification which is obvious on radiographs of the region.

Regarding treatment of these complications, the patient is advised to accept minor degrees of residual deformity, and stiffness. When there is gross prominence of the ulna causing symptoms, excision of the distal end of the bone may be advised. Ruptures of extensor pollicis longus are treated by tendon transfer (extensor indicis proprius is generally employed). Sudeck's atrophy generally requires intensive physiotherapy, and often other measures (which may include sympathetic blockade with guanethidine sulphate) if much permanent stiffness is to be avoided.

Ganglions

Ganglions are extremely common about the wrist and hand. In many cases they may have a tenuous communication with a carpal joint or tendon sheath. Some are spherical in shape, firm, and have no obvious connection to other structures. Tiny ganglions of this type are common in the fingers. Fluctuations in the size of ganglions and their rupture from trauma is well known, and diagnosis is not usually difficult unless the swelling is small. This applies in particular to small ganglions on the back of the wrist, arising from the radio-carpal joint; local swelling and tenderness may only be obvious when the wrist is palmar-flexed. This type of ganglion is often the cause of persisting wrist pain in young women; their symptoms are often labelled as functional when this difficulty in examination has not been appreciated. Excision of most ganglions is advised, and this is essential if the ganglion is producing nerve complications (e.g. if the ulnar nerve in the ulnar tunnel in the hand is producing motor and sensory loss).

de Quervain's disease

Tenosynovitis involving abductor pollicis longus and extensor pollicis brevis is known as de Quervain's disease. It occurs in the middle-aged. The walls of the fibrous tendon sheaths on the lateral aspect of the radius are greatly thickened, and there is often marked underlying swelling. The patient complains of pain on certain movements of the wrist, and weakness of grip. Treatment is by splitting the lateral wall of the sheath.

Extensor tenosynovitis

Acute frictional tenosynovitis occurs most frequently in the 20–40 age group, generally following a period of excess activity. Any or all of the extensor tendons may be involved. The condition has a benign course and usually settles if the wrist is immobilised in a cast for 3 weeks.

Osteoarthritis of the wrist

Osteoarthritis of the wrist is surprisingly uncommon considering the frequency with which the joint is involved in fractures. It is seen most often after avascular necrosis of the scaphoid following fracture of that bone, non-union of the scaphoid, comminuted fractures involving the articular surface of the radius, and Kienböck's disease (spontaneous avascular necrosis of the lunate).

Where symptoms are severe, fusion of the wrist (radio-carpal joint) is undertaken.

Rheumatoid arthritis

Rheumatoid arthritis of the wrist is common, and extensive synovial thickening of the joint and related tendon sheaths leads to gross swelling, increased local heat, pain and stiffness. Fluctuation can sometimes be transmitted from just above the wrist to the palm, the synovial fluid being displaced from one level to the other underneath the flexor retinaculum (compound palmar ganglion). With progressive joint involvement the carpus tilts into ulnar deviation and subluxes in a palmar direction. The head of the ulna displaces dorsally, disrupting the inferior radio-ulnar joint, and causing painful and reduced pronation and supination. Rarely, tuberculosis of the wrist may produce a similar clinical picture, but the multifocal nature of rheumatoid arthritis usually makes differentiation easy.

As far as treatment is concerned, local measures can include the use of night splints; later, synovectomy of the wrist and of the inferior radio-ulnar joints may be effective in slowing the progress of the condition. Where pronation and supination are particularly affected, excision of the distal end of the ulna may give worthwhile functional improvement. Where there is gross destruction of the joint and marked local symptoms, fusion may have to be considered.

Carpal tunnel syndrome

This condition occurs most commonly in women in the 30–60 age group. Basically, there is compression of the median nerve, which leads to symptoms and signs related to its distribution. In some cases premenstrual fluid retention, early rheumatoid arthritis with synovial tendon sheath thickening, and old Colles' or carpal fractures may be responsible by restricting the space left for the nerve in the carpal tunnel. The condition is sometimes seen in association with myxoedema, acromegaly and pregnancy; often, however, no obvious cause can be found. The patient complains of paraesthesia in the hand. Often all the fingers are claimed to be involved, although theoretically at least the little finger should always be spared. Paraesthesia may also radiate proximally to the elbow. There may be pain in the same areas, and weakness in the hand. The symptoms may become most marked in the early hours of the morning, often waking the patient from sleep and causing her to shake the hand or hang it over the side of the bed. In many cases the history and results of the clinical examination are unequivocal. In others it may be difficult to differentiate the patient's symptoms from those produced by cervical spondylosis, and indeed both conditions may be present at the same time. A trial period of immobilisation of the wrist in a cast or the use of a cervical collar may be helpful. Nerve conduction time tests, showing a delay at the wrist, may be used to confirm the diagnosis. These studies are being employed with increasing frequency in the practice of defensive medicine.

Most cases are treated quite simply by division of the flexor retinaculum which forms the roof of the carpal tunnel, thereby relieving pressure on the nerve. The procedure may be performed arthroscopically through a minimal incision. Conservative measures may be tried, especially in cases occurring in pregnancy when diuretics may be prescribed with success. Other measures include the use of night splints and injections of hydrocortisone.

Note that on rare occasions the median nerve may be compressed *proximal to the carpal tunnel*. Above the elbow this may be due to a supracondylar bony spur (obvious on radiographs); just distal to the elbow, by the origin of pronator teres; and in the proximal part of the forearm, by the sublimis. Proximal lesions of the median nerve give rise to the anterior interosseous nerve syndrome.

Ulnar tunnel syndrome

The ulnar nerve may be compressed as it passes through the ulnar carpal canal between the pisiform and the hook of the hamate. Both the sensory and motor divisions of the nerve may be affected, but often one only is involved. The symptoms therefore may include small muscle wasting and weakness in the hand, with sensory disturbance on the volar aspect of the little finger. The sensory supply to the dorsum of the hand is given off in the distal forearm, so that sensory disturbance on the dorsum of the hand and little finger excludes a lesion at this level. In all cases every effort should be made to exclude a more proximal cause for the patient's symptoms (e.g. ulnar neuritis at the elbow and cervical spondylosis). Nerve conduction studies are often of particular value in this situation. The commonest causes of nerve involvement at the wrist are ganglionic compression, occupational trauma, ulnar artery disease and old carpal or metacarpal fractures.

On the establishment of a firm diagnosis of a localised lesion in the ulnar tunnel, exploration and decompression of the nerve are carried out.

Ehlers-Danlos syndrome

This is the name given to a number of closely related connective tissue disorders which are due to a collagen abnormality. The condition is comparatively rare (50 000 cases are said to be affected in the UK), with a strong (autosomal dominant) hereditary tendency. It is found in association with Marfan's syndrome and osteogenesis imperfecta. *The skin* has a velvety feel, and is fragile and hyperelastic; when grasped, it can be raised and stretched by a remarkable amount. *Wound healing* is poor, leading to abnormal and somewhat keloid scarring, evidence of which may be widespread. Cases vary in severity, but in some healing may be so poor that surgery is contra-indicated. *The walls of blood vessels* are affected, and bruising is a common problem. *Ligaments* lose their resistance to stretching, so that there is usually a striking increase in the range of movements in the affected joints. This is often well in excess of the normal range (sometimes to a grotesque degree), and there may be instability, leading to sprains and dislocations. There is no effective treatment.

Tuberculosis of the wrist

Tuberculosis of the wrist is now rare in the UK. Marked swelling of the joint is followed by muscle wasting in the forearm, erosion, destruction and anterior subluxation of the carpus. The diagnosis is confirmed by synovial biopsy. Monarticular rheumatism is the only condition likely to cause difficulty in diagnosis.

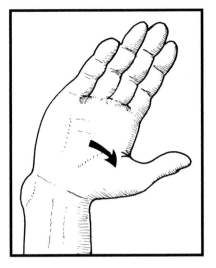

1. *Inspection: front* (1): Note any deformity of the wrist, e.g. radial deviation of the hand, common after Colles' fracture, and striking in congenital absence of the radius. Note any ulnar deviation, common in rheumatoid arthritis.

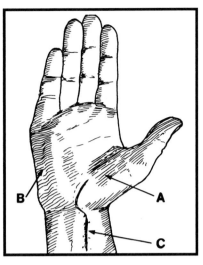

2. *Front* (2): Note (A) thenar wasting in hand; (B) hypothenar wasting; (C) scars suggestive of previous surgery or injury.

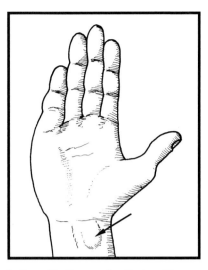

3. *Front* (3): Note any localised swellings suggestive of ganglion, rheumatoid nodule or tumour.

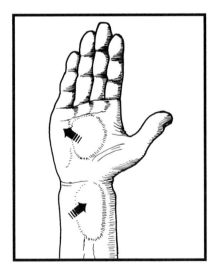

4. *Front* (4): If there is swelling at the wrist and also in the palm, try to demonstrate cross fluctuation. This occurs in compound palmar ganglion, seen most often in rheumatoid arthritis and tuberculosis.

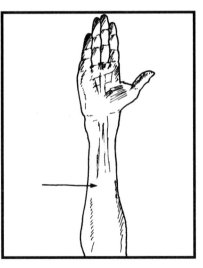

5. *Front* (5): Note the presence of muscle wasting in the forearm, also suggestive of rheumatoid arthritis and tuberculosis. Widespread, bilateral wasting is common in many neurological conditions (e.g. after cervical spine injuries, multiple sclerosis etc.) and in the muscular dystrophies.

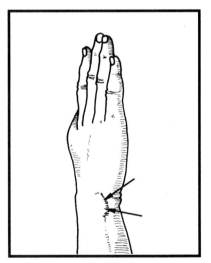

6. *Inspection: side* (1): Note any undue prominence of the ulna (common after Colles' fracture or Madelung deformity), any anterior tilting of the plane of the wrist (e.g. after Smith's fracture), backward tilting (post-Colles') or anterior subluxation (rheumatoid arthritis, old carpal injury or infective arthritis).

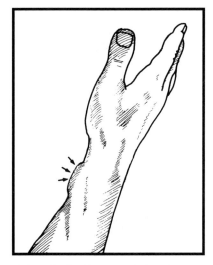

7. *Side* (2): Swelling over the lateral aspect of the distal radius occurs in de Quervain's tenosynovitis. If this is present, carry out additional tests (6, 34).

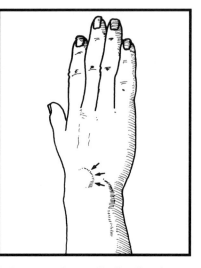

8. *Inspection: dorsum* (1): Ganglions in relation to the wrist, carpus and extensor tendons may be quite obvious on inspection.

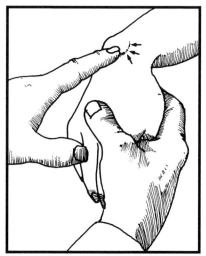

9. *Dorsum* (2): Palmar flex the wrist and compare one side with the other. Small ganglions between the radius and carpus are a common source of obscure wrist pain. Palmar flexion makes such ganglions obvious, and local tenderness confirms the diagnosis.

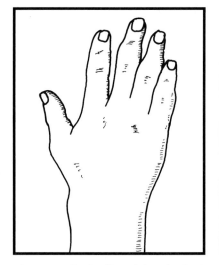

10. *Dorsum* (3): Swelling of the wrist, hand and fingers, with a glazed appearance of the skin, diffuse tenderness, pain and stiffness is typical of Sudeck's atrophy which may occur as a sequel to Colles' fracture or carpal injury.

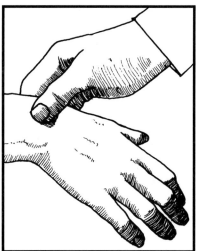

11. *Palpation* (1): Pain in the wrist persisting after a Colles' fracture, and due to disruption of the inferior radio-ulnar joint is always associated with well-localised tenderness at that site.

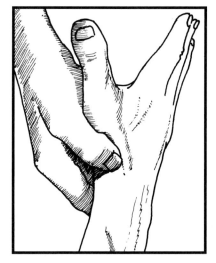

12. *Palpation* (2): Tenderness in the anatomical snuff box occurs classically after scaphoid fractures, but in fact is present after many wrist sprains and other minor injuries.

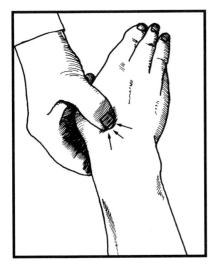

13. *Palpation* (3): To help distinguish a sprain from fracture palpate the dorsal surface of the scaphoid. Tenderness here is usually present after fractures but not sprains. Scaphoid radiographs and plaster fixation are necessary in all cases of suspected fracture.

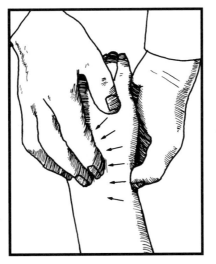

14. *Palpation* (4): Diffuse tenderness is common in all inflammatory lesions (e.g. rheumatoid arthritis and tuberculosis of the wrist) and in Sudeck's atrophy.

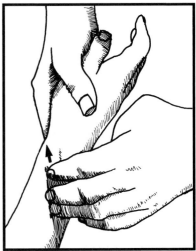

15. *Palpation* (5): Tenderness localised to the sheaths of abductor pollicis longus and extensor pollicis brevis is found in de Quervain's tenosynovitis. There is often striking local thickening of the tendon sheaths over the dorso-lateral aspect of the radius.

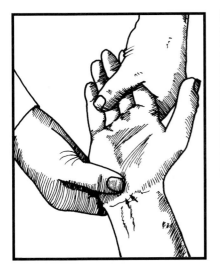

16. *Palpation* (6): Tenderness over the median nerve, with the production of paraesthesia in the fingers and lateral side of the hand is suggestive of the carpal tunnel syndrome. (See also 6, 36 et seq.)

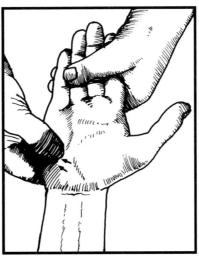

17. *Palpation* (7): In the same way, tenderness with paraesthesia on pressure over the ulnar nerve is suggestive of the ulnar tunnel syndrome.

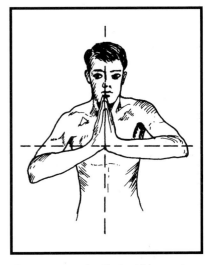

18. *Movements: dorsiflexion* (1): *screening test:* Ask the patient to press the hands together in the vertical plane, and to raise the elbows to the horizontal. Loss of any dorsiflexion should be obvious. The commonest cause is stiffness after a Colles' fracture.

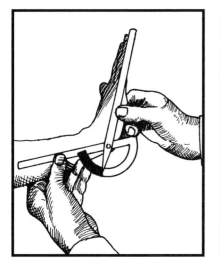

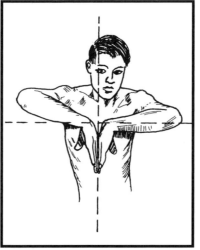

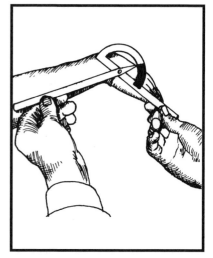

19. *Dorsiflexion* (2): Dorsiflexion may be measured with a goniometer. *Normal range: 75°.* Hypermobility is not uncommon in women. If hypermobility is gross, however, other joints should be examined.

20. *Palmar flexion* (1): *screening test:* Ask the patient to put the backs of the hands in contact, and then to bring the forearms into the horizontal plane. Loss of palmar flexion should be obvious.

21. *Palmar flexion* (2): Palmar flexion may be measured with the goniometer. *Normal range: 75°.* If the range exceeds this, look for other signs of wrist (and other joint) hypermobility as described in the following figures.

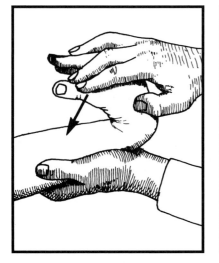

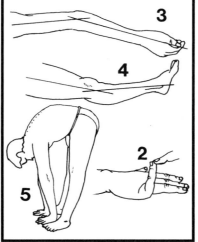

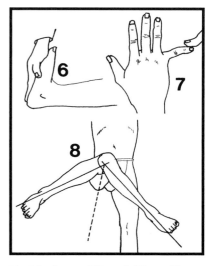

22. *Joint hypermobility* (1): Try to bring the thumb into contact with the forearm, and measure any gap. The average separation is 4.5 cm at age 17½, and it increases with age (as the ligaments lose some of their elasticity). While the thumb contacting the forearm suggests hypermobility, this is nevertheless said to occur in 56% of normal subjects.

23. *Joint hypermobility ctd:* (2) Test if the little finger can be passively dorsiflexed to 90° or more. (3) Check the elbow and (4) the knee to see if they can hyperextend by 10° or more. (5) Check if the spine can be flexed so that the palms of the hands can be placed on the floor. Joint laxity is diagnosed if any three of these tests (1–5) are present.

24. *Joint hypermobility ctd:* Other evidence of hypermobility includes (6) hyperextension of the ankle beyond 45°; (7) an abnormal range of abduction of the little finger; (8) an increase in hip rotation in children (from 90–93° to about 110°), with the centre of the range internally rotated. Joint hypermobility is a feature of the Ehlers-Danlos syndrome, Marfan's disease, osteogenesis imperfecta and Morquio-Brailsford's disease.

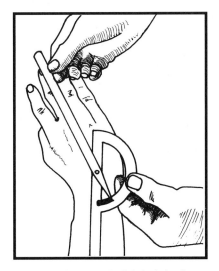

25. *Radial deviation:* Radial deviation is measured as the angle formed between the forearm and the middle metacarpal. This test is best carried out in the mid-position of the pronation/supination range. *Normal range: 20°.*

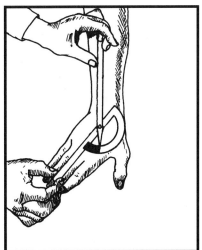

26. *Ulnar deviation:* Ulnar deviation is measured in the same general way. *Normal range: 35°.*

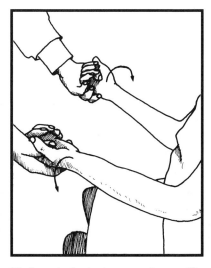

27. *Pronation/supination: screening test* (1): Ask the patient to hold the elbows firmly at the sides. Grasp the hands and turn them so that the palms are uppermost. Compare the amount of supination in both sides.

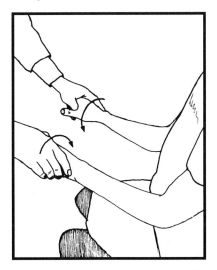

28. *Pronation/supination: screening test* (2): Repeat, turning the palms downwards to assess pronation. If no obvious cause for loss of pronation or supination is found at the wrist, then the forearm and elbow must be carefully examined.

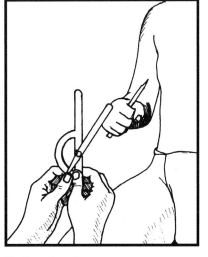

29. *Pronation:* For accurate measurement, give the patient a pen to hold. Ask the patient to keep the elbows firmly at the sides and to pronate the wrist. Measure the angle between the vertical and the held pen. *Normal range: 75°.*

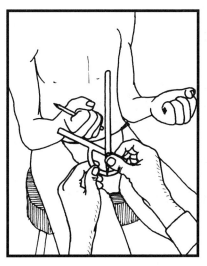

30. *Supination:* Supination may be measured in the same general way. *Normal range: 80°.*

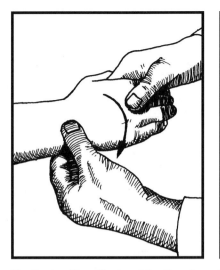

31. *Crepitus* (l): *radio-ulnar joint:* Place the index and thumb over the joint and pronate and supinate the wrist. Crepitus is common when the joint is disorganised, especially after a Colles' fracture.

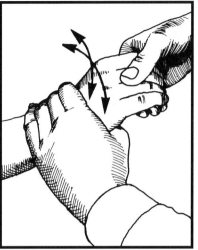

32. *Crepitus* (2): *radio-carpal joint:* Encircle the wrist with the hand and ask the patient to dorsiflex, palmar flex, radial deviate and ulnar deviate the wrist. Osteoarthritis of the wrist is uncommon, but occurs after scaphoid and distal radius fractures, Kienböck's disease etc.

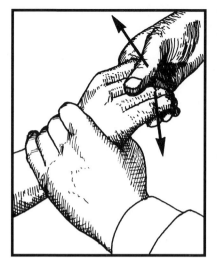

33. *Crepitus* (3): While grasping the wrist, flex and extend the fingers. Ask the patient to repeat these movements on his own. Crepitus, fine in character, occurs in tenosynovitis of the extensor tendons. Auscultation over the tendons may reveal characteristic grating sounds.

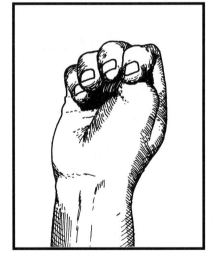

34. *de Quervain's tenosynovitis* (of abductor pollicis longus and extensor pollicis brevis): Where this is suspected from the history, local swelling and tenderness, confirm the diagnosis with the following test. Ask the patient to flex the thumb and close the fingers over it.

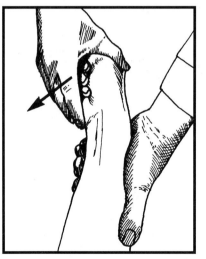

35. *de Quervain's tenosynovitis:* Now move the hand into ulnar deviation. Excruciating pain accompanying this manoeuvre occurs in de Quervain's tenosynovitis.

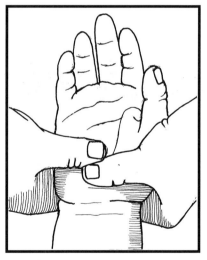

36. *Carpal tunnel syndrome* (1): Where this is suspected, apply very firm, steady pressure with both thumbs for 30 seconds over the median nerve as it runs within the carpal tunnel. Note the interval between the application of pressure and the onset of numbness, pain or paraesthesia in the median distribution (average 16 seconds in carpal tunnel syndrome). *This is the most reliable test.*

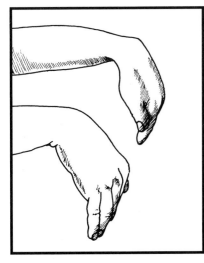

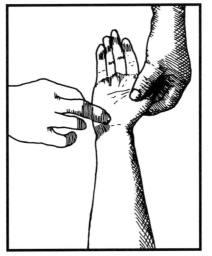

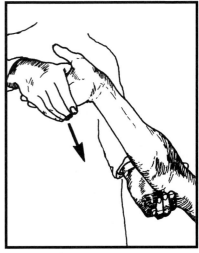

37. *Carpal tunnel syndrome* (2): *Phalen test:* Ask the patient to hold both wrists in a fully flexed position for 1–2 minutes. The appearance or exacerbation of paraesthesia in the median distribution is suggestive of the carpal tunnel syndrome, and is positive in 70% of cases.

38. *Carpal tunnel syndrome* (3): *Tinel's sign:* the test is positive if gentle finger percussion over the median nerve produces paraesthesia in its distribution. This test is said to be positive in 56% of cases of carpal tunnel syndrome.

39. *Carpal tunnel syndrome* (4): Note any pain and paraesthesia on stretching the nerve by the manoeuvre of extending the elbow and dorsiflexing the wrist.

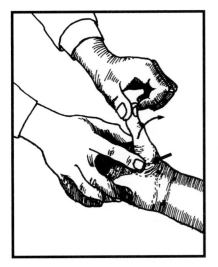

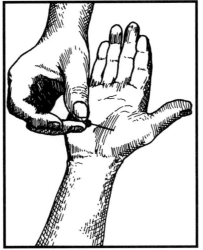

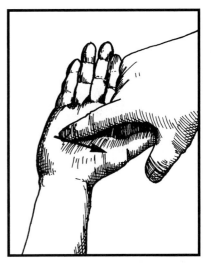

40. *Carpal tunnel syndrome* (5): Test the motor division of the median nerve. Note the resistance offered by the patient as you try to push the vertically held thumb into the plane of the palm. Feel the thenar tone. (See also 2, 59–70.)

41. *Carpal tunnel syndrome* (6): Look for sensory impairment in the median distribution.

42. *Carpal tunnel syndrome* (7): Slide the tip of the index across the palm noting frictional resistance and temperature. Increased thenar resistance (from lack of sweating) and temperature rise (vaso-dilatation) may occur with median involvement.

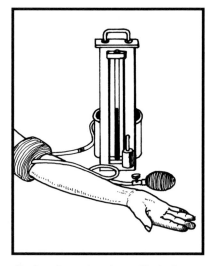

43. *Carpal tunnel syndrome* (8): Apply a tourniquet and inflate to just above the systolic blood pressure for 1–2 minutes. The appearance or exacerbation of symptoms again suggests the carpal tunnel syndrome. This test should be interpreted with caution.

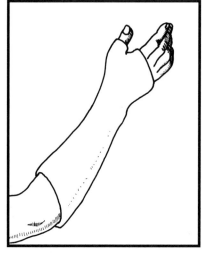

44. *Carpal tunnel syndrome* (9): If there is still doubt, apply a scaphoid plaster for 7–10 days. Improvement of symptoms while in plaster, and deterioration on removal is suggestive of the carpal tunnel syndrome. Nerve conduction studies which show impairment of conduction at the level of the tunnel are virtually diagnostic, and are used by many to counter litigation.

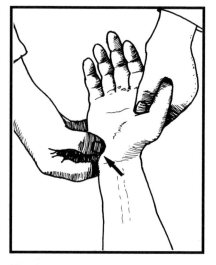

45. *Ulnar tunnel syndrome* (1): Look for tenderness over the tunnel, and for signs of ulnar nerve involvement (hypothenar wasting, abduction of the little finger, early clawing of the ring and middle fingers (see also 2, 44).

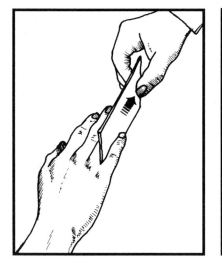

46. *Ulnar tunnel syndrome* (2): Test for involvement of the motor distribution of the nerve. The power of adduction of the little finger is a useful screening test. Note that weakness of *adduction*, with normal power of *abduction*, is one early sign of cervical spinal myelopathy.

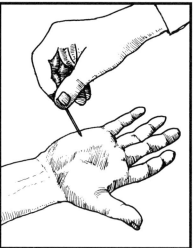

47. *Ulnar tunnel syndrome* (3): Test for sensory impairment in the common area of sensory distribution of the nerve.

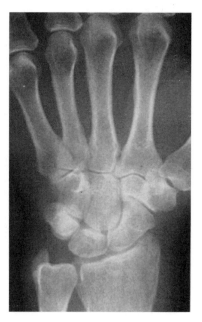

48. *Radiographs* (1): Normal antero-posterior radiograph of the wrist.

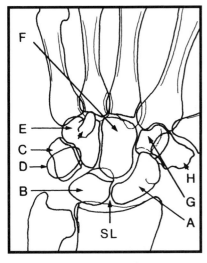

49. *Radiographs* (2): In the antero-posterior, identify the carpal bones and note their shape, density and position. (A) Scaphoid; (B) lunate; (C) triquetral; (D) pisiform; (E) hamate with hook; (F) capitate; (G) trapezoid; (H) trapezium. Note the gaps between the various carpal bones, particularly between the scaphoid and lunate (SL).

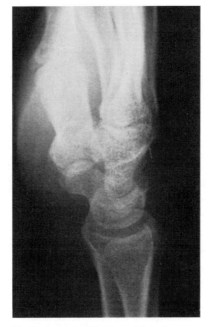

50. *Radiographs* (3): Normal lateral radiograph of the wrist.

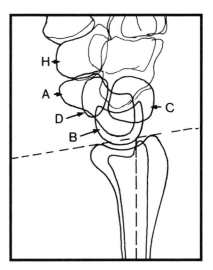

51. *Radiographs* (4): It is usually possible to make out in the lateral, in spite of superimposition, (H) trapezium, (A) tubercle and mass of scaphoid, (D) pisiform, (B) crescent of lunate and (C) triquetral. Note that the plane of the wrist joint normally has a 5° anterior tilt.

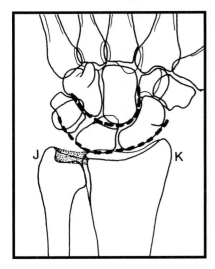

52. *Radiographs* (5): In the antero-posterior view, note the smooth curves formed by both proximal and distal margins of scaphoid, lunate and triquetral. Note that the distal end of the ulna stops short of the radius to make room for the triangular fibro-cartilage. (J) Ulnar styloid; (K) radial styloid.

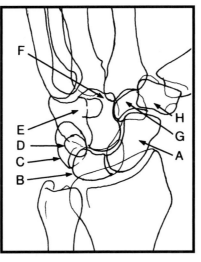

53. *Radiographs* (6): When the carpus is suspect, at least one, but preferably two oblique views should be taken in addition to the routine antero-posterior and lateral. These are of particular value in detecting hairline crack fractures of the carpal bones. (The labelling is the same as in previous figures.)

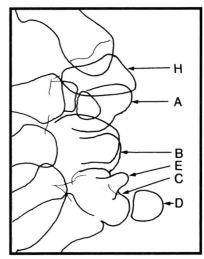

54. *Radiographs* (7): In suspected carpal tunnel syndrome, a tangential projection of the tunnel should be obtained. This view occasionally shows osteoarthritis lipping or other causal pathology. (A) Scaphoid; (B) lunate; (C) triquetral; (D) pisiform; (E) hook of hamate; (H) trapezium.

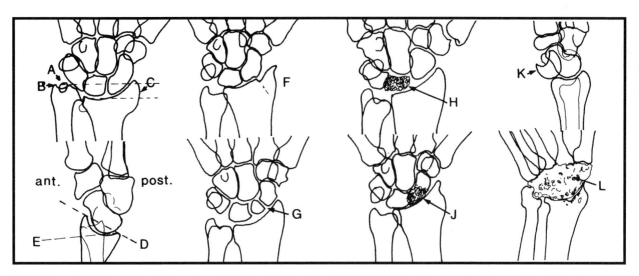

55. *Radiographs* (8): Look for evidence of previous injury. In the mal-united Colles' fracture there may be (A) non-union of the ulnar styloid; (B) prominence of the distal ulna secondary to (C) distortion and resorption at the radial fracture. The joint line (D) may be tilted away from (E) the normal. Osteoarthritic changes are uncommon after Colles' fracture, but are seen after (F) radial styloid fractures. Osteoarthritis may not always follow (G) non-union of a scaphoid fracture. Note increased bone density and deformity in (H) Kienböck's disease of the lunate or in (J) avascular necrosis of the scaphoid, both of which are almost invariably accompanied by osteoarthritis. Note any carpal mal-position (K), dislocation of the lunate being the most common. Gross porotic changes are seen most often in rheumatoid arthritis and in Sudeck's atrophy, while gross destructive changes are seen in (L) tuberculosis and other infections.

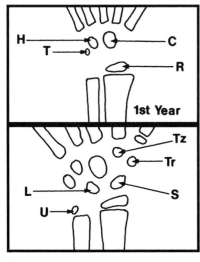

56. *Ossification:* In the first year of life, the capitate (C) and hamate (H) appear at 2 months, the radius (R) at 6 months, and the triquetral (T) at 10 months. After the first year, the lunate (L) appears at 2, the trapezium (Tr) at 2½, the trapezoid (Tz) and scaphoid (S) at 3, and the distal ulna (U) at 4½ years.

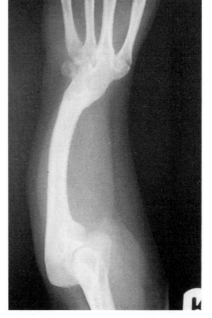

57. *Wrist radiographs: examples of pathology* (1): The radiograph shows a congenital deformity of the upper limb in which there is absence of the radius and thumb, along with failure of carpal differentiation.

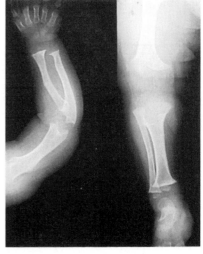

58. *Pathology* (2): The radiographs show an upper and lower limb in achondroplasia. The width of the bones is normal, but they are proportionately short, contributing to the dwarfism associated with this hereditary abnormality. The metaphyses are wide, and there is defective modelling of the shafts.

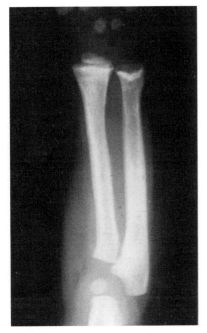

59. *Pathology* (3): There is a little metaphyseal widening and irregularity, with ulnar metaphyseal cupping (from pressure transmitted in crawling), all typical of rickets.

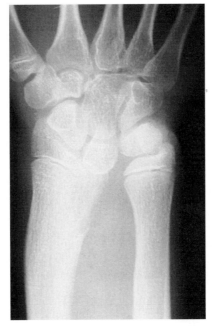

60. *Pathology* (4): There are deformities of the distal radius and ulna which are splayed. There is relative lengthening of the ulna, which is unduly prominent at the side and back of the wrist. This is a Madelung deformity of the wrist.

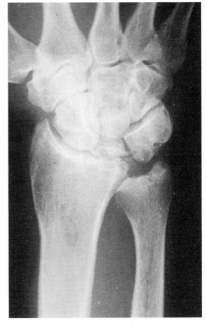

61. *Pathology* (5): There is gross distortion and collapse of the lunate typical of Kienböck's disease.

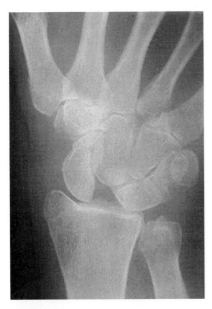

62. *Pathology* (6): There is a wide gap between the scaphoid and lunate typical of scapho-lunate dissociation. Suspect the possibility of this condition where the history suggests a severe sprain or possible scaphoid fracture. *In doubtful cases the condition may be unmasked if the antero-posterior radiograph is taken with the fist tightly clenched.*

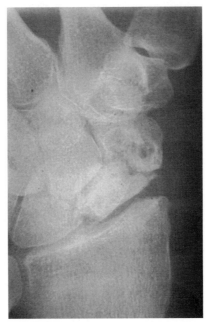

63. *Pathology* (7): The radiograph shows the unusual combination of non-union and avascular necrosis of the scaphoid following a fracture of the wrist. Note the increased density of the proximal pole of the scaphoid.

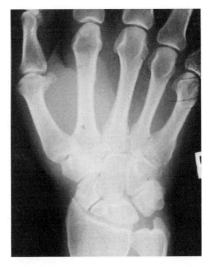

64. *Pathology* (8): This shows long-standing, established non-union of the scaphoid following fracture. There is some arthritic narrowing of the joint space between the proximal pole of the scaphoid and the radius.

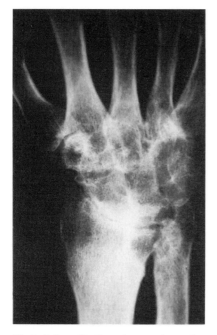

65. *Pathology* (9): There is gross destruction of the carpal and wrist joints, with fibrous ankylosis typical of the late appearances of an infective arthritis (in this case due to tuberculosis).

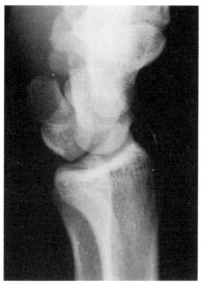

66. *Pathology* (10): The radiograph shows two bones lying proud of the rest of the carpus at the front of the wrist: one is the normally situated pisiform; the other semilunar in shape and lying more proximal, is a dislocated lunate. If this condition is not rapidly reduced, or is missed, median nerve symptoms commonly ensue.

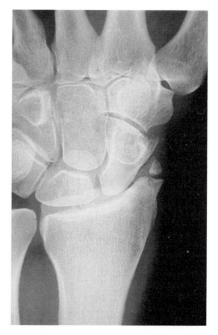

67. *Pathology* (11): The tip of the radial styloid process has been fractured at some time, and there is established non-union. Such a condition may be symptom-free, or give pain if secondary arthritic changes develop between the radius and scaphoid.

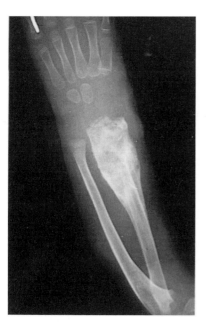

68. *Pathology* (12): This radiograph of a child's wrist and forearm shows gross distortion of the distal radius due to osteitis. There are large bone abscesses and new bone formation. In this case the causal organism was the tubercle bacillus. (*NB:* Most tuberculous infections have their principal effects on the joints rather than the shafts of the long bones.)

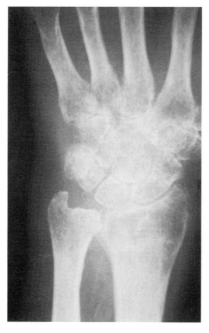

69. *Pathology* (13): There is widespread decalcification due to Sudeck's atrophy following a minor local injury. The radiological appearances are similar to those found in rheumatoid arthritis.

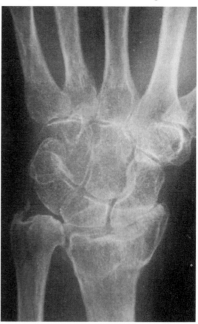

70. *Pathology* (14): This antero-posterior radiograph shows distortion of the inferior radio-ulnar joint, relative lengthening and prominence of the ulna, and widening of the radius as a result of mal-union in a Colles' fracture. The patient complained of pain in the wrist (radio-ulnar joint), and restriction of pronation/supination movements.

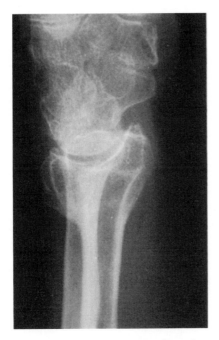

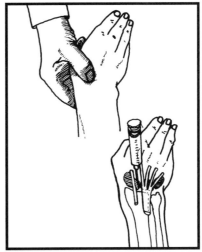

71. *Pathology* (15): The lateral radiograph of the same case shows marked alteration in the plane of the radio-carpal joint, again due to mal-union; this, apart from the deformed appearance, has the effect of seriously restricting palmar flexion.

72. *Aspiration of the wrist joint:* With the thumb, feel for the depression at the back of the wrist which lies between the distal end of the radius and scaphoid in the vertical plane, and between extensor digitorum communis and extensor carpi radialis brevis in the plane at right angles to it. After infiltration of the skin with local anaesthetic, incline the aspirating needle at 60°, with the tip directed cranially.

7. The hand

Note that the separation of conditions into those affecting the wrist and those affecting the hand has been done for convenience, and that in many cases examination of both regions is necessary.

Dupuytren's contracture

In this condition there is nodular thickening and contracture of the palmar fascia. The palm of the hand is affected first, followed at a later stage by the fingers. The ring finger is most frequently involved, followed by the little and middle fingers. The index and even the thumb may be affected. In some cases there is corresponding thickening of the *plantar* fascia. The progressive flexion of the affected fingers interferes with the function of the hand and may be so severe that the fingernails dig into the palm. The condition mainly affects men over the age of 40. There is a definite genetic predisposition in 60–70% of cases, and in some cases there may be an association with epilepsy, diabetes or alcoholic cirrhosis. There is a distinct geographical distribution: it is rare in Africa, India and China. Below the age of 40, and in either sex, its onset may be precipitated by trauma. Under these circumstances it may pursue a particularly rapid course.

As far as treatment is concerned, a waiting policy may be pursued if the condition is confined to the palms. When the fingers are affected, surgical treatment is usually advised, but this is complicated by a number of factors. If the fingers have been held in a flexed position for a long time, secondary changes in the interphalangeal joints may prevent finger extension even after the involved tissue has been removed. In the case of the little finger, amputation in these circumstances may be the best line of treatment. The digital nerve sheaths may blend with the fascia so that dissection is tedious and difficult; involvement of the skin may necessitate Z-plasties or other plastic procedures; and the patient's age and general health may be adverse factors. In most cases, wide excision of the affected fascia is advised. When this is not possible, improvement in function, often lasting for some years, may follow simple division of the contracted fascia in the palm.

Vibration syndromes

Prolonged exposure to high-frequency vibration (such as may be experienced from the use of jack hammers or hand-held buffing, riveting and caulking machines) may affect bone, nerves and blood vessels. *Bone* is rarely affected to a significant degree, but new bone formation and hairline fractures (which are slow to heal), are sometimes seen. Involvement of the *peripheral nerves* may lead to pain and paraesthesia, numbness, tremor, loss of fine touch sensation, proprioception and discrimination. There may be muscle denervation and weakness involving especially the small muscles of the hand. In the case of the *peripheral blood vessels* there is disturbance of their autonomic control, and the arterioles of the hand become hypersensitive to cold and vibration. In the typical case there are attacks in which one or more fingers turn white on exposure to cold ('episodic blanching'), with reactive hyperaemia on warming; and there is usually associated discomfort and clumsiness of the hand during attacks. As the condition progresses, more fingers become involved, attacks occur both in summer and in winter, and hand function becomes permanently disturbed. The hand becomes weak and clumsy, and with impaired sensation and proprioception the patient has difficulty in dressing (e.g. doing up buttons and shoelaces), handling small objects (e.g. coins, nuts and screws), and carrying out many other tasks (e.g. tying fishing hooks). The differential diagnosis includes Raynaud's disease, cervical rib and the costo-clavicular syndrome, cervical spondylosis, and sensitivity to beta-blockers.

There are a number of classifications of the stages of the condition, and the long-established Taylor-Pelmear scale is still widely used (Table 7.1). Well-established cases are recognised as one of the Prescribed Diseases under the Social Security Act, and the qualifying criteria are clearly stated. (The condition must occur throughout the year, involve at least three fingers of one hand (with the middle and/or proximal phalanges being affected), and be due to exposure to vibrating tools.) No treatment is effective, but deterioration may be slowed or prevented by avoiding further exposure to vibration.

Table 1   The Taylor-Pelmear scale

Stage	Condition of digits	Work and social interference
0	No blanching of digits	No complaints
0T	Intermittent tingling	No interference with activities
0N	Intermittent numbness	No interference with activities
1	Blanching of one or more fingertips, with or without tingling or numbness	No interference with activities
2	Blanching of one or more fingers, with numbness. Usually confined to winter	Slight interference with home and social activities; no interference at work
3	Extensive blanching. Frequent episodes, summer and winter	Definite interference at work, at home, and with social activities. Restriction of hobbies
4	Extensive blanching. Most or all fingers affected. Frequent episodes, summer and winter	Occupation changed to avoid further exposure to vibration because of severity of signs and symptoms

Tendon and tendon sheath lesions

See also under rheumatoid arthritis in this section.

1. Mallet finger. In a mallet finger the distal interphalangeal joint is held in a permanent position of flexion; the deformity may be moderate or complete. The patient is either not at all able to extend the distal joint of the finger or can extend it incompletely. The problem is that the extensor tendon, usually as a result of trauma, either ruptures close to its insertion in the distal phalanx, or it avulses its bony attachment. Healing may occur spontaneously over a 6–12-month period, but it is usual practice to treat these injuries for 6 weeks with a light splint which holds the distal interphalangeal joint in hyperextension.

2. Mallet thumb. Delayed rupture of the extensor pollicis longus tendon may follow Colles' fracture (see Chapter 6) or rheumatoid arthritis, and repair by tendon transfer (using extensor indicis proprius) is usually advised. If the tendon is damaged by an incised wound, repair by direct suture is undertaken.

3. Boutonnière deformity. Flexion of the interphalangeal joint of a finger with extension of the distal interphalangeal joint characterises this deformity. It is due to detachment of the central slip of the extensor tendon which is attached to the base of the middle phalanx. This may follow incised wounds on the dorsum of the finger and avulsion injuries, but is commonly seen in rheumatoid arthritis. Surgical repair of the extensor band is often undertaken for isolated lesions of this type.

4. Extensor tendon division in the back of the hand. Extensor tendons divided by wounds on the back of the hand carry an excellent prognosis and are treated by primary suture and splintage for approximately 4 weeks.

5. Profundus tendon injuries.

(a) Isolated avulsion injuries, which are uncommon, may be treated by surgical re-attachment of the tendon.

(b) Profundus tendon division in open wounds: in the palm, repair by direct suture is usually feasible. In the flexor tendon sheaths, there is considerable risk of adhesions spoiling function. In uncontaminated wounds where good facilities are available, primary flexor tendon repair may be undertaken; otherwise free flexor tendon grafting is usually advised. Accompanying digital nerve divisions may also be dealt with by primary repair.

6. Trigger finger and thumb. This condition results from thickening of a fibrous tendon sheath or nodular thickening in a flexor tendon.

In young children, the thumb is held flexed at the metacarpo-phalangeal (MP) joint, and a nodular thickening in front of the MP joint is palpable. Not infrequently, the deformity is wrongly considered to be of congenital origin and untreatable.

In adults, the middle or ring finger is most frequently involved. When the fingers are extended, the affected finger lags behind and then quite suddenly straightens. Nodular thickening, always at the level of the MP joint, may also be palpable. Division of the sheath at the level of the MP joint gives an immediate and gratifying cure.

Rheumatoid arthritis

Rheumatoid arthritis, as is well known, very frequently affects the hand, and as it progresses may involve joints, tendons, muscles, nerves and arteries, producing most severe deformities and crippling effects on hand function.

In the earliest phases the hands are strikingly warm and moist; later the joints become obviously swollen and tender. Synovial tendon sheath and joint thickening with effusion, muscle wasting, and deformity then become apparent. Tendon ruptures and joint subluxations are the main factors leading to the more severe deformities.

The surgery of the rheumatoid hand is highly specialised, requiring particular skills and experience in judgement, timing and technique, and is difficult to summarise with any accuracy.

In the earliest stages of the disease, analgesic and anti-inflammatory drugs are advised, with the judicious use of physiotherapy and splintage to alleviate pain, preserve movement and minimise deformity. When there is much synovial thickening at a stage before joint destruction has advanced, synovectomy is often helpful in alleviating pain and delaying local progress of the condition. In a few well-selected cases, where there is severe joint destruction and progressive deformity, joint replacement may be helpful. Some cases of major tendon involvement may benefit from repair and other procedures.

Osteoarthritis of the interphalangeal joints

Nodular swellings situated dorsally over the bases of the distal phalanges (Heberden's nodes), or less commonly over the bases of the middle phalanges (Bouchard's nodes) are a sign of osteoarthritis of the finger joints. They occur most frequently in women after the menopause, and are often familial. They are not related to osteoarthritis elsewhere. In many cases they are symptom-free, but they may be associated with progressive joint damage which does cause pain.

Carpo-metacarpal joint of the thumb

Osteoarthritic changes are common between the thumb metacarpal and the trapezium, and they may give rise to disabling pain and impaired function in the hand. There may on occasion be a history of a previous Bennett's fracture or of occupational overuse. Several surgical procedures (e.g. excision of the trapezium) are available which give relief of pain, sometimes at the expense of some functional loss.

Tumours in the hand

Tumours in the hand are not uncommon. Most involve the soft tissues and are simple, but it need hardly be stressed that where the diagnosis is uncertain a full investigation is essential. Among the commonest tumours are the following:

1. Ganglions. These occur in the fingers, most commonly along the volar aspects. They are small, spherical, and tender to the touch. They are generally treated by excision.

2. Implantation dermoid cysts. These occur along the volar surfaces of the fingers and palms. They are treated by excision.

3. Glomus tumours. Less common, these small, vascular, exquisitely tender tumours are seen most often in the region of the nail beds. They are also treated by excision.

4. Mucous cysts. These always occur on the dorsal surface of a distal interphalangeal joint. Excision is best avoided unless their rupture has led to a synovial fistula.

5. Osteoid osteoma. This tumour may involve a distal phalanx (or a carpal bone), and has a typical X-ray appearance. If there is doubt about the diagnosis, an isotope bone scan will show it up as a 'hot spot'. Spontaneous resolution may occur, but if symptoms are marked the tumour should be excised.

6. Chondroma. This is a very common benign tumour which occurs in the metacarpals and phalanges. It is generally confined to bone (enchondroma) and may give rise to a pathological fracture, or to gross swelling and deformity. It is often solitary, but multiple tumours of a similar nature are found in Ollier's disease, which has a hereditary diathesis. Tumours of this type may be treated by excision and bone grafting of the defect.

7. Metastatic tumours. These are uncommon, but have a tendency to involve the distal phalanges. Lung and breast are the commonest primary sites. The treatment is dependent on the nature of the primary and spread elsewhere.

Infections in the hand

1. Paronychia. This is the commonest of all infections in the hand, and occurs between the base of the nail and the cuticle.

2. Apical infections. These occur between the tip of the nail and the underlying nail bed.

3. Pulp infections. These occur in the fibro-fatty tissue of the fingertips, and are extremely painful. If unchecked, infection frequently leads to involvement of the terminal phalanx.

These three common infections are treated along well-established lines, using antibiotics and surgical drainage if frank pus is formed.

4. Tendon sheath infections. Infection within a tendon sheath (Figure 7.A) leads to rapid swelling of the finger and build-up of pressure within the tendon sheath; there is always a serious risk of tendon sloughing or disabling adhesion formation. In the case of the little finger there may be retrograde spread of infection to involve the ulnar bursa in the hand. In the case of the thumb, infection may also spread proximally to involve the radial bursa. In either case, swelling appears in the palm and in the wrist proximal to the flexor retinaculum. It should also be noted that in 70% of cases there is a connection between these two bursae, allowing spread from one to the other.

5. Web space infections. Web space infections are usually accompanied by great pain and systemic upset. There is redness and swelling in the affected web space. Infection may spread along the volar aspects of the

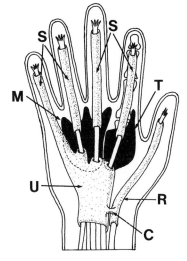

Fig. 7.A Some potential sites of infection in the hand and fingers. S = synovial tendon sheaths; U = ulnar bursa; R = radial bursa; M = mid-palmar space; T = thenar space. *Note:* C = communication between the radial and ulnar bursae.

related fingers or to adjacent web spaces across the anterior aspect of the palm. If seen early, most web space infections respond to antibiotics, splintage and elevation, but drainage is sometimes necessary.

6. Mid-palmar and thenar space infections. These two compartments of the hand lie between the flexor tendons and the metacarpals. Infection may spread to them from web space or tendon sheath infections; dissemination through the hand is then rapid and potentially crippling. In either case, there is usually gross swelling of the hand and a severe systemic upset. Unless there is a rapid response to antibiotics, elevation and splintage, with early drainage is essential for the preservation of function in the hand.

It should be noted that where splintage of the hand is advocated, and if functional recovery is to be hoped for, the fingers should be held in a position of right-angled flexion at the MP joints and extension in the interphalangeal joints.

7. Tuberculosis and syphilis. On rare occasions either of these two infections may produce spindle-shaped deformity of a finger. Spindling of a finger is much more common, however, in rheumatoid arthritis, gout or collateral ligament trauma.

8. Occupational infections. Superficial infections are common in certain trades and the following may be noted:

(a) Pilo-nidal sinus in barbers
(b) Erysipeloid in fishmongers and butchers
(c) 'Butcher's wart' (tuberculous skin lesions) in butchers and pathologists
(d) Malignant pustule (anthrax) in hide sorters and tanners.

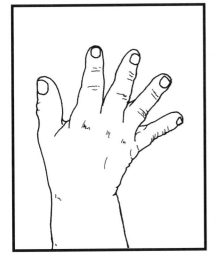

1. *Inspection* (1): Look first at the general shape of the hand and its size in proportion to the rest of the patient; e.g. the fingers are short and stumpy in achondroplasia. The hand is large and coarse in acromegaly. In myxoedema, the hand is often podgy and the skin dry.

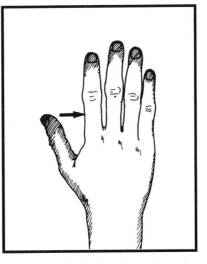

2. *Inspection* (2): In Marfan's syndrome the proximal phalanges in particular are long and thin. In Turner's syndrome the ring metacarpal is often very short. In hyperparathyroidism the fingertips may be short and bulbous, while in Down's and Hurler's syndromes the little fingers are incurved.

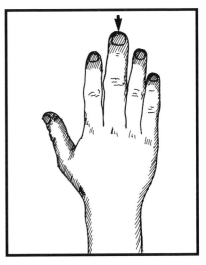

3. *Inspection* (3): Note the presence of any hypertrophy of a finger. This may occur in Paget's disease, neurofibromatosis and local arteriovenous fistula.

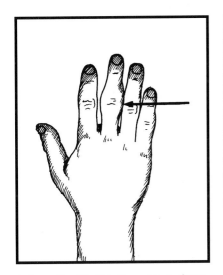

4. *Inspection* (4): Note the presence of any fusiform swelling. The commonest causes are collateral ligament tears and rheumatoid arthritis. Less commonly it is seen in syphilis, TB, sarcoidosis and gout. In psoriatic arthritis, the distal joint is usually involved.

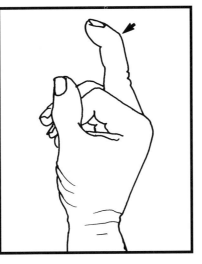

5. *Inspection* (5): *mallet finger:* The distal interphalangeal joint is flexed. The patient cannot extend the terminal phalanx, although the joint can usually be extended passively. It is caused by rupture or avulsion of the extensor tendon, usually from trauma or rheumatoid arthritis.

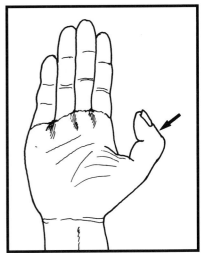

6. *Inspection* (6): *mallet thumb:* Loss of active extension in the interphalangeal joint of the thumb is due to rupture of extensor pollicis longus. This is seen as a late complication of Colles' fracture, from rheumatoid arthritis or wounds of the wrist or the thumb with tendon division.

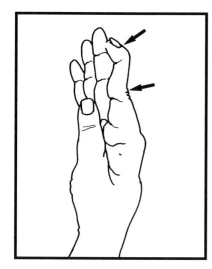

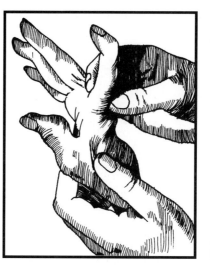

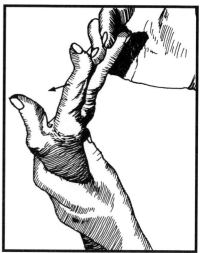

7. *Inspection* (7): *swan-neck deformity* (1): The distal interphalangeal joint is flexed amd the proximal interphalangeal joint is hyperextended. It is seen most often in rheumatoid arthritis, and may be produced by a number of different factors.

8. *Inspection* (8): *swan-neck deformity* (2): Extend the metacarpo-phalangeal joint of the affected finger. Improvement in the deformity indicates that shortening of extensor digitorum communis is a factor. If the deformity is made worse, tight interossei are likely to be responsible.

9. *Inspection* (9): *swan-neck deformity* (3): Hold all the fingers in an extended position, but leave the affected finger free. Ask the patient to flex it. If he cannot, this indicates rupture of flexor digitorum sublimis as the cause of the deformity.

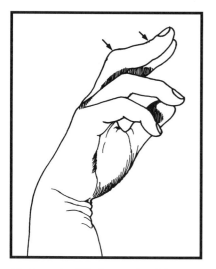

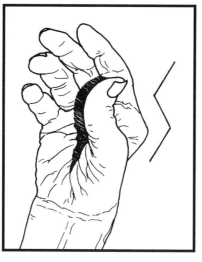

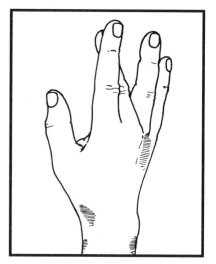

10. *Inspection* (10): *boutonnière deformity:* The proximal interphalangeal joint is flexed and the distal joint extended. It occurs when the central extensor tendon slip to the middle phalanx is affected, by a wound on the dorsum of the finger, by traumatic avulsion, or rupture in rheumatoid arthritis.

11. *Inspection* (11): *Z-deformity of the thumb:* The thumb is flexed at the metacarpo-phalangeal joint and hyperextended at the interphalangeal joint. The deformity is seen in rheumatoid arthritis secondary to displacement of the extensor tendons or rupture of flexor pollicis longus.

12. *Inspection* (12): Flexion of a finger at the metacarpo-phalangeal joint, with inability to extend, follows rupture or division of the extensor tendon in the back of the hand or at the wrist.

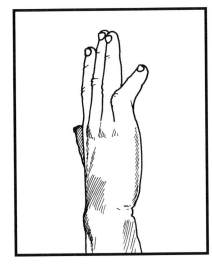

13. *Inspection* (13): Flexion of the little finger, mainly at the proximal interphalangeal joint, is seen in congenital contracture of the little finger.

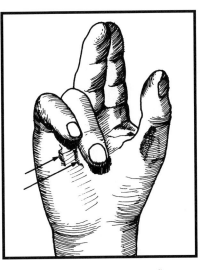

14. *Inspection* (14): Flexion of the fingers at the metacarpo-phalangeal and interphalangeal joints, associated with nodular thickening in the palm and fingers, is characteristic of Dupuytren's contracture. The thumb is occasionally involved.

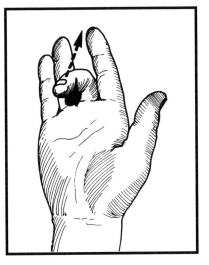

15. *Inspection* (15): Flexion of the middle or ring finger at the proximal interphalangeal joint, with sudden extension on effort or with assistance, is seen in trigger finger. There is usually a palpable nodular thickening over the corresponding metacarpo-phalangeal joint.

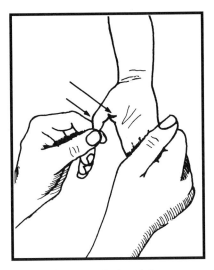

16. *Inspection* (16): Flexion of the interphalangeal joint of the thumb in infants and young children is usually due to stenosing teno-vaginitis involving flexor pollicis longus. A nodular thickening is usually palpable over the metacarpo-phalangeal joint. The condition is said to be acquired (i.e. it is not congenital) and triggering is not a feature.

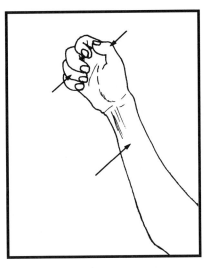

17. *Inspection* (17): In Volkmann's ischaemic contracture (which usually occurs as a sequel to brachial artery damage in a supracondylar fracture) there is clawing of the thumb and fingers and forearm wasting. The fingers can be extended if the wrist is flexed.

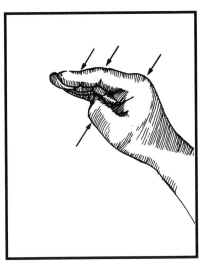

18. *Inspection* (18): Ischaemic contracture of the small muscles of the hand (usually as a result of swelling within a tight forearm plaster) leads to fingers which are flexed at the metacarpo-phalangeal joints and extended at the interphalangeal joints. The thumb is adducted into the palm.

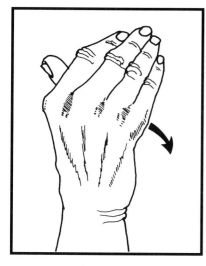

19. *Inspection* (19): Ulnar deviation of the fingers at the metacarpo-phalangeal joints occurs in rheumatoid arthritis. In the later stages the metacarpo-phalangeal joints may dislocate.

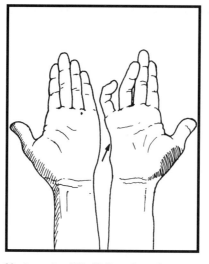

20. *Inspection* (20): Unilateral wasting suggests a root, plexus or nerve lesion. Widespread involvement necessitates a full examination to exclude disorders such as generalised peripheral neuropathy, syringomyelia, multiple sclerosis and the muscular dystrophies.

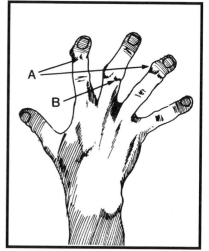

21. *Inspection* (21): *swellings* (1): Note (A) Heberden's nodes on the dorsal surface of the distal interphalangeal joint. (They are often associated with deviation of the distal phalanx and are a sign of osteoarthritis of the fingers.) (B) The proximal interphalangeal joints may be similarly affected (Bouchard's nodes).

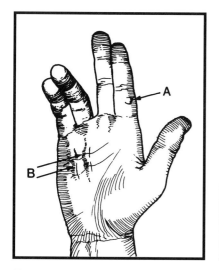

22. *Inspection* (22): *swellings* (2): Note (A) firm, pea-like ganglions are common along the line of the tendon sheaths. (B) Nodular swellings of the palm and fingers accompany Dupuytren's contracture.

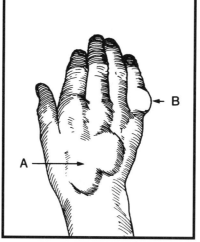

23. *Inspection* (23): *swellings* (3): Note (A) isolated rheumatoid nodules or synovial swellings. (B) Enchondroma (sometimes multiple) is one of the commonest bone tumours occurring in the hand. If small, it may declare itself only by pathological fracture.

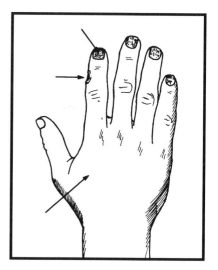

24. *Inspection* (24): Note the nutrition of the skin and nails. In the case of the nails, note any disturbance of growth, deformity, evidence of fungal infection or psoriasis. In the skin, note the presence of finger burns or trophic ulceration, suggestive of neurological disturbance. Note any alteration of skin colour, suggesting circulatory involvement from local arterial or sympathetic supply disturbance.

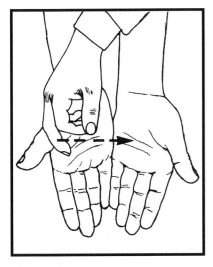

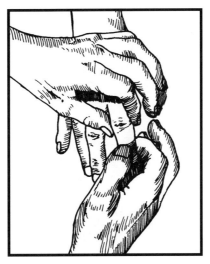

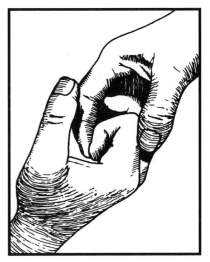

25. *Palpation* (1): Note any generalised or local disturbance of temperature or sweating in the palm or volar surfaces of the fingers. The other hand may be used for comparison.

26. *Palpation* (2): Palpate the individual finger joints between the finger and thumb, looking for thickening, tenderness, oedema and increased local heat. Note that in gouty arthritis a single joint only may be affected, especially in the early stages.

27. *Palpation* (3): Try to tuck each finger into the palm, and ask the patient to repeat this unaided. Loss of active movements only is usually due to nerve or tendon discontinuity while passive loss may be due to joint or tendon adhesions or arthritis.

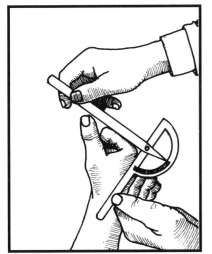

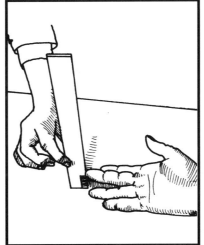

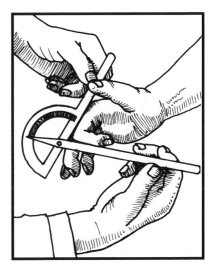

28. *Movements* (1): Where indicated for continued assessment or medico-legal purposes, both the active and passive range in an affected finger should be recorded. The normal active range in the metacarpo-phalangeal joints is 0–90°. The metacarpo-phalangeal joints can be passively hyperextended by up to 45°.

29. *Movements* (2): Extension loss may also be recorded by noting linear discrepancy. When passive extension is possible, loss of active extension suggests division, rupture or displacement of the extensor tendons, or a posterior interosseous palsy if all are affected.

30. *Movements* (3): The normal range in the proximal interphalangeal joints is 0–100°.

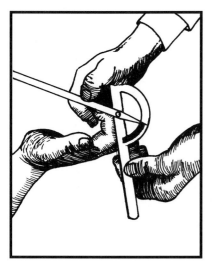

31. *Movements* (4): In the distal interphalangeal joints the normal range is 0–80°.

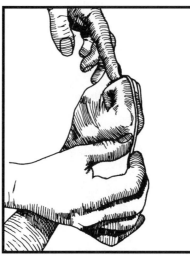

32. *Movements* (5): An alternative method involves moulding a length of malleable wire over the finger (14G, solder wire, approximately 2 mm in diameter, is suitable).

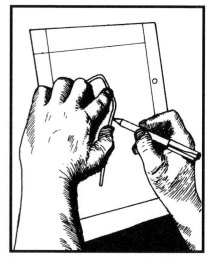

33. *Movements* (6): The wire is then transferred to the case record, and an outline drawn round it. The finger and date should be noted. An additional record of extension may be superimposed. Subsequent assessment of progress is easily made by repeating the process.

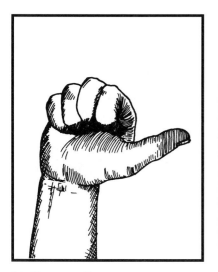

34. *Movements* (7): *composite movement:* As all the joints of all the fingers are involved in grasping and holding, ask the patient to make a fist. Normally the distal phalanges should 'tuck in', touching the palm at right angles.

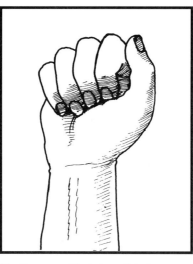

35. *Movements* (8): Only a slight loss at any level is sufficient to prevent 'tuck-in'. All the fingers may be involved as shown. If a single finger is affected its prominence will be obvious. This screening test may be carried out earlier in the examination if desired.

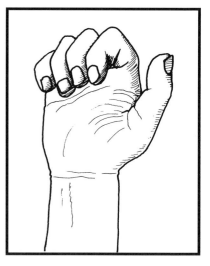

36. *Movements* (9): Greater reduction in movements will prevent the fingers from reaching the palm, and indicate more serious impairment of the patient's ability to grasp and hold.

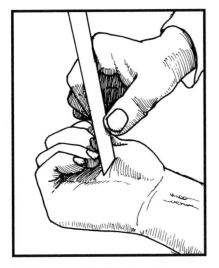

37. *Movements* (10): This important restriction of functional ability may be measured by noting the distance that the fingers stand proud of the palm on maximum flexion.

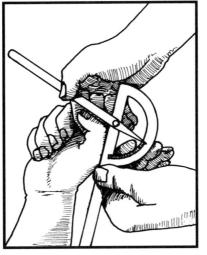

38. *Movements* (11): *the thumb:* The normal interphalangeal joint can be flexed 80° and extended 20° (both actively and passively) beyond the neutral position, giving a total range of 100°.

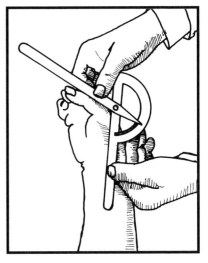

39. *Movements* (12): The normal range of flexion in the metacarpo-phalangeal joint is approximately 55°. The joint may be extended passively 5° beyond the neutral position.

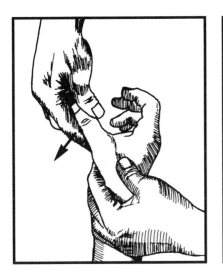

40. *Movements* (13): At this stage, test the stability of the metacarpo-phalangeal joint in a side-to-side plane. Extend the joint and stress the medial collateral ligament. Compare the sides. Excess mobility follows tears ('gamekeeper's thumb') and rheumatoid arthritis, and can be very disabling.

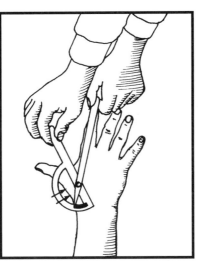

41. *Movements* (14): *carpo-metacarpal joint:* Test extension (abduction parallel to the plane of the palm) by placing the hand palm down, and measuring the range from a position in contact with the index to its fully extended position. *Normal range: 20°.*

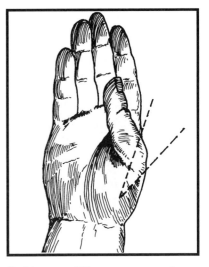

42. *Movements* (15): *carpo-metacarpal flexion:* From the neutral position with the thumb in contact with the index, the normal thumb can flex 15°. This angle is difficult to measure, and an inaccurate assessment is seldom of value.

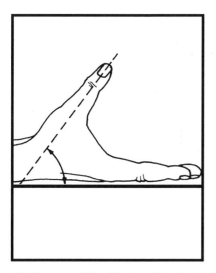

43. *Movements* (16): *abduction of the thumb in a plane at right angles to the palm:* The patient attempts to point the thumb at the ceiling, with the back of the hand resting on a table. *Normal range: 60°.*

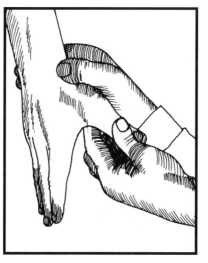

44. *Movements* (17): While examining the carpo-metacarpal joint of the thumb, note any crepitus from the joint. This finding is common in osteoarthritis and rheumatoid arthritis of this joint, and there is often prominence of the base of the metacarpal.

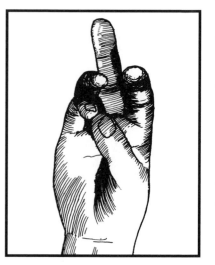

45. *Movements* (18): *opposition* (1): This movement involves abduction at right angles to the palm, flexion and rotation. Normally the thumb should be able to touch the tip of the little finger.

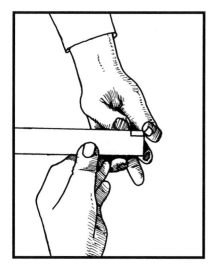

46. *Movements* (19): *opposition* (2): Loss of opposition may be assessed by measuring the distance between the tip of the thumb and little finger.

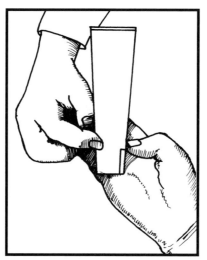

47. *Movements* (20): *opposition* (3): Alternatively, the distance between the tip of the thumb and the metacarpo-phalangeal joint of the little finger may be recorded.

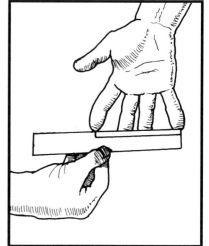

48. *Movements* (21): Finger abduction may be assessed by measuring the spread between index and little fingers, or the spread between individual fingers. Excessive abduction of the little finger is found in the Ehlers-Danlos syndrome (see 6, 22).

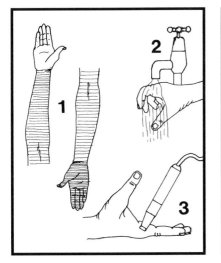

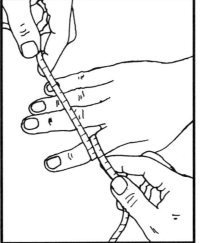

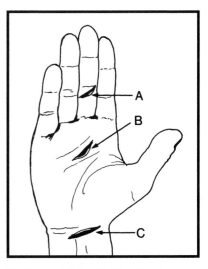

49. *Vibration syndromes:* In vibration white finger, although little clinical abnormality may be found, (1) note if the hand becomes pale on elevation, and the speed with which it pinks up on depression; (2) see if an attack is precipitated by holding the hand under cold water for 2 minutes; (3) check the flow in the digital vessels with a Doppler flowmeter. Note that the peripheral circulation may be disturbed by oral anti-hypertensives.

50. *Joint thickening and swelling:* The activity of the inflammatory process in a swollen joint is sometimes assessed by measuring the joint circumference from time to time. Accuracy without special equipment is difficult to achieve, and the results are of limited value.

51. *Tendon injuries* (1): Note first the position of any wound, and try to work out the structures at risk, e.g. (A) flexor profundus, (B) sublimis, and if deeper, profundus, (C) median nerve, flexor carpi radialis longus, sublimis, and more deeply profundus tendons.

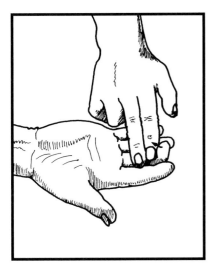

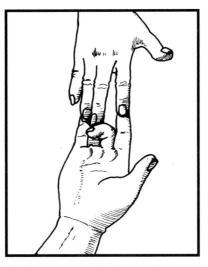

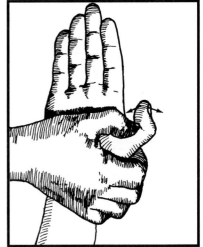

52. *Tendon injuries* (2): If the *profundus* tendon is suspect, support the finger and ask the patient to bend the tip. Loss of the ability to flex the terminal phalanx occurs when the flexor digitorum profundus tendon is divided.

53. *Tendon injuries* (3): If the *sublimis* tendon is suspect, hold all the fingers except the suspect one in a fully extended position to neutralise the effect of flexor profundus. If the patient is able to flex the finger at the proximal interphalangeal joint then sublimis is intact.

54. *Tendon injuries* (4): *flexor and extensor pollicis longus:* Support the proximal phalanx and ask the patient to flex and extend the tip.

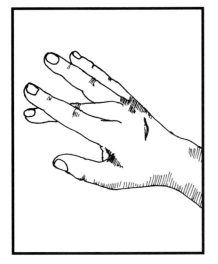

55. *Tendon injuries* (5): *extensor digitorum communis:* Ask the patient to extend the fingers. Any extensor tendon divided on the dorsum of the hand or finger will be obvious by the lack of extension in the finger, assuming the finger joints have been checked for mobility. To assess the distal slips, grasp the middle phalanx and ask the patient to try to extend the distal IP (DIP) joint.

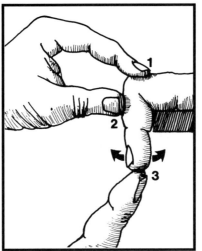

56. *Tendon injuries* (6): *Elson's middle slip test:* Flex the proximal IP (PIP) joint of the finger over the edge of a table, and steady the proximal phalanx (1). Ask the patient to try to extend the PIP joint, and feel for any activity (2): this occurs if the middle slip is intact, and the DIP joint will be *flail* (3). If the middle slip is ruptured, extension at the PIP joint does *not* occur, *and* the DIP joint *stiffens* and *extends.*

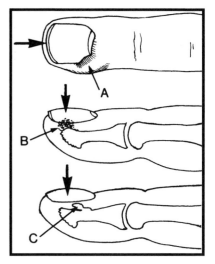

57. *Infections* (1): (A) Paronychia is the commonest infection. Pain is aggravated by pressure on the end of the nail. (B) Apical infections give pain which is aggravated by downward pressure on the nail. A subungual exostosis (C) (which can be confirmed by radiographs) may sometimes cause confusion.

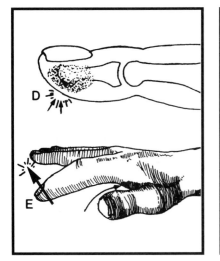

58. *Infections* (2): (D) Pulp infections are exquisitely tender and may lead to destruction of the distal phalanx. (E) Tendon sheath infections lead to a fusiform flexed finger. Straightening causes pain. Tenderness is marked and localised (usually to the base of the sheath).

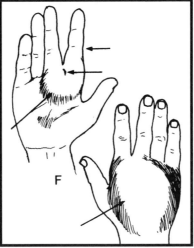
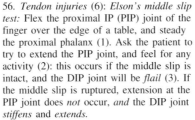

59. *Infections* (3): (F) In web space infections, there is usually marked swelling of the back of the hand and web, with spreading of the fingers. Note the site of any causal wound.

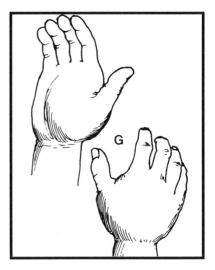

60. *Infections* (4): (G) In thenar and mid-palmar space infections there is gross swelling of the hand involving both the dorsal and palmar surfaces. In the case of the thenar space, the swelling may be more pronounced on the radial side of the palm.

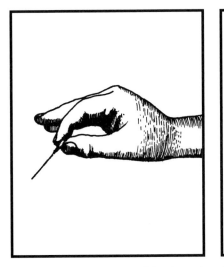

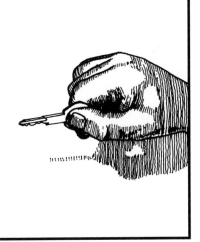

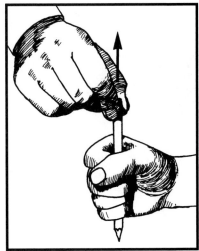

61. *Assessment of the principal functions of the hand* (1): *pinch grip:* Ask the patient to pick up a small object between the tips of the thumb and index. Intact sensation is necessary for a satisfactory performance. The patient should be asked to repeat the test with his eyes closed.

62. *Hand function* (2): *thumb to side of index grip:* The patient should be asked to grip a key between the thumb and side of the index in the normal fashion. Test the firmness of the grip by attempting to withdraw the key, using your own pinch grip.

63. *Hand function* (3): *grasp:* Ask the patient to grasp a pen firmly in the hand, using the thumb and fingers. Attempt to withdraw the pen and note the resistance offered. Where finger flexion is restricted, repeat using an object of greater diameter.

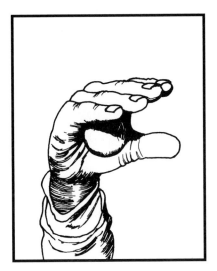

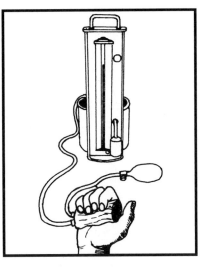

64. *Hand function* (4): *palmar grasp:* Test the cupping action of the hand by asking the patient to grasp a small ball in the palm of the hand. Note the patient's ability to resist the ball being withdrawn.

65. *Hand function* (5): *grip strength:* This may be tested using a dynamometer; alternatively, inflate a rolled sphygmomanometer cuff to 20 mm of mercury and ask the patient to squeeze it as hard as he can. A reading of 200 mm or over should be achievable with the normal hand.

66. *Hand function* (6): *bilateral function:* While the function in one hand may be assessed as described, it is important to note that impairment of function in one hand may clearly affect many activities which normally involve both performing together. The degree of overall functional impairment may be investigated by enquiring about, or testing, the patient's ability to perform certain tasks. When progress is being measured, each of these may be scored on a scale (0–5 or 0–10) and summed. The following list (adapted from tests devised by Lamb et al) may be found to be helpful, either selected or as a whole:

1. Unscrew top from bottle.
2. Fill cup and drink.
3. Open tin with tin-opener.
4. Remove match from box and light it.
5. Use knife and fork for eating.
6. Apply paste to toothbrush and clean teeth.
7. Put on jacket.
8. Do up buttons.
9. Fasten belt round waist.
10. Tie shoe laces.
11. Sharpen pencil.
12. Write messages.
13. Use dial telephone.
14. Staple papers together.
15. Wrap string round parcel.
16. Use playing cards.

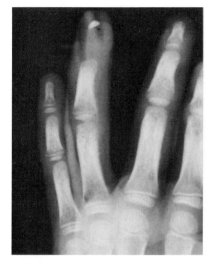

67. *Hand radiographs: examples of pathology* (1): A pyogenic infection of the pulp of the ring finger in a child leading to osteitis and destruction of the terminal phalanx.

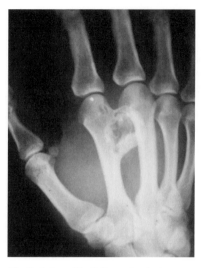

68. *Pathology* (2): Solitary (benign) enchondroma involving the neck of the index metacarpal.

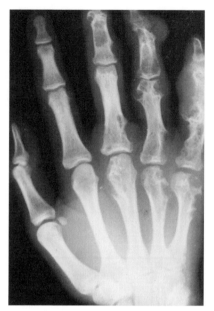

69. *Pathology* (3): The thumb and index are normal, but there are multiple enchondromata involving the other rays, typical of Ollier's disease (multiple enchondromatosis).

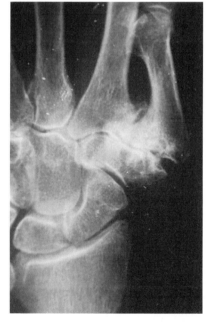

70. *Pathology* (4): There is distortion of the proximal end of the thumb metacarpal and narrowing of the joint space typical of advanced osteoarthritic changes in the carpo-metacarpal joint of the thumb.

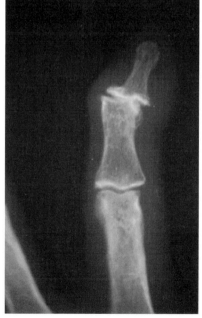

71. *Pathology* (5): There is narrowing of the distal interphalangeal joint and subluxation of the distal phalanx of this finger, typical of osteoarthritis. Heberden's nodes were present clinically.

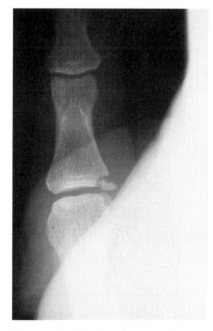

72. *Pathology* (6): There is an avulsion fracture of the base of the proximal phalanx of the thumb associated clinically with instability in the metacarpo-phalangeal joint (gamekeeper's thumb).

8. The thoracic and lumbar spine

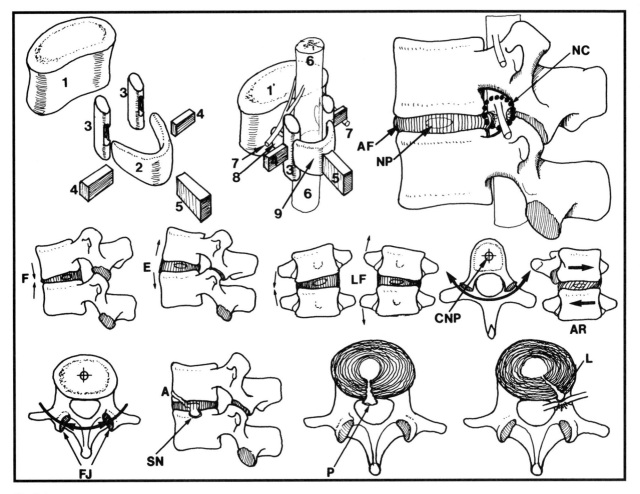

Fig. 8.A

The spine: anatomical features

The complex relationships of the components of a typical vertebra may be illustrated by an exploded diagram (shown here after Kapandji). The bony elements comprise the vertebral body (1), composed of cancellous bone covered with an outer shell of cortical bone, the horseshoe-shaped neural arch (2), two articular masses or processes (3) which take part in the facet (interarticular) joints, the transverse processes (4), and the spinous processes (5).

When these components are brought together they form a protective covering for the cord (6) and issuing nerve roots (7). The neural arch (2) is divided by the articular processes (3) into pedicles (8) and laminae (9).

Each vertebra articulates with the one above and below by means of the facet joints and the intervertebral discs. Each disc, lying between the hyaline cartilage end-plates of adjacent vertebral bodies, is composed of a nucleus pulposus (NP) surrounded by concentric sheets of fibrous tissue (annulus fibrosis) (AF).

Movements between the vertebrae are possible in several planes, and the axes of these movements pass through the approximate centres of the intervertebral discs. At all levels of the spine, flexion (F) and extension (E), and lateral flexion (LF) to both sides are possible. In the thoracic spine, the plane of the facet joints lies in the arc of a circle which has its centre in the nucleus pulposus (CNP); as a result, (axial) rotation (AR) is possible in this part of the spine. In contrast, the orientation of the facet joints (FJ) in the lumbar region is such that rotation is blocked, i.e. *virtually no vertebral rotation occurs in the lumbar spine.*

As a result of the elasticity of annulus, the nucleus pulposus is under constant pressure, and may (uncommonly) herniate into a vertebral body anteriorly (A) or centrally (Schmorl's node) (SN). A much more common occurrence is for the annular fibres to tear (as a result of trauma or degenerative changes) so that the nucleus bulges posteriorly (P) or laterally (L): 'slipped discs' — central or lateral protrusions. A posterior (central) disc protrusion may affect the cord directly (or the cauda equina in the lower lumbar spine); this may lead to bilateral lower limb signs with or without bladder involvement. With lateral protrusions, the neurological disturbance usually results from pressure on one or two nerve roots only — so that the effects are more localised and usually predominate on one side. In the neural canals (NC, circled, top right) the space for the segmental nerves is restricted, and in this region symptoms may be caused not only by a disc prolapse, but by any pathology in the neural canals (e.g. arthritic facet joint lipping).

Back pain

Back pain is one of the commonest and most troublesome of complaints; its causes are legion and an exact diagnosis is often difficult. The disability with which it is usually associated is often severe and prolonged; therapy is often ineffective, and the anxious, impatient and dissatisfied sufferer often resorts to lines of treatment which are unproved, illogical and irrational. In this difficult area it is not possible to provide a guide to pathology and diagnosis which is simple and at the same time comprehensive and foolproof. Nevertheless, it may be helpful to consider this subject under three headings:

1. Back pain found in association with spinal pathology such as vertebral infections, tumours, ankylosing spondylitis, polyarthritis, Paget's disease and primary neurological disease.
2. Back pain associated with nerve root pain; the commonest causes are intervertebral disc prolapse and compression of nerve roots within the neural canals.
3. Back pain caused by disturbance of the mechanics of the spine (mechanical back pain). This is the largest group of conditions causing back pain. In a number of cases the mechanical disturbance is clear (e.g. osteoporotic spinal fractures, senile kyphosis, spondylolisthesis, Scheuermann's disease (spinal osteochondrosis) and sometimes osteoarthritis. In other cases, although the symptoms may be identical in character, the cause cannot be determined with any accuracy; these

cases of mechanical back pain formerly attracted many emotive but valueless names (such as lumbago, low-back strain etc.).

In taking a history, examining and investigating a patient suffering from back pain, possible extra-spinal causes should be excluded, and an attempt should be made to place the patient in one of the three groups described above. Thereafter, and if possible, a more precise diagnosis may be attempted.

Important points in history-taking

1. Note the patient's age and occupation(s): both may be relevant.
2. Ask about the onset of the pain:
    (a) When did the symptoms commence?
    (b) Was the onset slow and insidious, rapid, or sudden? The latter is strongly suggestive of mechanical factors.
    (c) Was there a history of an injury, such as, for example, a sudden twist or strain, or a sneeze occurring when the patient was in a flexed position? (This is a common history in cases of intervertebral disc prolapse.)
3. Ask about any directly relevant previous history:
    (a) Is there a history of a previous similar attack?
    (b) Is there a history of any previous trouble with the spine?
4. Ask about the site and nature of the pain:
    (a) Where is the pain situated? Is it well localised or is it diffuse?
    (b) Is the pain always present or does it disappear at times? The latter is suggestive of a mechanical cause.
    (c) Are there any factors which aggravate or alleviate the pain? Note that with mechanical back pain, bending or sudden movement may make the pain worse, while lying flat, particularly on a hard surface, or applying local heat, or even sitting may relieve the pain. In the case of backache associated with spinal pathology — particularly in the case of tumour, infections or inflammatory disease — the patient may be unable to find a position of rest; constant night pain (as distinct from short-lived pain when turning in bed) is a feature.
5. Ask about radiation of the pain:
    (a) Does the pain radiate into the legs?
    (b) If so, exactly how far down does the pain go, and what area is involved? (Note that the commonly affected roots of the sciatic nerve (L4, L5, S1) supply skin *below* the knee.)
    (c) What is the pain like?
    (d) Is there paraesthesia?
    Note that pain radiating into the legs is not necessarily due to nerve root involvement; it seems the case that irritation of facet joints, ligaments and muscles may produce dull, aching pain in the buttocks and backs of the thighs. In contrast, pain arising from nerve roots is usually sharp and knife-like, and in addition, in the case of the commonly affected L5 and S1 roots, it often extends below the knee to the ankle or foot. In the common situation where there is involvement

of one or at the most two nerve roots, the whole limb cannot be affected. Instead, the area of sensory disturbance should correspond with the relevant dermatome(s), and it should be noted if paraesthesia occurs within the same restricted territory.

6. Ask about motor involvement:
   (a) Has the patient noted any weakness in the lower limbs, or any muscle wasting or fibrillation?
   (b) Has there been any disturbance of gait or balance, any tendency to giving-way of the legs, any sign of drop foot?
7. Make enquiries in the following areas:
   (a) Has there been any malaise, fever or involvement of other joints?
   (b) Has there been any weight loss?
   (c) Has the patient had any large bowel or other gastro-intestinal problem?
   (d) Have there been any genito-urinary symptoms, especially retention or incontinence?
   (c) Has the patient had any respiratory difficulty?
   (f) Has the patient any symptoms suggestive of a major neurological disturbance?

A positive answer to any of these questions will generally necessitate appropriate further investigation. The possibility of an invasive primary tumour or metastatic lesion must always be kept in mind, and examination of the abdomen, rectum and common sites of primary tumour is wise if there is any likelihood of malignancy.

The spine should then be examined clinically; if the symptoms have remained unchanged over a 2-week period, radiological examination and estimation of the sedimentation rate should be carried out. At this stage any well-defined spinal pathology should be detected (such as spondylolisthesis, ankylosing spondylitis, osteitis of the spine etc.). If conditions such as these have been eliminated, the question of whether the symptoms are due to a prolapsed intervertebral disc should be considered. The history, clinical findings and plain radiographs of the spine should be in harmony before it is reasonable to make this diagnosis. By the process of elimination, if a diagnosis has not yet been made, the patient is likely to be suffering from mechanical back pain; but note that both the history and findings should be in accord with this. If not, caution must be exercised, close surveillance should be maintained, and further investigation may be indicated.

Scoliosis

Scoliosis is a lateral curvature of the spine. In the management of any case, the first and most important decision to make is whether there is any deformity of the vertebrae (structural scoliosis). If the vertebrae are normal (non-structural scoliosis), the deformity is usually due to one of the following conditions: it may be *compensatory*, resulting from tilting of the pelvis from real or apparent shortening of one leg. It may be *sciatic*, and due to unilateral protective muscle spasm, especially that accompanying a prolapsed intervertebral disc. *Postural scoliosis* occurs most commonly in adolescent girls and generally resolves spontaneously.

In *structural scoliosis* there is alteration in vertebral shape and mobility, and the deformity cannot be corrected by alteration of posture. A careful history and examination is required to find a cause and give a prognosis, the two factors on which treatment depends. Structural scoliosis may be *congenital*, the deformity being due, for example, to a hemivertebra (only half of a single vertebra is fully formed), fused vertebrae, or absent or fused ribs.

In *paralytic scoliosis* the deformity is secondary to loss of the supportive action of the trunk and spinal muscles, nearly always as a sequel to anterior poliomyelitis.

Neuropathic scoliosis is seen as a complication of neurofibromatosis, cerebral palsy, spina bifida, syringomyelia, Friedreich's ataxia and neuropathic conditions. Primary disorders of the supportive musculature of the spine are responsible for *myopathic scoliosis* (e.g. in muscular dystrophy, arthrogryphosis). *Metabolic scoliosis* is uncommon, but occurs in cystine storage disease, Marfan's syndrome and rickets.

Idiopathic scoliosis is the commonest and by far the most important of the structural scolioses, and its cause remains obscure. Several vertebrae at one or less commonly two distinct levels are affected (*primary curve*). In the area of the primary curve there is loss of mobility (the fixed curve) and rotational deformity of the vertebrae (the spinous processes rotate into the concavity, and the bodies which carry the ribs in the thoracic region rotate into the convexity). Above and below the fixed primary curves, *secondary curves* which are mobile develop in an effort to maintain the normal position of the head and pelvis. The spinal deformity is accompanied by shortening of the trunk (which may be assessed by using anthropometric tables) and there is often impairment of respiratory and cardiac function. In severe cases this may lead to invalidism. Cor pulmonale may feature in cases where the primary curve exceeds 80°.

Once scoliosis has appeared in the growing child the natural tendency is to deterioration. The prognosis of a given case is dependent on the age of onset, the level of the spine affected, the size and number of the primary curves, and the type of structural scoliosis (e.g. idiopathic or congenital). Deterioration may stop when skeletal maturity is reached, but sometimes continues as a result of disc degeneration and vertebral subluxation; 17° deterioration in 70° thoracic curves, and 20° deterioration in 30° lumbar curves have been recorded. Generally speaking, the higher the level of the spine involved in the primary curve, and the younger the patient, the worse the prognosis. There is the notable exception that in some cases occurring in infancy there is spontaneous recovery, which is as remarkable as its mysterious onset. Favourable factors are left-sided curves occurring in the first year of life in males, where there is a rib–vertebral angle of less than 20°. Life expectancy may be reduced in congenital and paralytic scolioses, but not it is said in idiopathic scoliosis.

In all cases of structural scoliosis appropriate investigation, radiographic measurement of the curves and careful observation are essential. Note in particular:

1. Syringomyelia is present in 25% of cases of juvenile idiopathic scoliosis. As decompression may lead to improvement, and failure to decompress before attempted surgical correction or stabilisation may lead to neurological complications, an MRI scan is mandatory in all cases occurring within this group.
2. Scoliosis is not normally at onset a painful condition. When there is pain (especially night pain relieved by aspirin), the commonest cause in the adolescent is an osteoid osteoma of a pedicle.

Treatment may be advised in the face of a poor prognosis, evidence of rapid deterioration, or for cosmesis. (Curves are not usually considered for attempted surgical correction unless they are in excess of 25–30°.) The methods available are highly specialised, as is the decision regarding their use and timing. Deterioration in a curve may be controlled by use of a Milwaukee brace (a device incorporating moulded supports for the chin, occiput and pelvis, interconnected by vertical metal struts). This support is employed in older children approaching skeletal maturity who have just-acceptable curves, or it may be used in the young child until an age suitable for spinal fusion (10 or over) is reached. Other patterns of support are available, although none has been shown to have a statistical superiority (and recently some doubts have been cast on their overall effectiveness). Fusion of the entire primary curve is aimed at preventing further deterioration and at allowing braces to be discarded. Prior to fusion it is necessary to correct the primary deformity as much as is possible. Often a hinged plaster spica (Risser jacket) or the surgical insertion of internal apparatus (e.g. Harrington instrumentation) is employed.

Kyphosis

Kyphosis is the term used to describe an increased convexity of the thoracic spine. This is usually obvious when the patient is viewed from the side. (Diminution of the lumbar concave curve is referred to as loss of lumbar lordosis or flattening of the lumbar curvature; in extreme cases there is reversed lordosis, or posterior convexity of the lumbar curve.) Kyphosis generally affects a major part of the thoracic spine (i.e. several vertebrae are affected), and the increased curvature is then said to be *regular*. In *angular* kyphosis, which must be carefully distinguished from regular kyphosis, there is an abrupt alteration in the thoracic curvature which is usually accompanied by undue prominence of a spinous process (gibbus).

Where mobility is normal in the kyphotic spine, the deformity is most frequently postural in origin; this is often seen (as is postural scoliosis) in adolescent girls. In some cases the deformity is secondary to an increased lumbar lordosis (which in turn may be due to abnormal forward tilting of the pelvis, sometimes from flexion contracture of the hips or congenital dislocation of the hips). Less commonly, kyphosis may result from muscle weakness secondary to anterior poliomyelitis or muscular dystrophy.

When the thoracic curvature is not mobile but fixed, the most frequent causes are Scheuermann's disease, ankylosing spondylitis, senile kyphosis and Paget's disease. When there is an angular kyphosis, the most common causes are tuberculous or other infections of the spine, fracture (traumatic or pathological — e.g. secondary to osteoporosis) or tumours. In adults the commonest tumour is the metastatic deposit, and in children, the eosinophilic granuloma.

Scheuermann's disease (spinal osteochondrosis)

This condition (whose exact aetiology is unknown although there is a strong familial tendency) results in a growth disturbance of the thoracic vertebral bodies which in lateral radiographs of the spine are seen to be narrower anteriorly than posteriorly (anterior wedging). The diagnostic protocol for the condition specifies that not less than three adjacent vertebrae should have at least 5° of anterior wedging. The epiphyses of the vertebral bodies are often irregular and may be disturbed by herniation of the nucleus pulposus. Nuclear herniation may occur between the epiphyses and bodies anteriorly, or into the centre of the bodies (Schmorl's nodes). Mobility is impaired, thoracic kyphosis is regular and often quite marked, and there is a compensatory increase in lumbar lordosis. Secondary osteoarthritic changes may supervene in the thoracic and lumbar spine.

The normal upper limit of the convexity of the thoracic spine (as measured by the Cobb method) is reckoned to be 45°, and cases of Scheuermann's disease in adolescence with curves of 50° or less should be observed. Where the curve is in excess of this, a Milwaukee brace, worn continuously for not less than 12–18 months (and afterwards till skeletal maturity) may be advised in an attempt to prevent deterioration. If the curve cannot be controlled, and reaches 75°, correction by surgical instrumentation should be considered. In the adult with uncontrollable pain and a curve in excess of 60°, surgical fusion may be performed.

Calvé's disease

Back pain in children may be accompanied by gross flattening of a single vertebral body. Symptoms resolve spontaneously. In many cases the pathology is due to an eosinophilic granuloma.

Ankylosing spondylitis

In this disease there is progressive ossification of the joints of the spine. Its aetiology is unknown, but there is a hereditary tendency, with the overall risk of children developing the condition being 1 in 6. The incidence is greatest in males during the third and fourth decades. Unlike rheumatoid arthritis to which it is often related, it is comparatively rare in women.

The joints between D12 and L1 are often first affected, but the rest of the thoracic and lumbar spine is rapidly involved. The costo-vertebral joints are usually involved, leading to a reduction in chest expansion and vital capacity; pulmonary tuberculosis is sometimes found as a complication. Stiffness of the back and pain are the presenting symptoms in the majority of cases, but on occasion involvement of the knees or hips may first attract attention. There may be pain at the insertions of the Achilles tendons or the plantar fascia (enthesopathy).

The disease is progressive, and although it sometimes arrests spontaneously at an early stage it usually leads to complete ankylosis of the spine, with characteristic changes in the radiographs (bambooing of the spine). Progressive flexion of the spine may be severe, so that forward vision becomes impossible. The sacro-iliac joints are almost invariably involved at an early stage, and there may be fusion of the manubrio-sternal joint. There may be a history of iritis or its sequelae. The sedimentation rate is high (40–120 mm), rheumatoid factor is not present, and estimations of HLA-B27 are usually positive. There is often associated anaemia, muscle wasting and weight loss.

The progress of ankylosing spondylitis may be controlled by anti-inflammatory drugs, and sometimes deep X-ray therapy (in spite of the risks of aplastic anaemia) is used. Where deformity of the spine is gross, spinal osteotomy is occasionally undertaken to give the patient a tolerably erect posture. Replacement arthroplasty of the hips or knees is often employed if these joints have progressed to fusion.

Diffuse idiopathic skeletal hyperostosis (DISH)

This comparatively benign condition, also known as Forestier's disease, is sometimes mistaken for ankylosing spondylitis. It is characterised and diagnosed by the presence of flowing calcification and ossification along the antero-lateral borders of at least four contiguous vertebral bodies. The disc spaces are however preserved (unlike in ankylosing spondylitis), without loss of height or other degenerative changes, and the sacro-iliac and the facet joints do not ankylose. Most cases are asymptomatic, or have mild or moderate restriction of movements in the parts of the spine affected. No treatment is effective.

Senile kyphosis

In true senile kyphosis, the ageing patient becomes progressively stooped and shorter in stature through degenerative thinning of the intervertebral discs. Pain may occur if there is associated osteoarthritis.

In elderly women, the kyphosis may be aggravated by senile osteoporosis or osteomalacia, which lead to anterior vertebral wedging and often pathological fracture. There is usually radiographic evidence of decalcification, the serum chemistry may be disturbed, and pain is a feature if fracture is present.

Treatment is directed towards controlling the underlying osteoporosis or osteomalacia. Thoracic spinal supports are not particularly effective and cannot be tolerated by the elderly, but often a simple lumbar corset is helpful in relieving pain arising from the associated increase in lumbar lordosis.

Paget's disease

Paget's disease of the spine is comparatively uncommon and although the diagnosis is made on the radiographic findings, it may be suggested clinically by other stigmata of the disease. Paget's disease may lead to disturbance of cord function which may often be successfully treated with biphosphonates (e.g. etidronate and pamidronate).

Tuberculosis of the spine

Bone and joint tuberculosis is uncommon in the UK, but the incidence is increasing. The factors responsible include the increase in numbers of immuno-suppressed individuals, the development of drug-resistant strains of the organism, and an ageing population. HIV is the leading risk factor for the reactivation of latent tuberculous infection. The World Health Organization reckons that a third of the global population is infected with the organism (*Mycobacterium tuberculosis*), and that it is the commonest cause of death and disability on a world-wide basis. About a fifth of newly diagnosed cases are extra-pulmonary, and the spine is involved in 50% of cases of bone and joint tuberculosis.

The onset of spinal tuberculosis is often slow, with aching pain in the back and stiffness of the spine. There may be fever and weight loss. Radiographs taken in the earliest stages of the disease show narrowing of a single disc space; later, as the anterior portions of the vertebral bodies become progressively involved, they collapse, leading to anterior and sometimes lateral wedging of the spine. This may produce angular kyphotic or scoliotic deformities. The local abscess may expand and track distally.

The spinal cord may be compromised extrinsically or intrinsically, and weakness of the limbs or paraplegia may ensue. *Extrinsic* causes include caseous abscesses, granulation tissue and fluid, sequestered bone or disc material, and spinal angulation leading to kinking of the cord over an internal gibbus. *Intrinsic* causes include the spread of tuberculous inflammation through the cord and meninges.

Initial investigation should include radiographs of the chest, culture of urine and any sputum, Mantoux testing, brucellosis complement fixation testing, and in the case of the lumbar spine at least, intravenous pyelography (IVP) (renal spread being not uncommon). CAT and MRI scans of the spine are also invaluable in demonstrating the extent of bone and soft tissue involvement.

The clinical and radiological features of tuberculosis of the spine are mimicked in the early stages by other infections (especially those due to *Staphylococcus aureus*) and the only certain method of establishing the diagnosis in the majority of cases seen at this stage is by obtaining specimens for histological and bacteriological examination. Computed tomography-guided needle aspiration biopsy may be employed if this facility is available. Again, as the abscess is small at first and the early removal of necrotic bone and pus is generally of value from the point of view of accelerating healing, many surgeons combine these procedures. In the later stages where there is gross bone destruction, minimal new bone formation and the formation of large abscesses, the diagnosis is seldom in doubt.

The aim of treatment is to overcome the infection, to eliminate abscesses and sequestra, and to promote sound fusion in the affected spinal segment (to help prevent any recrudescence of the disease). The mainstay of treatment is the use of the anti-tuberculous drugs, although the emergence of resistant strains is causing problems. Sensitivity testing is advisable, and drugs should not be used in isolation. Drug therapy for periods of up to 2 years was formerly advised, but it has been shown that regimes employing the combination of rifampicin and isoniazid for 6 months only seem equally effective. This is of particular importance where compliance is low.

Conservative treatment alone leads to a comparatively low fusion rate, and in about 70% of adult cases there is a deterioration in the kyphosis. In those parts of the world where resources are good, there is at present a trend to early surgical intervention to achieve or accelerate the healing process and assist fusion by early drainage of abscesses and bone grafting. Where paraplegia is due to intrinsic causes, it may resolve following anti-tuberculous therapy, but in many cases the causes are extrinsic, and surgery is indicated to decompress the cord. An MRI scan may give valuable assistance in selecting cases and delineating the scope of the surgery required. If adequately dealt with in the early stages (i.e. within 6–9 months of the onset of paraplegia) complete cure is often achieved. In paraplegia of late onset, where the cord is often acutely angled over an internal gibbus, surgical intervention should always be carried out, but the prognosis here is less good.

Pyogenic osteitis of the spine

Pyogenic osteitis of the spine is relatively uncommon. In the early stages of the disease differentiation from tuberculosis of the spine is often extremely difficult, so that the diagnosis may not be clearly established unless material is provided for bacteriological examination. Specimens may be obtained by needle biopsy with the use of an image intensifier, or by exploration. At a later stage (and many cases may delay in their presentation) exuberant new bone formation in the region of the lesion may favour this diagnosis. The presenting features are of pain and stiffness in the back, often of insidious onset but sometimes occurring quite rapidly. Nearly all cases resolve with prolonged treatment with the appropriate antibiotic (the majority are due to a staphylococcal infection, but *Salmonella*, *Bacillus typhosus* and other organisms are sometimes causal).

Metastatic lesions of the spine

Metastatic disease of the spine is seen particularly in the elderly and may be complicated by paraplegia. The diagnosis is established by relevant radiographs. Treatment of the uncomplicated lesion is dependent on the nature of the primary tumour; in some cases deep X-ray therapy and supportive measures may help the local lesion and give relief of pain. Where paraplegia is present, decompression should be undertaken unless the case is terminal. Primary tumours of the spine are rare; the common types are mentioned in Chapter 3.

Spondylolysis, spondylolisthesis

In the erect position, there is a tendency for the body of the fifth lumbar vertebra (carrying the weight of the trunk) to slide forwards on the corresponding surface of the sacrum, as the plane of the L5–S1 disc is not horizontal but slopes downwards anteriorly. This movement is usually prevented by the downward projecting inferior articular processes of the fifth lumbar vertebra impinging on the corresponding upward projecting articular processes of the sacrum. This mechanism may fail if there is a fracture or defect in the part of the fifth lumbar vertebra lying immediately anterior to its inferior articular process. A defect in this region, if unaccompanied by any significant forward movement of the vertebral body, is known as spondylolysis. The defect may be unilateral or bilateral. When forward slip occurs, the condition is known as spondylolisthesis. Less commonly, the fourth lumbar vertebra may be involved, the slip occurring between L4 and L5.

Both congenital and developmental factors have been recognised in the causation of the condition. There is a higher incidence in the families of those affected (30–70%, with dominant transmission), in certain Inuit tribes (where it reaches 54%), and amongst the Japanese. The lowest incidence is in black females (1.1%), and in white males it is 6.1%. Defects are rare at birth and before the age of 5, but the incidence in the population goes on increasing up to the end of the fourth decade. Fractures due to trauma or fatigue are thought to be the most likely cause, and this explains the high incidence amongst gymnasts, weightlifters, labourers, loggers and backpackers. It may be associated with sacral spina bifida and Scheuermann's disease.

Both spondylolysis and spondylolisthesis give rise to low back pain which radiates into the buttocks. In adolescents, the majority of whom are active in sports, resolution of symptoms (and the healing of hairline fractures) may be achieved in 80% of cases by the avoidance of sports and the use of a corset support. In more severe cases, where there is significant forward slip, a local spinal fusion (without reduction of the deformity) is the treatment of choice.

A number of patients may suffer from neurological disturbances in the lower limbs, either initially or as an uncommon complication of a local fusion. In the *cauda equina syndrome* there is usually low back pain with radiation into the buttocks, spinal stiffness, hamstring spasm, gait abnormalitites, and disturbance of bladder and bowel control. This may be due to an associated disc protrusion, or be caused by the cauda equina and roots of the lumbo-sacral plexus being stretched over the prominent upper edge of the fifth lumbar vertebra or the sacrum. These complications should be dealt with by an immediate decompression procedure.

Osteoarthritis (osteoarthrosis)

Primary osteoarthritis of the spine is extremely common, especially in the elderly, and is often asymptomatic. In the majority of cases there are no obvious causes, apart from those associated with the degenerative processes of age. Sometimes obesity and excessive use of the spine by manual workers may be factors. In secondary osteoarthritis, previous pathology in the spine accelerates normal wear and tear processes.

Occasionally osteoarthritis may be localised to one spinal level, at for example the site of a previous fracture or a prolapsed intervertebral disc. Often, however, many vertebral levels are affected, particularly where there is some alteration in the normal curves of the spine; for example secondary osteoarthritic changes may occur in the lumbar spine when lumbar lordosis is increased as a sequel to Scheuermann's disease of the thoracic spine.

Osteoarthritis of the spine may be accompanied by disc degeneration, anterior and posterior lipping of the vertebral bodies, narrowing and lipping of the facet joints, and sometimes abutment of the vertebral spines (kissing spines) due to disc degeneration bringing the vertebrae nearer together.

When osteoarthritis gives rise to symptoms, these are usually of pain and stiffness in the back; once other conditions have been eliminated, the radiological appearances are diagnostic. Treatment is by weight reduction where applicable, spinal exercises to improve the back musculature, and analgesics. Short-wave diathermy is sometimes helpful. In the commonest area, the lumbar spine, a corset support is a widely used and generally very helpful line of treatment. Only rarely is spinal fusion indicated, but this is sometimes considered in the younger patient suffering from secondary osteoarthritis localised to a single level of the spine.

Rheumatoid arthritis

Rheumatoid arthritis may affect the spine; other peripheral sites are normally involved, so that the diagnosis is not normally difficult. Radiographs of the spine in rheumatoid arthritis generally show widespread osteoporosis, disc space narrowing, narrowing of the facet joints, and often reduction in the height of vertebral bodies. The treatment is that of generalised rheumatoid arthritis; locally, corset supports may give considerable relief of symptoms.

Spina bifida

Spina bifida is a condition in which there is a congenital failure of fusion of the posterior elements of the spine, through which the contents of the spinal canal may herniate. The grosser forms in the newly born child present no difficulty in diagnosis. A number require and are amenable to immediate surgery, which may prevent early death from ascending meningitis and ameliorate the frequently concomitant neurological and hydrocephalic problems. The residual neurological defect may unfortunately be profound and the selection of cases for surgery is specialised and to some extent controversial.

The older child or adult may present with spina bifida occulta, which is diagnosed by radiological examination, although it may be suspected by the presence of a hairy patch, naevus, fat pad or dimpling of the skin at the site of the abnormality. Many cases are symptom-free. In some the only manifestation may be the presence of pes cavus. In others there may be progressive bladder dysfunction, weakness and incoordination of the legs, or trophic changes in the feet.

Spinal stenosis

A decrease in the sagittal diameter of the spinal canal, perhaps associated with narrowing of the nerve root tunnels, may give rise to symptoms of vague backache and morning stiffness. Occasionally there may be temporary motor paralysis or neurogenic claudication where there are lower limb pains, cramps and paraesthesia related to walking or exercise. There may be weakness or giving-way of the legs. The claudication distance is variable and pain may be rapidly relieved by forward flexion of the spine or by sitting. The sensory loss is segmental, and impulse symptoms are usually present. (In claudication due to vascular insufficiency, the claudication distance is constant, the peripheral pulses are usually absent, and the sensory loss generally of stocking type.) The average age of presentation is 65. Clinically the straight-leg-raising test is hardly ever affected, but motor disturbances and absence of the knee jerks(s) are common.

Spinal stenosis is common in achondroplasia, but is more often seen as a complication of osteoarthritis of the lumbar spine, spondylolisthesis, Paget's disease, previous fracture or spinal surgery. In others the condition may be suspected on clinical grounds. Analysis of the dimensions of the pedicles and the spinal canal in the plain radiographs may be helpful in establishing the diagnosis, but CAT and MRI scans reliably demonstrate the space available within the spinal canal for the neurological structures.

If symptoms are marked and the patient is otherwise fit, gratifying relief is often achieved by a decompression procedure.

The prolapsed intervertebral disc

In the commonest pattern of intervertebral disc prolapse, a tear in the annulus allows protrusion of the semi-liquid nucleus pulposus. This may be limited by intact fibres at the periphery of the annulus (*contained prolapse*). In other cases extrusion of the nucleus is usually more extensive, and the prolapsed material may be cut off from its source (*sequestered disc prolapse*). Lumbar disc prolapses are by far the most common, and the diagnosis is usually made on the clinical evidence alone. Confirmation may be obtained by means of non-invasive procedures such as CAT and MRI scans. Discography often yields valuable information, as does radiculography. Nevertheless it is most important to note that the investigative findings must be interpreted in conjunction with the history and clinical findings. (In a recent study of a control group completely free from symptoms, abnormalities were found in the MRI scans in 57%; 36% had evidence of disc prolapse, and 21% had spinal stenosis!)

The disc between L5 and S1 is most commonly involved, followed in order by L4–L5, and that between L3 and L4. In a typical case there is a history of a flexion injury which tears the annulus fibrosus, allowing the nucleus pulposus to herniate through. Back pain is produced by the annular tear and protective lumbar muscle spasm may contribute to it. Pain is felt in the lumbar region. There is usually tenderness between the spines at the affected level, and sometimes at the side over muscles in spasm. Muscle spasm often leads to loss of the normal lumbar lordotic curve, to restriction of movements in the lumbar spine, and a protective scoliosis. The extruding nucleus frequently presses on a lumbar nerve root, giving rise to sciatic pain, paraesthesia in the leg, and sometimes muscle weakness, sensory impairment, and diminution or abolition of the ankle jerk. At higher levels, the knee jerk may be lost. The neurological disturbance is *segmental in pattern, and is dependent on the level of the prolapse*. Impulse symptoms are common. When the prolapse is large and central, the cauda equina may be affected, producing bladder disturbance, diminished perineal sensation and even paraplegia. Such an occurrence is a surgical emergency, and immediate exploration imperative.

When a disc prolapse occurs in the adolescent, there is striking restriction of movements in the lumbar spine. In the older patient, where degenerative changes have occurred in the annulus, symptoms may be produced by an extensive backward bulging of the disc without there being a frank localised annular tear.

Disc prolapses in the thoracic spine are rare, and have a variety of presentations, often with a confusing clinical picture. There may be band-like chest pain, scoliosis, bizarre neurological disturbances with peripheral temperature changes, altered reflexes, and weakness of the limbs. A number are misdiagnosed as multiple sclerosis or amyotrophic lateral sclerosis. The diagnosis is established by MRI scan.

In the long term, the extrusion of disc material from between the vertebral bodies leads to narrowing of the disc space. The facet joints are disturbed, and tend to develop secondary arthritic changes which decrease the mobility of the spine at that level, and may themselves be a source of pain and sometimes nerve root irritation.

Occasionally, in the young in particular, the nucleus may herniate into the substance of the vertebral bodies, giving rise to mild backache without root symptoms. This pattern of herniation (Schmorl's nodes) is diagnosed radiographically.

Apart from the large central prolapse, all cases of acute disc prolapse are first treated by conservative methods. In the majority of cases symptoms subside with a 2-week period of strict bed rest on a firm bed. Analgesics are essential initially. If the response is good, the patient is then allowed up although he is warned to avoid lifting and bending in case of recurrence. In some centres spinal extension exercises may be advocated at this stage. If the response has only been moderate, a number of surgeons nevertheless allow the patient to become ambulant wearing a corset back support. If there is no response to 2 weeks' bed rest, the case must be carefully re-assessed before further treatment by bed rest is continued. Where ultimately there is an unsatisfactory response, or where residual symptoms are severe, further investigation by CAT scan and/or myelography is usually undertaken, with a view to treatment of the lesion by surgical methods (e.g. excision). The results of treatment, particularly as far as return to work is concerned, are surprisingly little affected by either the physical findings, the extent of the local pathology, or the effects of surgery. (Social or work-related factors have the greatest influence on the results.)

Mechanical back pain

Although usually suspected following history-taking, clinical examination and the study of appropriate radiographs, the diagnosis is made largely by a process of elimination: it is back pain which is not due to a prolapsed intervertebral disc or any other clearly defined pathology. The patient is usually in the 20–45 age group, and complains of dull backache aggravated by activity. There is often a history of morning stiffness which is gradually relieved as the patient moves about. Extensive radiation of pain is not a feature; physical signs are often slight, and positive neurological signs are not a feature.

Acute cases may be precipitated by a traumatic incident, such as the flawed lifting of a heavy weight, a fall, or a head-on impact pattern road traffic accident. There may be intense protective muscle spasm. Symptoms may resolve completely over a 4–6-week period with physiotherapy, analgesics and other conservative measures, but in a number of cases they become prolonged, with the impatient sufferer often trying any of the large number of alternative medicine treatments now so widely available.

In chronic cases there is often a long history of intermittent low back pain over a number of years. The cause is often obscure, although degenerative changes in the spine are not uncommonly present. Resistance to treatment is a frequent problem, and many are ultimately referred to pain clinics. Sometimes a change of employment to work of a lighter character may have to be contemplated.

Coccydynia

In patients with this complaint of pain in the coccygeal area, there is often a history of a fall in the seated position on to a hard surface; consequently in a number of cases radiographs may reveal a fracture of the end piece of the sacrum, or show the coccyx to be subluxed into the anteverted position. Symptoms of pain on sitting and defecation are often protracted for 6–12 months, but tend to resolve spontaneously. It was formerly thought that if symptoms proved persistent, either a disc lesion in the lumbar spine (with distal referral) or a functional problem was likely to be the cause, but this is now discounted.

In stubborn cases conservative treatment should invariably be first employed (short-wave diathermy, ultrasound, injection of long-acting local anaesthetics or steroids, or coccygeal manipulation). If there is complete failure to respond to a substantial period of conservative treatment, excision of the coccyx is reported as being successful in 80% of cases.

Commoner causes of back complaints in the various age groups

Children	Scoliosis
	Spondylolisthesis
	Pyogenic or tuberculous infections
	Calvé's disease
Adolescents	Scheuermann's disease
	Scoliosis (idiopathic and postural)
	Mechanical back pain
	Adolescent intervertebral disc syndrome
	Pyogenic or tuberculous infections
Young adults	Mechanical back pain
	Prolapsed intervertebral disc
	Spondylolisthesis
	Spinal fracture
	Ankylosing spondylitis
	Coccydynia
	Pyogenic or tuberculous infections
	Spinal stenosis
Middle-aged	Mechanical back pain including primary osteoarthritis
	Prolapsed intervertebral disc
	Scheuermann's disease and old fracture
	Spondylolisthesis
	Rheumatoid arthritis
	Spinal stenosis
	Paget's disease
	Coccydynia
	Spinal metastases
	Pyogenic osteitis of the spine
Elderly	Osteoarthritis, primary and secondary
	True senile kyphosis
	Osteoporosis ⎱ with or without
	Osteomalacia ⎰ fracture
	Spinal metastases

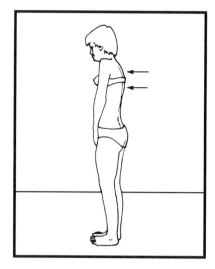

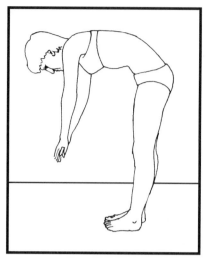

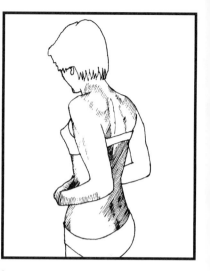

1. *Inspection* (1): *from the side:* Ask the patient to stand and look at the spine from the side. Although normal posture is difficult to define, try to make an assessment of the thoracic curvature, noting whether the curve is quite regular and if apparently increased.

2. *Inspection* (2): It is valuable to know if the thoracic spine is mobile, especially if there is a kyphosis. Ask the patient to bend forwards, carefully examining the flow of movement in the spine, and whether the curvature increases. (As the range of flexion in the thoracic spine is small, it may also help to check rotation — see 8, 29.)

3. *Inspection* (3): Now ask the patient to stand upright, and brace back the shoulders to produce extension. An increased curvature (kyphosis) which is regular and mobile is found in postural kyphosis.

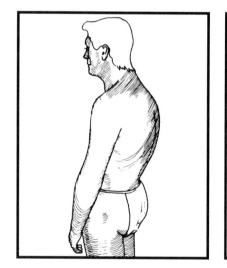

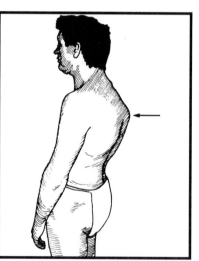

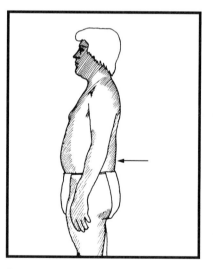

4. *Inspection* (4): If a regular but fixed kyphosis is found, the commonest causes are senile kyphosis (sometimes with osteoporosis, osteomalacia or pathological fracture), Scheuermann's disease and ankylosing spondylitis.

5. *Inspection* (5): If there is an angular kyphosis, with a gibbus or prominent vertebral spine, the commonest causes are fracture (traumatic or pathological), tuberculosis of the spine, or a congenital vertebral abnormality.

6. *Inspection* (6): Note the lumbar curvature. Flattening or reversal of the normal lumber lordosis is a common finding in prolapsed intervertebral disc, osteoarthritis of the spine, infections of the vertebral bodies, and ankylosing spondylitis. Flexion of the spine, hips and knees (simian stance) is suggestive of spinal stenosis.

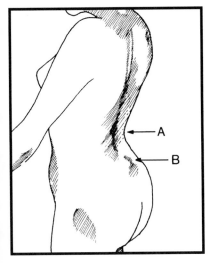

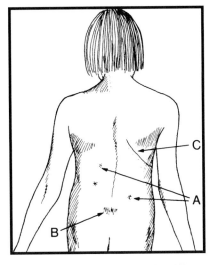

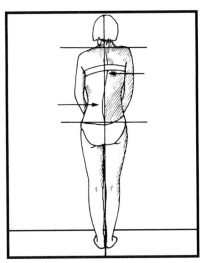

7. *Inspection (7):* (A) Increase in the lumbar curvature may be normal (especially in women) or be found with prominence of the spine of L5 and the sacrum (B) in spondylolisthesis. It may be *secondary* to an increased thoracic curvature or to flexion deformity of the hip(s). Always screen-test the hips.

8. *Inspection (8): from behind:* Note (A) café-au-lait spots which may suggest neurofibromatosis and associated scoliosis; (B) a fat pad or hairy patch suggestive of spina bifida; (C) scarring suggestive of previous thoracotomy (and possible thoracogenic scoliosis) or spinal surgery.

9. *Inspection (9):* Note the presence of any lateral curvature (scoliosis). The commonest scoliosis is a protective scoliosis or list in the lumbar region secondary to a prolapsed intervertebral disc. Note whether the shoulders and hips are level.

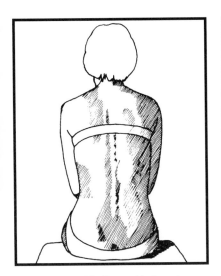

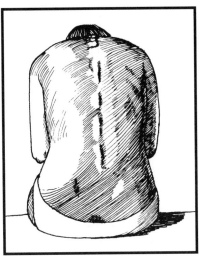

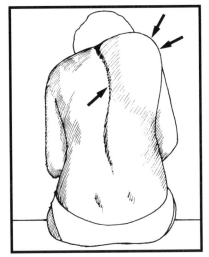

10. *Inspection (10):* In considering other causes of scoliosis, examine the spine with the patient sitting. Obliteration of an abnormal curve suggests that the scoliosis is mobile and secondary to shortening of a leg. Check relative leg lengths (see 10, 5).

11. *Inspection (11):* If on sitting the scoliosis persists, ask the patient to bend forwards. If the curve disappears, this suggests that it is quite mobile and most likely to be postural in origin.

12. *Inspection (12):* If the curvature remains, this suggests that the scoliosis is fixed (structural scoliosis). If a *rib hump* is present, this confirms the diagnosis. Note should be made of its severity. (Goniometers for measuring the angle of the hump are available.) Remember that syringomyelia is present in about a quarter of cases of juvenile idiopathic scoliosis, and an MRI scan is mandatory.

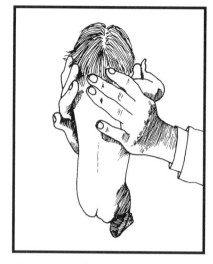

13. *Inspection* (13): In the case of infantile scoliosis, assess the ridigity of a curvature by noting any alterations as the child is lifted by the armpits.

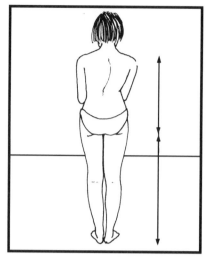

14. *Inspection* (14): Note that where there is an idiopathic scoliosis with double fixed (primary) curves, the deformity may not be obvious on first inspection. There will however be shortening of stature, with a trunk which is short in proportion to the limbs. (If desired this may be assessed using the anthropometric tables of Aldegheri and Agostini.)

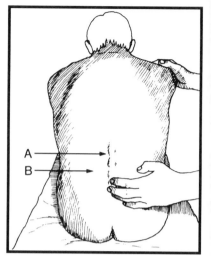

15. *Palpation* (1): Ask the patient to lean forwards if possible. Look for tenderness (A) between the spines of the lumbar vertebrae and lumbo-sacral junction (common in prolapsed intervertebral disc) and (B) over the lumbar muscles (common in prolapsed intervertebral disc and in cases of mechanical back pain).

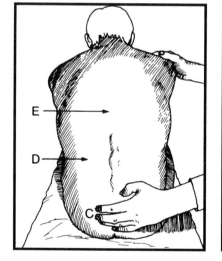

16. *Palpation* (2): Tenderness over the sacro-iliac joints (C) may also occur in cases of mechanical back pain and in sacro-iliac joint infections. Re-examine with the patient prone. Renal tenderness (D) must be investigated fully. Look also for tenderness higher in the spine (E) e.g. from vertebral body infections.

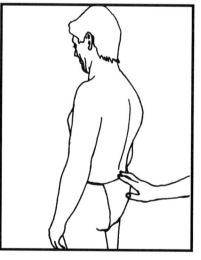

17. *Palpation* (3): With the patient standing. slide the fingers down the lumbar spine on to the sacrum. A palpable step at the lumbo-sacral junction is a feature of spondylolisthesis. Note any other curve irregularity (e.g. gibbus). Note also any change in friction (due to alterations in sweating patterns) which may help localisation of any pathology.

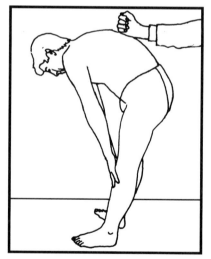

18. *Percussion:* Ask the patient to bend forwards. Lightly percuss the spine in an orderly progression from the root of the neck to the sacrum. Marked pain is a feature of tuberculous and other infections.

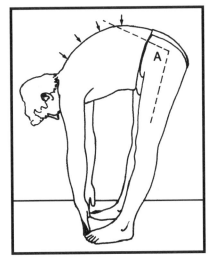

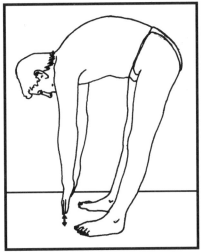

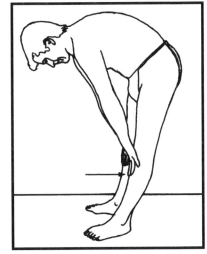

19. *Movements: flexion* (1): Ask the patient to attempt to touch his toes while you closely watch the spine for smoothness of movement and any areas of restriction. Note that (A) hip flexion plays an important part, and can account for apparent motion in a rigid spine.

20. *Movements: flexion* (2): Flexion may be recorded in several ways, the commonest being to note the distance between the fingers and the ground, e.g. 'the patient flexes to within 10 cm from the floor.' This is an indication of the summation of thoracic, lumbar and hip movements; it does not distinguish between them, and is under voluntary control.

21. *Movements: flexion* (3): Flexion may also be recorded, e.g. 'the patient flexes so that the fingertips reach mid-tibia' — or other appropriate level. The majority of normal patients can reach the floor or within 7 cm from it. (Actual maximum range flexion is approximately 45° thoracic, 60° lumbar.) Again, this does not indicate the relative contributions of the hips and spine.

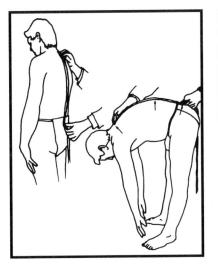

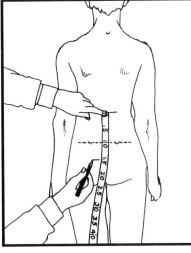

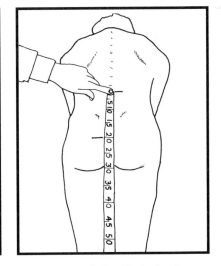

22. *Movements: flexion* (4): When the spine flexes, the distance between each pair of vertebral spines increases. By measuring the spine when the patient is erect, and then when bent forwards, any gain is clear evidence of spinal flexion. In practice this is used most frequently in assessing movements in the lumbar spine (where flexion is greatest, and pathology more common).

23. *Movements: flexion* (5): In *Schober's method*, a 10-cm length of lumbar spine is used as a base. Greater accuracy is claimed for the *modified Schober's method* (most often used in the UK), where a 15-cm length of spine is employed. Begin by positioning a tape measure with the 10-cm mark level with the dimples of Venus (which mark the posterior superior iliac spines). Mark the skin at 0 and 15 cm.

24. *Movements: flexion* (6): Anchor the top of the tape with a finger, and ask the patient to flex as far forward as he can. Note where the 15-cm mark strikes the tape, and work out the increment which is entirely due to lumbar spine flexion. This is normally about 6–7 cm. Less than 5 cm is indicative of organic spinal pathology.

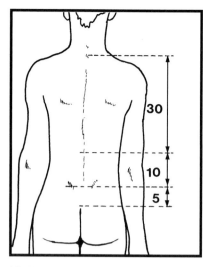

25. *Movements: flexion* (7): Flexion in the thoracic spine may be measured with the upper point 30 cm from the previous zero mark. Thoracic flexion is not great, and is normally in the order of 3 cm. *NB:* To exclude the possibility of overlay, repeat these measurements with the patient distracted, sitting up, and leaning forwards on the examination couch.

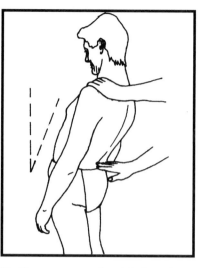

26. *Movements: extension:* Ask the patient to arch his back, assisting him by steadying the pelvis and pulling back on the shoulder. Pain is common in prolapsed intervertebral disc. Accurate measurement with a goniometer is difficult. Maximum theoretical range is thoracic 25°, lumbar 35°. Normal probably about 30° total. The decrease in the L1–S1 distance on extension may also be measured with a tape.

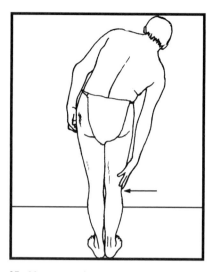

27. *Movements: lateral flexion* (1): Ask the patient to slide the hands down the side of each leg in turn, and record the point reached, either in centimetres from the floor, or the position that the fingers reach in the legs.

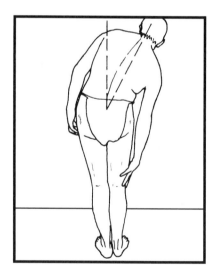

28. *Movements: lateral flexion* (2): Alternatively, measure the angle formed between a line drawn through T1, S1 and the vertical. The average range is 30° to either side, and the contributions of the thoracic and lumbar spine are usually equal.

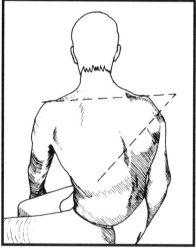

29. *Movements: rotation:* The patient should be seated and asked to twist round to each side. Rotation is measured between the plane of the shoulders and the pelvis. The normal maximum range is 40°, and is almost entirely *thoracic.* (Lumbar 5° or less.) Some claim a more accurate assessment if the test is carried out with the patient's arms across the chest.

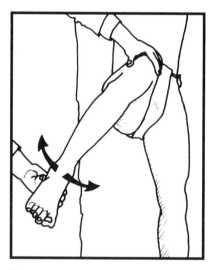

30. *Suspected prolapsed intervertebral disc:* Always start by screening the hips. Osteoarthritis of the hip and prolapsed intervertebral disc are frequently confused. A full range of rotation in the hips with absence of pain at the extremes is generally all that is required to eliminate the former.

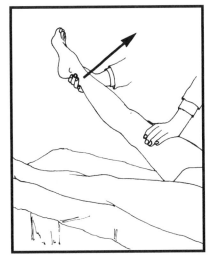

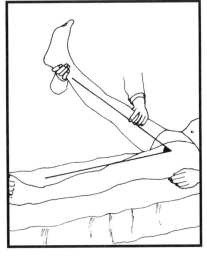

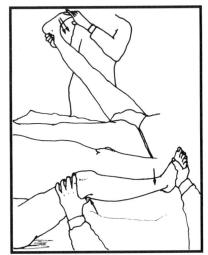

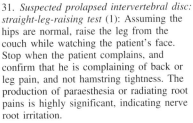

31. *Suspected prolapsed intervertebral disc: straight-leg-raising test* (1): Assuming the hips are normal, raise the leg from the couch while watching the patient's face. Stop when the patient complains, and confirm that he is complaining of back or leg pain, and not hamstring tightness. The production of paraesthesia or radiating root pains is highly significant, indicating nerve root irritation.

32. *Straight-leg raising* (2): Note the result (e.g. SLR (R) +ve at 60° or straight-leg raising (R) full (no pain)). Note the site of pain — back pain suggests a central disc prolapse, leg pain a lateral protrusion. Distinguish and ignore hamstring tightness. Repeat on the good side. If well-leg raising produces pain and paraesthesia on the affected side, this is highly suggestive of root irritation. Note that pain *must be below the knee* if the roots of the sciatic nerve are involved.

33. *Straight-leg raising* (3): Passive dorsiflexion of the foot increases tension on the nerve roots, generally aggravating any pain or paraesthesia; try this, and record the response. Alternatively, once the level of pain has been reached, slightly flex the knee and apply firm pressure with the thumb in the popliteal fossa over the stretched tibial nerve: radiating pain and paraesthesia in the leg suggest nerve root irritation (*bowstring test*).

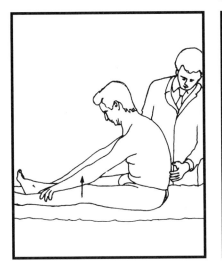

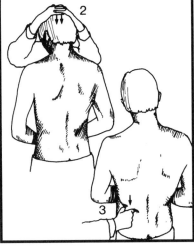

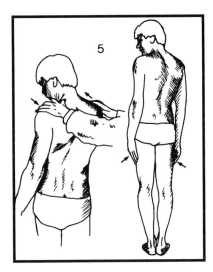

34. *Straight-leg raising* (4): If there is some doubt regarding the severity or genuineness of the patient's complaints, ask him to sit up under the pretext of examining the back from behind. (Flexion of the spine may also be remeasured in this position.) The malingerer will have no difficulty, but the genuine patient will either flex the knees or fall back on the couch with pain (*flip test*).

35. *Suspected prolapsed intervertebral disc: functional overlay ctd:* (2) Apply pressure to the head. Overlay is suggested if this aggravates the back pain. (3) Pinch the skin at the sides. Such superficial stimulation should not produce deep-seated back pain. (4) Any motor or sensory disturbance should be segmental and localised. Widespread weakness and/or stocking anaesthesia also suggest overlay (but do carry out a thorough neurological and circulatory examination).

36. *Suspected prolapsed intervertebral disc: functional overlay ctd:* (5) Note the amount of rotation required to produce pain in the back. Now ask the patient to keep his hands firmly at his sides and repeat; the major part of the movement will now take place in the legs. Pain occurring with the same amount of apparent rotation again suggests overlay. In many centres, if three or more of the preceding tests are positive, surgery is considered to be contra-indicated.

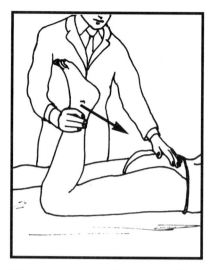

37. *Suspected prolapsed intervertebral disc: reverse Lasegue test* (1): The patient should be prone. Flex each knee in turn. This gives rise to pain in the appropriate distributions (by stretching of femoral nerve roots) in *high lumbar disc lesions*.

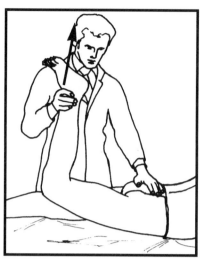

38. *Reverse Lasegue* (2): The pain produced in such a test, if positive, is normally aggravated by extension of the hip, and this should be noted. High disc lesions are rare compared with those affecting the L5–S1 and L4–L5 spaces. Note also that pain in the *ipsilateral buttock or thigh* on full knee flexion may occur in more distally situated disc prolapses.

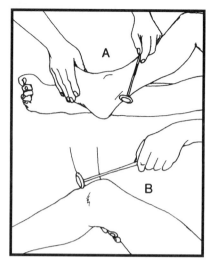

39. *Suspected prolapsed intervertebral disc ctd:* Look for further evidence of neurological involvement. A reduced or absent (A) ankle jerk (S1, 2) or (B) knee jerk (L3, 4) is a highly significant finding accompanying a positive straight-leg-raising or positive reverse Lasegue test. In practice, however, confirmatory findings of this nature may not be present.

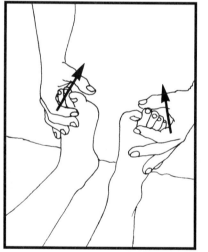

40. *Suspected prolapsed intervertebral disc:* Root pressure from a disc may affect myotomes and dermatomes in a rather selective fashion (see Chapter 9). Note the presence of any muscle wasting. Ask the patient to dorsiflex both feet. Now attempt to force them into plantar flexion against his resistance (L4, 5).

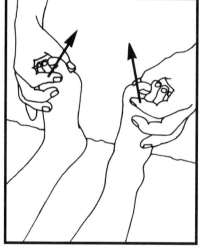

41. *Suspected prolapsed intervertebral disc:* Shift the grip to the great toes and test the power of dorsiflexion. Repeat with the lesser toes (L4, 5). Now test the power of plantar flexion of the great and lesser toes (S1, 2).

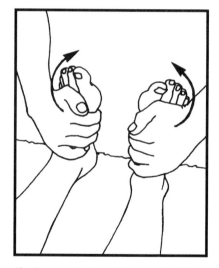

42. *Suspected prolapsed intervertebral disc:* Encircle the feet with the hands, and test the power of the peronei against the patient's resistance (L5, S1). Test the power of the quadriceps (L3, 4) when a high disc lesion is suspected.

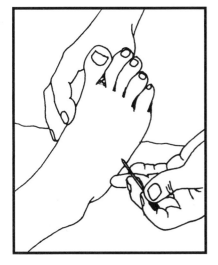

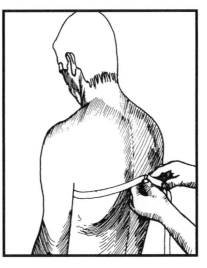

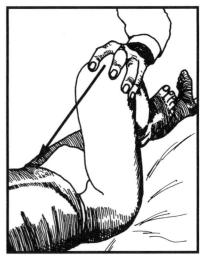

43. *Suspected prolapsed intervertebral disc:* Test sensation to pinprick in the dermatomes of the lower limb. Diminution of sensation at the side of the foot (S1) is one the commonest findings (see also Chapter 9).

44. *Suspected ankylosing spondylitis:* Check the patient's chest expansion at the level of the fourth interspace. The normal range in an adult of average build is at least 6 cm. Less than 2.5 cm is regarded as highly suggestive of ankylosing spondylitis. In addition, look for evidence of iritis, which is often associated with this condition.

45. *Suspected sacro-iliac joint involvement* (1): Flex the hip and knee, and forcibly adduct the hip. Pain may accompany this manoeuvre in early ankylosing spondylitis, tuberculosis and other infections, and Reiter's syndrome, but many false positives do occur with this test.

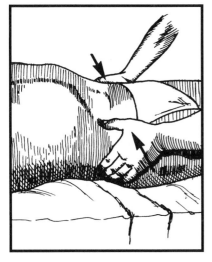

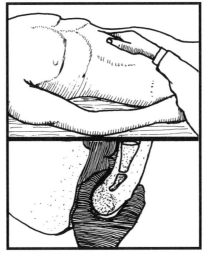

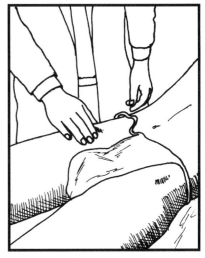

46. *Suspected sacro-iliac involvement* (2): Note if pain is produced by pelvic compression or by trying to 'open out' the pelvis with the thumb hooked round the anterior spines. Alternatively, with the patient in the prone position, place the side of one hand over the sacrum and upper natal cleft; press down hard, using the other hand to assist. True sacro-iliac pain may occur in women shortly before and after childbirth.

47. *Abdominal examination:* This is an essential part of the investigation of all cases of back pain. Rectal or vaginal examination may be required on the indication of the history and any other elements in the case. The *sacro-coccygeal joint* may be examined by first grasping the coccyx between the index (in the rectum) and the thumb outside, and then gently moving the joint. In coccydynia, marked pain normally accompanies this manoeuvre.

48. *Circulation:* The peripheral pulses and circulation should also be checked in all cases. Back and leg pain caused by arterial insufficiency are usually aggravated by activity, and absence of femoral pulsation is of particular significance.

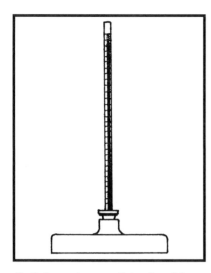

49. *Sedimentation rate:* Estimation of the sedimentation rate is a valuable screening test in the investigation of all spinal complaints. It is normal in prolapsed intervertebral disc, low back strain and Scheuermann's disease, but elevated in ankylosing spondylitis, many infections and neoplasms. It is best if 25 mm is taken as the upper limit of normal. False positives are not uncommon, but false negatives are rare.

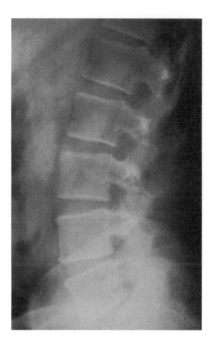

50. *Radiographs* (1): Normal lateral lumbar spine.

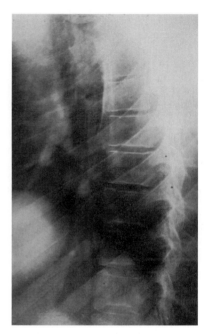

51. *Radiographs* (2): Normal lateral thoracic spine.

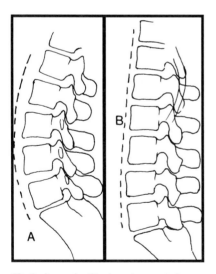

52. *Radiographs* (3): An antero-posterior and lateral are the standard projections for both the lumbar and thoracic spine. Localised views of the lumbo-sacral junction are a useful addition. In the lateral note first the lumbar curve: (A) typical normal; (B) loss of lordosis (most often seen in prolapsed intervertebral disc as a result of protective muscle spasm).

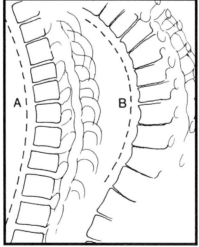

53. *Radiographs* (4): In the thoracic spine note (A) a typical normal curve; (B) an increased but regular curve typical of senile kyphosis. Scheuermann's disease is another frequent cause of a regular dorsal kyphosis. Kyphosis may be measured with the technique used for assessing scoliosis (Cobb method, 8, 79). *45° is taken as the upper limit of normal.*

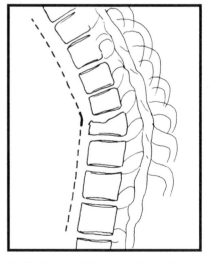

54. *Radiographs* (5): In both the lumbar and thoracic spine note any sharp alteration in the curvature, found typically where there is pathology restricted to one or two vertebral bodies, e.g. from fractures, tuberculosis or other infections, tumour, and osteomalacia with local collapse.

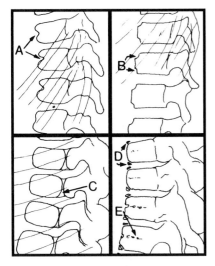

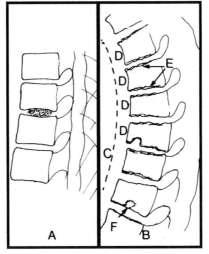

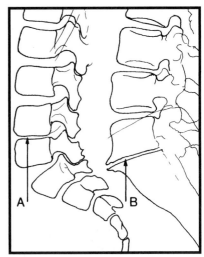

55. *Radiographs* (6): Now look at the shape of the bodies and the size of the discs. Compare with the bodies and disc spaces above and below. The following are normal in the child's spine: (A) anterior clefts; (B) anterior notches; (C) incomplete fusion of elements; (D) epiphyses; (E) vascular tracks (which may persist).

56. *Radiographs* (7): Note (A) disc calcification; (B) the typical appearance of Scheuermann's disease, with (C) kyphosis; (D) anterior wedging of not less than 5° involving at least three sequential vertebrae; (E) ragged appearance of the epiphyses. Note (F) a central disc herniation (Schmorl's node); this is not always associated with Scheuermann's disease.

57. *Radiographs* (8): Note (A) disc narrowing at any level in the spine is the earliest evidence of tuberculosis and other infections. (B) Narrowing at L5–S1 and less commonly in the two spaces above occurs in long-standing disc lesions and is often associated with anterior lipping.

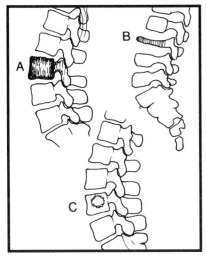

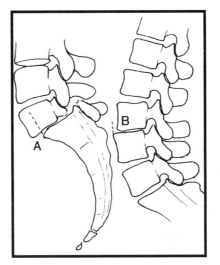

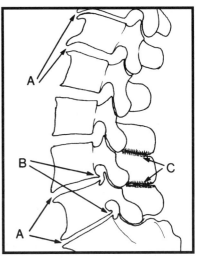

58. *Radiographs* (9): Note (A) increased density and 'picture-frame' appearance of vertebrae seen in Paget's disease; (B) marked narrowing and density seen in Calvé's disease (vertebra plana); (C) space-occupying lesion in body usually due to tumour or infection (but note Schmorl's nodes).

59. *Radiographs* (10): Note the relationship of each vertebra to its neighbour. In particular note (A) spondylolisthesis (see also 8, 71); (B) retrospondylolisthesis (usually associated with disc degeneration).

60. *Radiographs* (11): Lipping is seen in chronic disc lesions, mainly at L5–S1, but also at the other rarer disc prolapse sites. Note (A) anterior lipping; (B) posterior lipping. Lipping is also the main feature (at all levels) of osteoarthritis. Note (C) impingement of spinous processes ('kissing spines').

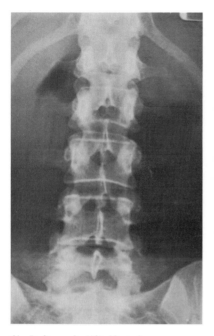

61. *Radiographs* (12): Normal antero-posterior view of the lumbar spine.

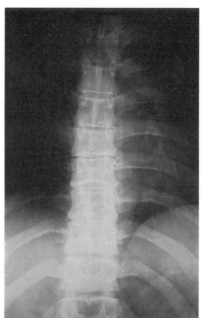

62. *Radiographs* (13): Normal antero-posterior view of the thoracic spine.

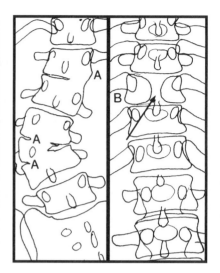

63. *Radiographs* (14): In the antero-posterior view note the presence of any congenital abnormalities such as (A) congenital vertebral fusion, often associated with a congenital scoliosis; (B) anterior spina bifida in which there is failure of fusion of the vertebral body elements (usually symptom-free).

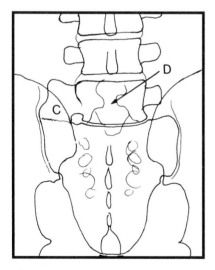

64. *Radiographs* (15): Note also any anomalies of the lumbo-sacral articulation such as (C) partial sacralisation of the fifth lumbar vertebra, a possible cause of low back pain. Note also (D) the presence of (posterior) spina bifida.

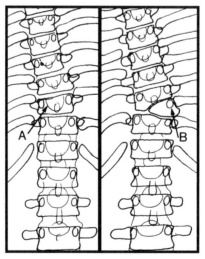

65. *Radiographs* (16): Note also the presence of any localised lateral angulation of the spine (A) due to lateral vertebral collapse, e.g. from fracture, infection, tumour, osteoporosis or other causes. (B) Hemivertebra, a common cause of congenital scoliosis (note extra rib).

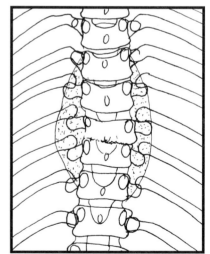

66. *Radiographs* (17): Look at the soft tissue shadows at the sides of the vertebrae, observing, for example, fusiform increased density typical of a tuberculous abscess. Note disc obliteration and early lateral wedging.

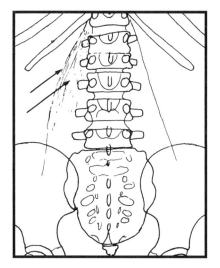

67. *Radiographs* (18): Examine the psoas shadows for symmetry. Lateral displacement of the edge of the shadow and increased density within the main area occupied by psoas suggest a psoas abscess, typically found in tuberculosis of the lumbar or lowermost thoracic spine.

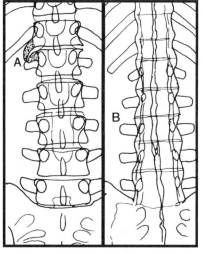

68. *Radiographs* (19): Look for lateral lipping. (A) At D12–L1, it may be an early sign of ankylosing spondylitis, but there and elsewhere it usually indicates osteoarthritis. 'Bamboo spine' (B) is diagnostic of ankylosing spondylitis. Note the body and facet joint fusions and ligament calcification.

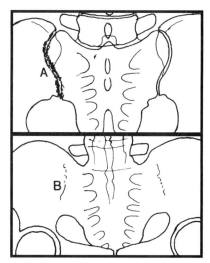

69. *Radiographs* (20): Look at the sacro-iliac joints. (A) Unilateral involvement (sclerosis, obliteration) may occur in tuberculosis and other infections. Any asymmetry should be investigated by oblique projections and if necessary, tomography. Bilateral involvement (B) is common in ankylosing spondylitis.

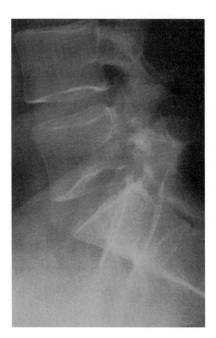

70. *Radiographs* (21): Normal localised lateral view of the lumbo-sacral junction.

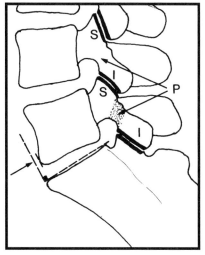

71. *Radiographs* (22): Look for evidence of spondylolisthesis. In the normal spine, the pars interarticularis (P) lying between (S) the superior and (I) the inferior articular facets is intact, and a vertical raised from the anterior margin of the sacrum lies in front of L5.

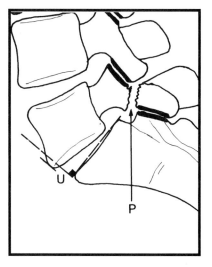

72. *Radiographs* (23): If spondylolisthesis is suspected, the lateral should always be taken with the patient standing. Note any defect (P) and forward slip (U). The deformity may occur between L5 and S1, and much less frequently between L4/L5 or L3/L4.

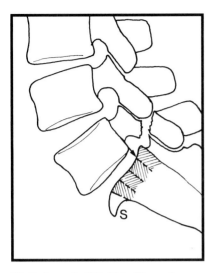

73. *Radiographs* (24): Note (S) new bone formation (buttressing) may make use of the anterior edge of the sacrum as a reference unreliable. Instead, note the relation of the *posterior* edge of the slipping vertebra to the one below. The example shows a forward slip of 25%.

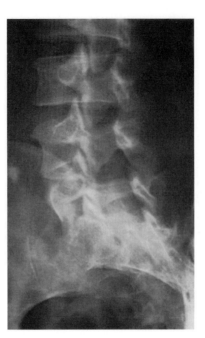

74. *Radiographs* (25): Normal oblique view of the lumbo-sacral junction.

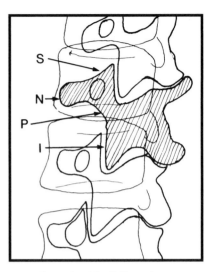

75. *Radiographs* (26): Oblique views are invaluable. In interpreting these, identify the 'Scotty dog' shadows. (N) The nose is formed by a transverse process, (S) the ear, by a superior articular process, (I) the front legs, by an inferior articular process, (P) the neck, by the pars interarticularis.

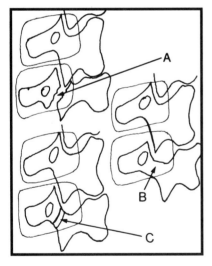

76. *Radiographs* (27): In spondylolisthesis (A) the 'dog' becomes decapitated due to forward slip and the inferior articular process of the vertebra above encroaches on the neck. In spondylolysis, where no slip has occurred, the neck (B) is elongated or (C) develops a collar.

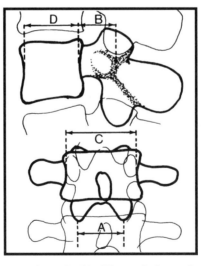

77. *Radiographs* (28): Where spinal stenosis is suspected, calculate the canal to body ratio, AB:CD, where A = interpedicular distance, B = spinal canal front-to-back (measure to root of spinous process), C = width of vertebral body, D = body, front-to-back. The normal range is from approximately 1:2 to 1:4.5. Values greater than 4.5 suggest spinal stenosis, but other investigations (e.g. CAT scanning, myelography) may be indicated.

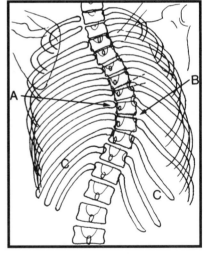

78. *Radiographs* (29): Note any structural scoliosis with (A) *on the concavity*, displacement of spines and narrowing of pedicles; (B) *on the convexity*, widening of disc spaces; (C) in the thorax, rib-cage distortion. Identify primary curves clinically or by lateral flexion radiographs.

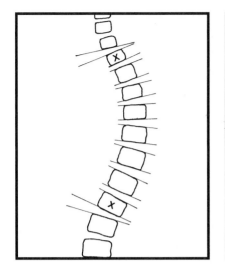

79. *Radiographs* (30): To assess the severity of a scoliotic curve and to allow its progress to be monitored, it is necessary to measure the deformity. The *Cobb method* is most popular. Firstly, find the upper and lower limits of the primary curve by drawing tangents to the bodies and noting where the disc spaces begin to become widened on the concavity of the curve.

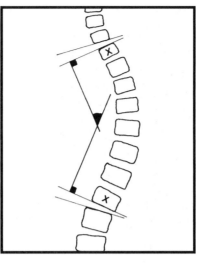

80. *Radiographs* (31): Now erect perpendiculars from the vertebrae which form the limits of the curve (marked 'X'). Note the angle between them. This is a measure of the primary curve, and can be used for comparison with past and future radiographs. Kyphotic curves may be measured in a similar way.

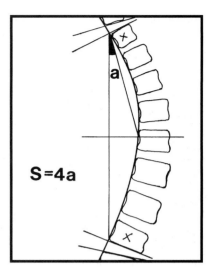

81. *Radiographs* (32): Although as yet not so widely established, *Capasso's method* of measuring scoliotic curves is said to be more sensitive and accurate. He determines the magnitude of the scoliotic curve (S) in degrees by multiplying by 4 the angle (a) subtended by a line joining the ends of the curves, with one running from the centre of the curve to one end of the curve: i.e. S = 4a.

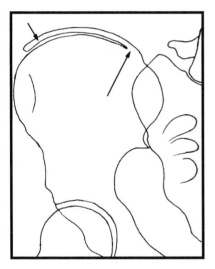

82. *Radiographs* (33): *Risser's sign:* In late adolescence the appearance and progressive fusion of the iliac apophysis from behind forwards heralds skeletal maturity. It would appear, however, that very slight growth may continue in the spine for up to 10 years after cessation of limb growth. This, along with disc degeneration and other factors, can lead to late deterioration in scoliotic curves, particularly those greater than 60°, so that this sign is of somewhat limited value.

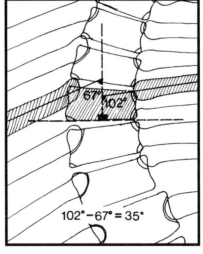

83. *Radiographs* (34): In *infantile scoliosis* note the difference in rib angles at the apex of the curve by the shown construction. A difference of 20° or more must be regarded as potentially progressive. An improvement over a 3-month period carries a good prognosis (Mehta). The best prognosis in infantile scoliosis is in males where the onset occurs in the first year of life and the RVAD (rib–vertebral angle difference) is less than 20°.

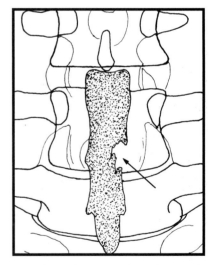

84. *Radiographs* (35): While myelography is invaluable in demonstrating filling defects in the coverings of the cord or cauda equina (as shown), or of the root sleeves, it has been superseded as a first-line investigative measure by CAT and MRI scans. These are non-invasive, and have the advantage of being able to visualise the suspect area in transverse section.

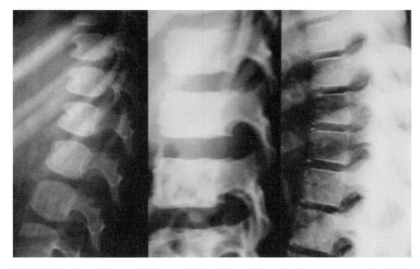

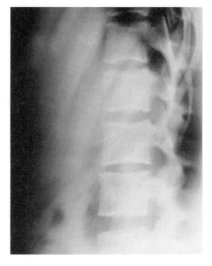

85. *Spinal radiographs: special features:* These three radiographs demonstrate anterior clefts, anterior notches, epiphyses and vascular tracks — normal features of the growing spine.

86. *Spinal radiographs: examples of pathology* (1): The radiograph shows narrowing of a single disc space. In most cases of spinal infections (including tuberculosis) this is the earliest sign.

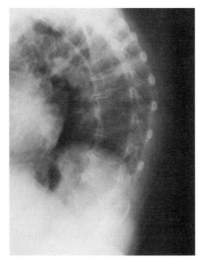

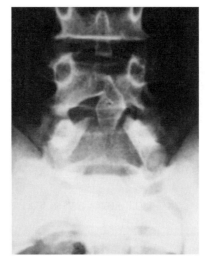

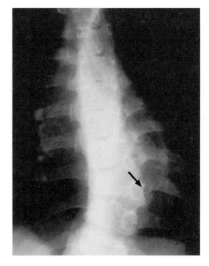

87. *Pathology* (2): The radiograph shows a regular dorsal kyphosis associated with anterior vertebral lipping and a degree of osteoporosis typical of senile kyphosis.

88. *Pathology* (3): The spinous process of L5 (and less obviously S1), along with associated posterior elements is absent; the patient has a spina bifida occulta. The only disturbance noted in the lower limbs was a bilateral pes cavus.

89. *Pathology* (4): The radiograph shows a dorsal scoliosis; the scoliosis is structural, and due to hemivertebra. There is an extra rib attached to the half-segment.

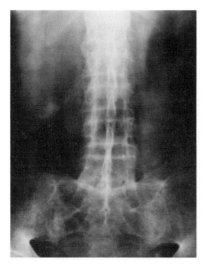

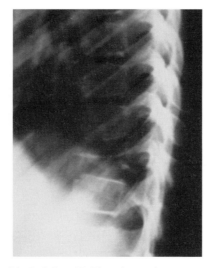

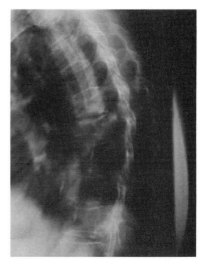

90. *Pathology* (5): The vertebral bodies throughout the thoracic and lumbar spine are fused, with early bambooing of the spine. The facet joints and the sacro-iliac joints are also fused. There is ossification of the interspinous ligaments.

91. *Pathology* (6): There is complete flattening of a single vertebral body, with preservation of the disc spaces above and below. These appearances, in a girl of 10 (note the vertebral notches), are typical of vertebra plana (Calvé's disease) due to eosinophilic granuloma).

92. *Pathology* (7): There is an angular kyphosis, with anterior wedging of D9 due to a pathological fracture associated with osteomalacia. Similar appearances are found in the presence of spinal metastases.

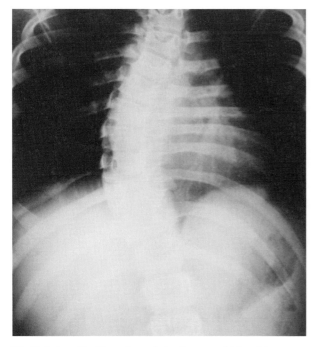

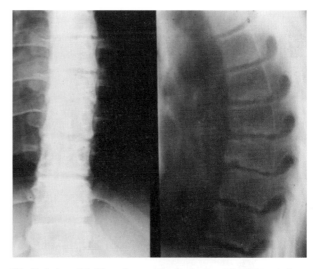

94. *Pathology* (9): There is a regular kyphosis, with slight anterior wedging of the vertebral bodies, irregularity of the disc margins and central disc herniation (Schmorl's nodes). The appearances are typical of Scheuermann's disease. Clinically the kyphosis was obvious and spinal movements greatly reduced.

93. *Pathology* (8): The radiograph is of a case of idiopathic scoliosis, with a fixed primary thoracic curve, convex to the right. Note the rib asymmetry.

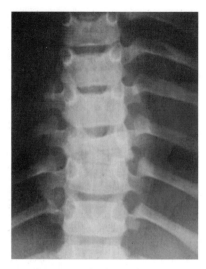

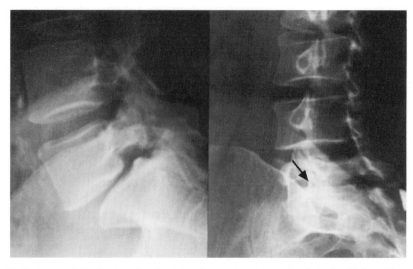

95. *Pathology* (10): There is loss of a disc space, slight vertebral wedging, and a fusiform abscess shadow on both sides of the spine. The appearances are typical of tuberculosis of the spine. In this 8-year-old boy there was associated back pain, malaise, night sweats, loss of spinal movements, and pain on percussion over the spine.

96. *Pathology* (11): The lateral radiographs show a chronic spondylolisthesis of L5 on S1, with less than 25% forward slip. There is an obvious defect in the pars interarticularis, and the 'Scotty dog' in the oblique projection has been decapitated. The complaint was of low back and buttock pain.

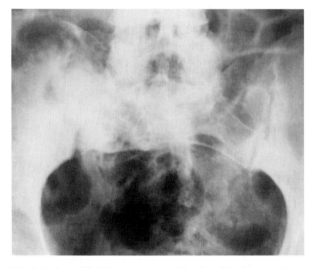

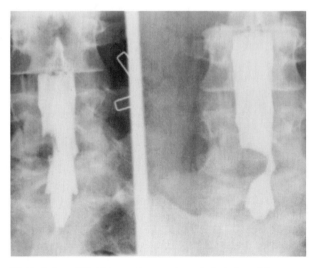

97. *Pathology* (12): There is increased density of the bony shadows in the region of the right sacro-iliac joint whose outline has become obscured. There was associated local pain, malaise and pyrexia. Attempts to spring the sacro-iliac joints produced great pain. The appearances are typical of an infective (pyogenic) arthritis of the sacro-iliac joint.

98. *Pathology* (13): This myelogram shows indentation of the contrast medium due to a prolapsed intervertebral disc. At operation the L5 root was found stretched over the prolapse. Before surgery there was weakness of dorsiflexion and eversion of the right foot, and there was some sensory impairment over the lateral aspect of the calf.

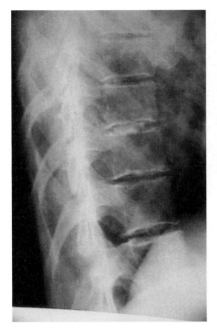

99. *Pathology* (14): There is calcification in an intervertebral disc with no significant narrowing of the corresponding disc space. This is an incidental finding, and is of no particular significance as a cause of back pain.

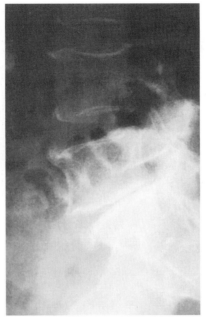

100. *Pathology* (15): There is narrowing of the L5–S1 disc space, with anterior lipping of these vertebrae, typical of degenerative disc disease and lumbo-sacral osteoarthritis.

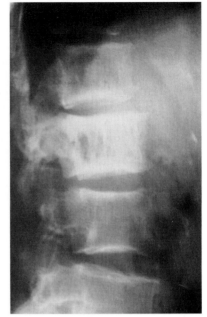

101. *Pathology* (16): There is striking alteration of bone texture affecting a single vertebra. The changes are typical of Paget's disease. At this site there would not necessarily be any associated symptoms.

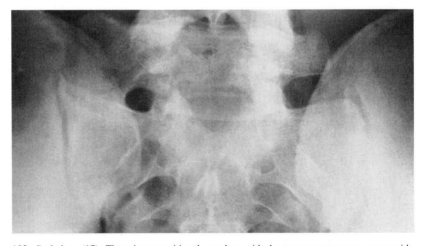

102. *Pathology* (17): There is a transitional vertebra, with the transverse process on one side articulating with both the sacrum and ilium. Some consider that this pattern of spinal anomaly, because it produces an asymmetrical distribution of local stresses, may be a cause of back pain.

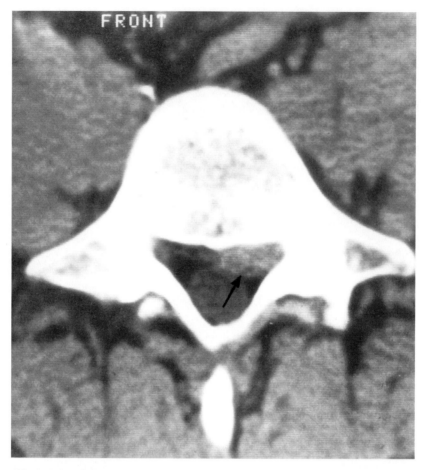

103. *Pathology* (18): There is a left-sided intervertebral disc prolapse (note the orientation to the *right* of the illustration), with distortion of the thecal shadow. It was associated with left-sided sciatic symptoms.

9. Segmental and peripheral nerves of the lower limb

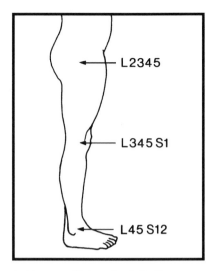

1. *Myotomes* (1) (see also 2, 2): Four consecutive spinal segments control each lower limb joint. The progression of control from hip to ankle is shown in the diagram.

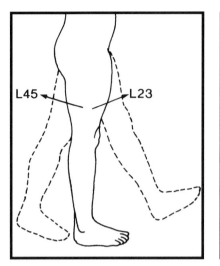

2. *Myotomes* (2): Flexion of the hip (mainly ilio-psoas) is controlled by L2, 3. Extension of the hip (mainly gluteus maximus and the hamstrings) is controlled by L4, 5. (L2, 3 also control internal rotation, and L4, 5 external rotation of the hip.)

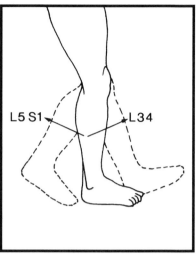

3. *Myotomes* (3): Extension of the knee and the knee jerk (quadriceps) is controlled by L3, 4. Flexion of the knee (mainly hamstrings) is controlled by L5, S1.

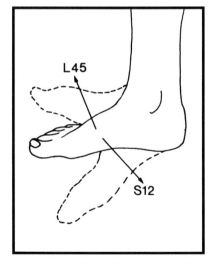

4. *Myotomes* (4): Dorsiflexion of the ankle is controlled by L4, 5 (mainly tibialis anterior and the long extensors of the hallux and toes). Plantar flexion is controlled by S1, 2 (mainly the muscles of the calf). The same segments control the ankle jerk.

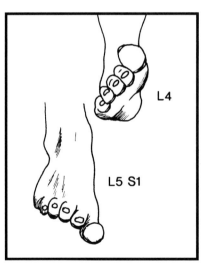

5. *Myotomes* (5): It is also useful to know that inversion (mainly tibialis anterior) is controlled by L4. Eversion is controlled by L5, S1 (the peronei).

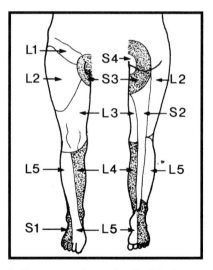

6. *Dermatomes:* Remember the following: the side of the foot, S1, is commonly involved in L5–S1 disc lesions. L5 sweeps from the medial side of the foot next to S1 to the lateral side of the leg. L4 occupies the medial side, L2, 3 occupy the thigh. S3 supplies the 'bed-pan' area.

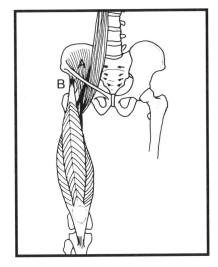

7. *Femoral nerve L2, 3, 4 (1): motor distribution:* (A) *Above* the inguinal ligament the femoral nerve supplies ilio-psoas. (B) *Below* the inguinal ligament it supplies the quadriceps (and also the sartorius and pectineus).

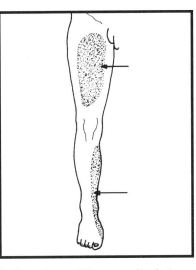

8. *Femoral nerve (2): sensory distribution:* On emerging below the inguinal ligament it supplies (through its cutaneous branches of thigh) the front of the thigh. The terminal part of the femoral nerve, known as the *saphenous nerve*, supplies the medial side of the leg below the knee and the medial side of the foot.

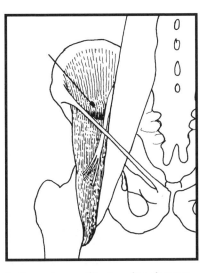

9. *Femoral nerve (3): sites of involvement:* Closed lesions of the femoral nerve are rare. Damage may occur when a haematoma is formed in the iliacus muscle causing local pressure. This is seen in haemophilia and in extension injuries of the hip.

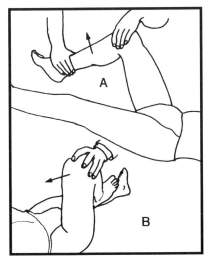

10. *Femoral nerve (4): tests:* (A) Test the quadriceps by asking the patient to extend the knee against resistance. (B) Test the ilio-psoas (hip flexion against resistance). The response to these tests should determine the level of any lesion. In doubtful cases, try to elicit the knee jerk. Observe any quadriceps wasting, and test for loss of sensation to pinprick in the area supplied by the nerve.

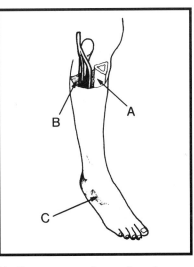

11. *Common peroneal nerve (lateral popliteal nerve) (1): L4, 5, S1, motor distribution:* (A) Muscles of the anterior compartment (tibialis anterior, extensor hallucis longus, extensor digitorum longus, peroneus tertius); (B) muscles of the peroneal compartment (peroneus brevis and longus); (C) on the foot, extensor digitorum brevis.

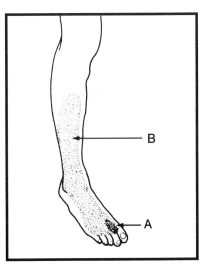

12. *Common peroneal nerve (2): sensory distribution:* (A) First web space (deep peroneal contribution); (B) dorsum of foot and front and side of leg (superficial peroneal contribution).

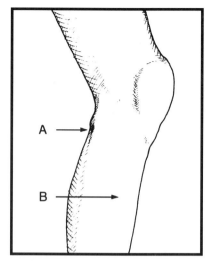

13. *Common peroneal nerve (3): sites of common involvement:* (A) Fibular neck — e.g. *trauma* (lateral ligament injuries of the knee, direct blows, pressure from plaster casts or the side irons of a Thomas splint), *ganglion, ischaemia* (e.g. tourniquet) and many neurological disorders; (B) the deep peroneal branch in anterior compartment syndrome.

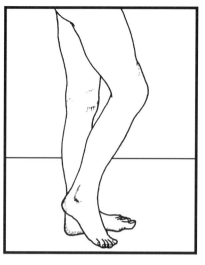

14. *Common peroneal nerve (4): deformity:* The patient will have a drop foot, and there will be disturbance of the gait; either the leg will be lifted high to allow the plantar flexed foot to clear the ground, or the foot will be slid along the ground with rapid wear of the shoe.

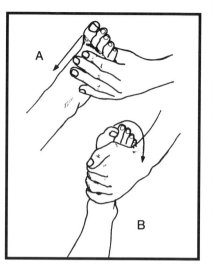

15. *Common peroneal nerve (5):* (A) Ask the patient to dorsiflex the foot (deep peroneal branch) and (B) to evert the foot (superficial peroneal branch). Test for sensation in the area of distribution of the nerve. Note any wasting of the front or side of the leg.

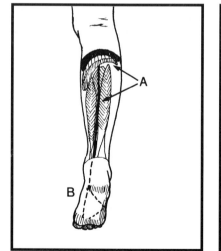

16. *Tibial nerve (posterior tibial nerve) (1): L4, 5, S1, 2, 3, motor distribution:* (A) Soleus and deep muscles of the posterior compartment (tibialis posterior, flexor hallucis longus, flexor digitorum longus); (B) all the muscles of the sole of the foot through the medial and lateral plantar nerves.

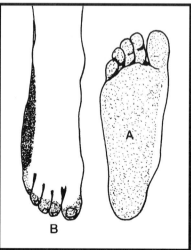

17. *Tibial nerve (2): sensory distribution:* (A) The sole of the foot through the medial and lateral plantar nerves, whose territory includes (B) the nail beds and distal phalanges. Note that the *side of the foot* is supplied by the *sural nerve* which is formed from branches from both the tibial and common peroneal nerves.

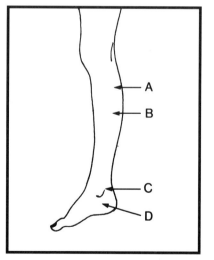

18. *Tibial nerve (3): common sites of involvement:* (A) When passing under the soleal arch, from tibial fractures; (B) ischaemic lesions of calf (e.g. posterior compartment syndrome from tight plasters) and diabetic neuropathy; (C) behind medial malleolus (lacerations and fractures); (D) in tarsal tunnel syndrome.

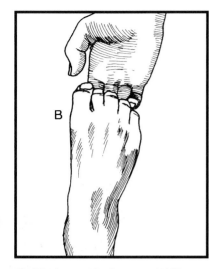

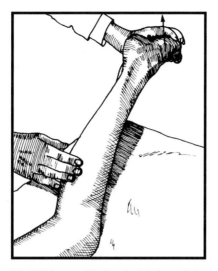

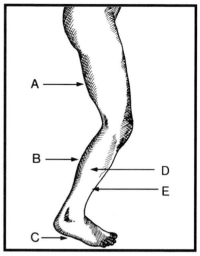

19. *Tibial nerve* (4): *diagnosis:* (A) Note any muscle wasting in the sole of the foot, clawing of the toes and trophic ulceration. (B) Test the power of toe flexion. (C) Look for sensory loss in the area supplied by the nerve.

20. *Tibial nerve* (5): Proximal lesions of the nerve (i.e. as it lies in the popliteal fossa) are uncommon due to the protection the nerve is afforded by the surrounding soft tissues, and the space available to accommodate expanding lesions. The findings are essentially the same as in distal lesions, but with wasting and loss of power of plantar flexion due to paralysis of gastrocnemius as well as soleus.

21. *Sciatic nerve* (l): *L4, 5, S1, 2, 3, motor distribution:* (A) The hamstrings in the thigh; (B) the superficial and deep muscles of the calf (by the tibial nerve); (C) the muscles of the sole of the foot (by the medial and lateral plantar nerves); (D) the peronei (by the superficial peroneal nerve); (E) the muscles of the anterior compartment (by the deep peroneal nerve).

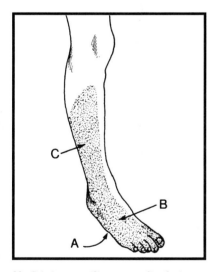

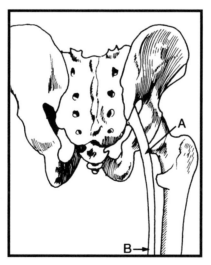

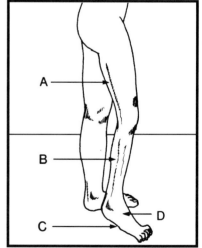

22. *Sciatic nerve* (2): *sensory distribution:* (A) The entire sole; (B) the dorsum of the foot; (C) the lateral aspect of the leg and lateral half of the calf. The medial side of the calf and foot are spared. If the posterior cutaneous nerve of the thigh is involved, there is loss of sensation at the back of the thigh.

23. *Sciatic nerve* (3): *sites involved:* (A) Behind the hip, e.g. after posterior dislocation of the hip, after some pelvic fractures (rare) and after hip surgery; (B) following deep wounds back of thigh (also uncommon). Do not confuse with root involvement in intervertebral disc prolapse.

24. *Sciatic nerve* (4): *diagnosis:* Note extensive wasting, (A) thigh, (B) calf and peronei, (C) sole of foot. Note (D) drop foot. Observe any trophic ulceration. Note loss of power in the hamstrings and all three compartments below the knee, absent ankle jerk and extensive sensory loss.

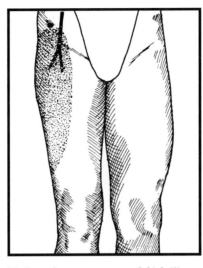 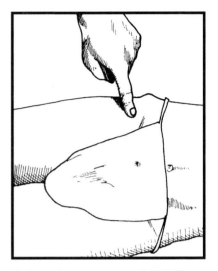

25. *Lateral cutaneous nerve of thigh* (1): *L2, 3:* The nerve pierces the lateral portion of the inguinal ligament and supplies the lateral aspect of the thigh. It may be compressed as it passes through the inguinal ligament, giving pain and paraesthesia in the leg (meralgia paraesthetica). Note that symptoms with the same distribution may occur secondary to spinal stenosis.

26. *Lateral cutaneous nerve of thigh* (2): *test:* Pressure over the nerve may give rise to paraesthesia in the thigh. Test for sensory impairment in the area supplied by the nerve.

10. The hip

Congenital dislocation of the hip (CDH)

Congenital dislocation of the hip is a term applied to a condition in which one or both hips are dislocated at birth, or dislocate in the first few weeks of life. It is much commoner in girls than boys; there is a familial tendency, and a well-established geographical distribution of the disorder. It is commoner after breech presentations, and it may occur in conjunction with other congenital defects.

It is now believed that there is a spectrum of conditions ranging from established dislocation, irreducible at birth, to simple neonatal instability of the hip which settles without treatment. An important group is one in which the hips are eccentrically placed; these may go on to acetabular dysplasia with subluxation. In the USA the present preference is to reject the term 'congenital dislocation of the hip' in favour of 'developmental dysplasia of the hip' (DDH).

CDH in the neonate

A simple test devised by Ortolani in the 1960s was found to show instability in the hips of some newborn children, and it was thought that this instability was directly related in every case to congenital dislocation of the hip. As a result it was considered that if all the newborn could be screened with this test, and treated promptly if instability were found, the condition would no longer pose a problem. Unfortunately, later experience showed that a number of children who had passed the screening test went on to develop hip dislocations. It also became clear that some unstable hips could resolve without treatment; and that treatment itself (in an abduction splint) was not free from complications (about 10% developing avascular necrosis).

X-ray examination of the hips is not of much diagnostic value at birth (due to skeletal immaturity), but can be helpful by about 3–4 months. Ultrasound screening leads to a dramatic increase in the number of apparently abnormal hips, most of which fortunately resolve without treatment. To accommodate these confusing facts, the following regime has been recommended:

1. All children should be examined on at least two occasions by those expert in the performance of the screening tests, during the first 3 months of life.
2. If the child is in a high-risk group (breech presentation, family history of CDH, clicking hip, the presence of other deformities), then

ultrasound screening should be added. If some doubt remains, the hips should be X-rayed at 3–4 months. If still negative, the hips should be re-examined clinically at 6 months and when weight-bearing commences.

3. If the hip is clearly dislocated, then splintage should be commenced immediately.

4. If the hip is not dislocated, but *can* be dislocated (Barlow's test), it should be re-examined at weekly intervals for 3 weeks.

If instability remains, then some recommend that splintage (in abduction) should then be commenced, although others prefer to have both X-ray and ultrasound confirmation. There are a number of splints available for the treatment of CDH (Malmö, van Rosen, Barlow, Pavlik harness, frog pattern plaster cast etc.); whatever is used is continued until the hip becomes stable (often by about 12 weeks).

CDH in the older child

This must be suspected in any child where there is disturbance of gait or posture, shortening of a limb, or indeed any complaint in which the hip might be implicated. If dislocation of the hip is diagnosed late, treatment is aimed at restoring the hip to as near normal as possible. Each case must be assessed on its own merits, but the general principles of treatment are common to all.

1. The head of the femur must be reduced into the acetabulum. This may be possible by manipulation alone, with or without a preliminary period of traction (to bring the femoral head down to the level of the acetabulum). An MRI scan can provide important information regarding any tissue which has the potential for preventing the femoral head from entering the socket (such as adhesion of the joint capsule to the ilium, an inverted limbus (the thickened acetabular labrum), or a displaced transverse ligament), and be a guide regarding the necessity for open reduction.

2. Once the hip has been reduced, the position must be maintained until stability is achieved; and from an early stage as much movement as possible should be allowed, to encourage concentric development of the head of the femur and the acetabulum. A popular method is to hold the hip in internal rotation by the application of a Batchelor plaster; this permits movements of the hip in other planes. Such a plaster is usually retained for about 12 weeks.

3. In a very high percentage of cases there is an associated anteversion deformity of the femoral neck. To help retain the femoral head in the acetabulum and encourage concentric development this is often corrected surgically by a rotational osteotomy of the proximal femur, performed at the end of the period of plaster fixation.

4. If the acetabular roof fails to develop properly and remains shallow, so that the femoral head is poorly contained (predisposing the joint to secondary osteoarthritic change), a Salter osteotomy of the pelvis may be advised at about the age of 4 or 5.

CDH in the adult

Where treatment in childhood has been unsuccessful, or even where the condition has not been diagnosed, a patient may seek help during the third and fourth decades of life. Symptoms may arise from the hips or the spine. In the hips, secondary arthritic changes occur in the false joint which may form between the dislocated femoral head and the ilium with which it comes into contact. In the spine, osteoarthritic changes are a result of long-standing scoliosis (in the unilateral case), increased lumbar lordosis (in both unilateral and bilateral cases), or excessive spinal movements which occur in walking. In a few cases hip replacement surgery may be considered, otherwise the treatment follows the lines for the conservative management of osteoarthritis of the hips and spine.

The dysplastic hip

Hip dysplasia is a condition in which the principal feature is that the femoral head is imperfectly contained by the acetabulum. The acetabular slope is frequently greater than normal, and the acetabulum may be relatively small in comparison with the femoral head. In early life this may be a major factor in congenital dislocation of the hip; even if the hip does not dislocate it may nevertheless give trouble later in life. In the dysplastic hip the central area only of the femoral head transmits the forces of weight-bearing to the acetabulum, increasing the joint loadings and predisposing the hip to osteoarthritis, and in some cases instability. The symptoms are those of osteoarthritis of the hip, and they may present during the second and third decades of life. Rapid deterioration is the rule. In the younger patient, a Chiari osteotomy of the pelvis, an acetabular shelf operation or a high femoral osteotomy may improve the containment of the femoral head, relieve symptoms, and slow the onset of osteoarthritis. In the older patient, replacement arthroplasty may be considered.

The irritable hip

In childhood there are a number of conditions affecting the hip which may be indistinguishable in their initial stages. They all give rise to a limp, restriction of movements, and sometimes pain in the joint (irritable hip). Children with this history are admitted routinely and treated by light traction until a firm diagnosis has been made. The commonest conditions responsible for irritable hip are transient synovitis, Perthes' disease, and tuberculosis of the hip.

Transient synovitis. This is the commonest cause of the irritable hip syndrome. The child presents with a limp, and there is sometimes a history of preceding minor trauma which in some cases at least is coincidental. Raised interferon levels have been found, which suggest that a viral synovitis may often be the cause. There is restriction of extension and internal rotation in the affected joint, but there is no systemic upset and the sedimentation rate is generally normal. Radiographs of the hip sometimes give confirmatory evidence of synovitis, as does ultrasound examination, but no other pathology is usually demonstrable. Aspiration and culture of synovial fluid (which is not routinely performed) generally fail to provide any evidence of bacterial infection. A full recovery after 3–6 weeks' bed rest is the rule. In a number of cases which have been slow to respond there have been positive faecal cultures of *Campylobacter*, and it is advised that this examination should be performed routinely.

Perthes' disease. In this condition there is a disturbance of the blood supply to the epiphysis of the femoral head so that a variably sized portion undergoes a form of avascular necrosis. The cause is unknown. It is commoner in boys than girls, there is an association with anteversion of the femoral neck, and one or both hips may be involved. When both hips are affected, they may be involved simultaneously or with an interval between them. Vague pain in the region of the hips, thighs or knees is a frequent accompaniment. Clinically, Perthes' disease may be suspected by the history, by the child's age and sex, and by the restriction of rotation in the affected hip. As a rule, radiological changes are well established by the time the child presents with symptoms, and these will confirm the diagnosis. (Ultrasound examination shows capsular distension due to synovial thickening, with *both* hips being generally affected at the earliest stages (as opposed to the findings in transient synovitis).)

The severity of the condition is dependent on the position and extent of the area of the femoral head involved. When a large part of the epiphysis is affected, there is a tendency to flattening and lateral subluxation of the femoral head; these changes are mirrored by the acetabulum, and the resultant deformity predisposes the hip to osteoarthritis later in life. If there is some doubt regarding the extent of these changes, an MRI scan will allow an accurate assessment. Thereafter, as a guide to management and prognosis, the investigative findings are used in an attempt to grade the case. This can be difficult in practice, and the results may be somewhat inconsistent. The most popular classification is that of Catterall, but those by Salter-Thompson and Herring have their advocates.

The aims of treatment have been summarised as the relief of symptoms, the containment of the femoral head, and the restoration of movements. The majority of patients, especially in the younger age groups (less than 6), make a good recovery. The long-term results are dependent on the growth of the femoral head, and it is unfortunately the case that treatment has not been shown to affect this materially, or to influence the ultimate outcome. Nevertheless it is accepted that in all cases the *acute* symptoms of pain and severe restriction of movements should be treated by bed rest and traction, followed by physiotherapy. In mild cases, where the prognosis by grading is judged to be good, no further treatment (apart from prolonged observation) is generally advocated, although some prescribe the use of a Snyder sling or calliper for a further period of some months to reduce the chances of weight-bearing stresses leading to further deformation of the femoral head. The results of intervention in those cases which are judged to carry a poor prognosis are perhaps less clear. The lines of treatment frequently advocated aim at improving the congruity of the femoral head and acetabulum, and improving the effective range of movements in the hip (e.g. by a varus osteotomy of the femoral neck or a Salter innominate osteotomy).

Tuberculosis. Tuberculosis of the hip is now rare in the UK. The affected child walks with a limp and often complains of pain in the groin or knee. Night pain is a feature. Rotation in the hip becomes limited, a fixed flexion deformity develops, and muscle wasting occurs. Radiographs of the hip in the early stages show rarefaction of bone in the region of the hip and widening of the joint space. As the disease advances, there is progressive joint destruction with abscess formation and sometimes dislocation. The diagnosis is usually confirmed by histological and bacteriological examination of synovial biopsy specimens, or by bacteriological examination of the aspirate.

In early cases complete resolution may be hoped for by anti-tuberculous therapy, bed rest and traction. In the advanced case, joint débridement is carried out with efforts to obtain a bony fusion of the joint.

Acute pyogenic arthritis of the hip

The *Staphylococcus* is the organism most frequently responsible for acute infections in the hip joint. The infection is blood-borne, and the diagnosis is seldom difficult. The onset is rapid, with high fever and toxaemia. All movements of the hip are severely impaired and accompanied by great pain and protective muscle spasm. The organism responsible may be isolated by blood culture or joint aspiration. Treatment is by use of the appropriate antibiotic in large doses to obtain a high local concentration. Bed rest and immobilisation are also essential.

Slipped femoral epiphysis

This is a disease of adolescence and is commoner in boys than girls. The attachment of the femoral epiphysis to the femoral neck loosens, so that the head appears to slide downwards on the femoral neck, giving rise eventually to a coxa vara deformity of the hip. The cause is unknown. In a number of cases there is a history of preceding trauma. A striking feature, however, is that in a high proportion of cases there is evidence of a hormonal disturbance. Many are fat, having the appearance of those suffering from the Frölich syndrome. Some cases have been noted to occur in association with hypothyroidism.

Pain may occur in the groin or knee, and if the onset is very acute, weight-bearing may become impossible. There is usually restriction of internal rotation and abduction in the affected hip. The diagnosis is confirmed radiographically, the earliest changes being seen in the lateral projections.

Slight degrees of slip are treated by internal fixation of the epiphysis without reduction. If there is a large amount of acute displacement, reduction may be attempted before fixation. If the slip is long-standing, osteotomy of the femoral neck (to correct the deformity) may be preferable to attempted reduction if the risks of avascular necrosis are to be reduced. During convalescence from surgery the other hip should be kept under surveillance in case it becomes involved but produces no symptoms. The incidence of this complication may be as high as 60%.

Primary osteoarthritis of the hip

Primary osteoarthritis of the hip occurs in the middle-aged and elderly, and is often associated with overweight and overwork, although in many cases no obvious cause may be found.

Pain is often poorly localised in the hip, groin, buttock or trochanter, and may be referred to the knee. There is increasing difficulty in walking and standing. Sleep is often disturbed and the general health of the patient becomes undermined as a result. Stiffness may declare itself in difficulty in putting on stockings and cutting the toe nails.

Fixed flexion and adduction contractures are common, with apparent shortening of the affected limb. In the early stages, weight reduction, physiotherapy and analgesics may be helpful; total hip replacement is the treatment of choice if the condition is advanced.

Secondary osteoarthritis of the hip

The symptoms of secondary osteoarthritis of the hip are identical to those of primary osteoarthritis. The condition occurs most frequently as a sequel to congenital dislocation of the hip, congenital coxa vara, hip dysplasia, Perthes' disease, tuberculous or pyogenic infections, slipped femoral epiphysis, and avascular necrosis secondary to femoral neck fracture or traumatic dislocation of the hip.

In secondary osteoarthritis, a younger age group is generally involved than in the case of primary osteoarthritis. In the young patient, where it is thought desirable to avoid the uncertain long-term morbidity of total hip replacement, a hip joint fusion may be considered in the unilateral case. Where pain is more a problem than stiffness, McMurray's osteotomy of the hip may sometimes be of value.

Rheumatoid arthritis

The hip joints are frequently involved in rheumatoid arthritis. When both hips and knees are affected, the disability may be profound. In the well-selected case, replacement of one or both hips may give a striking improvement in the patient's symptoms and mobility.

Other conditions affecting the hip

Of the rarer conditions affecting the hip joint, the following are not infrequently overlooked:

1. Ankylosing spondylitis may present as pain and stiffness in the hip in a young man. There may be no complaint of back pain, but there is almost invariably radiographic evidence of sacro-iliac joint involvement.
2. Reiter's syndrome may also first present in the hip.
3. Primary bone tumours are uncommon; of these, osteoid osteoma

involving the femoral neck may be a cause of persistent hip pain. As this tumour is always small, repeated radiographic examination with well-exposed films may be required to show it. The tumour may also be revealed as a 'hot spot' in isotope bone scans.

4. The snapping hip, involving 'clunking' sounds emanating from the region of the hip on certain movements, may be a source of annoyance to a patient. In most cases no more than reassurance should be offered, but where pain is a feature an effort should be made to trace the source, and if found, to consider surgery for the relief of the mechanical problem responsible. It is often due to part of the ilio-tibial tract flicking over the prominence of the greater trochanter, and is amenable to a Z-plasty.

The following important points should always be remembered in dealing with the hip joint:

1. The *commonest cause of hip pain in the adult is pain referred from the spine, e.g. from a prolapsed intervertebral disc.* Hip movements are not impaired, and there are almost invariably signs of the primary pathology, e.g. diminution of straight-leg raising.
2. *In the elderly, pain in the hip with inability to weight-bear is frequently due to a fracture of the femoral neck or of the pubic rami.* In an appreciable number of cases there is no history of injury, and radiographic examination is essential.
3. *Flexion contracture of the hip may result from psoas spasm secondary to inflammation or pus in the region of its sheath in the pelvis.* This is seen, for example, in appendicitis, appendix abscess or other pelvic inflammatory disease. Examination of the abdomen is essential.

Conditions associated with total hip joint replacements

Because of the success of hip joint replacement procedures, many of these operations have been performed, and complications, which occur in about 5% of cases, are being seen with increasing frequency.

The most widely used replacement is the Charnley low-friction arthroplasty (LFA) or one of its many variants. In it the socket is formed from high-density polyethylene, and the replacement head from stainless steel. Both components are anchored with quick-setting acrylic cement. If a lateral approach has been used, the greater trochanter is usually detached and replaced at the end of the operation using stainless steel wires.

There are a number of other replacements which vary in the design of the parts, the materials used, and the techniques of their insertion. In some, the components are inserted without the use of acrylic cement, and the surgical exposure may be made without detachment of the trochanter. Where the functional requirements are not expected to be high (e.g. after intra-capsular hip fractures in the very elderly), a hemi-arthroplasty may be performed, where the femoral head is replaced with a stemmed prosthesis, and the acetabulum is not interfered with.

Excluding complications which may arise in the immediate post-operative period, the problems which may occur include the following:

1. Dislocation. The stability of the replacement is dependent on the precision with which the components have been aligned during their insertion, the time that has elapsed since surgery, and the degree of violence to which the components have been subjected. After any hip replacement, the fibrous capsule which forms round the artificial joint thickens and strengthens as time progresses, leading to a progressive resistance to dislocation. In the first few months following surgery, a badly aligned joint may dislocate under comparatively minor stress; in other cases and at a later stage, considerable violence may be necessary. If dislocation occurs, weight-bearing suddenly becomes impossible, and there is usually marked pain. The limb shortens, and may be externally rotated. The diagnosis is confirmed by X-ray examination. Treatment is by reduction (which occasionally needs to be an open one), usually followed by a period of traction until the hip becomes stable. In those cases where there is a major problem of component malalignment, a revision procedure may have to be considered should the dislocation recur.

2. Component failure. Socket failure is rare, but the stem of the femoral prosthesis may occasionally fracture. This is most likely when the patient is overweight or the component has a varus alignment, or loosens. Generally there is immediate loss of the ability to weight-bear, and replacement of the fractured component becomes essential.

If the greater trochanter has been re-attached with wires, these may fracture and fragment, giving rise to local discomfort and sometimes episodes of sharp, jagging pain. This may be treated by removal of the broken wires. The trochanter itself may fail to unite and may displace. This may cause local discomfort and a Trendelenberg gait. Normally there is slow, spontaneous improvement, but in the early case where the fragment is large and displaced, re-attachment may be considered.

3. Component loosening and infection. When this occurs, it is usually at the interface between the cement and bone. It is commonest in the area of the femoral stem, although both components may be affected. The complaint is of pain and impairment of function, and the diagnosis is usually made on the basis of the radiological appearances. Loosening may be the result of infection; in some cases this may be frank, and in others organisms of low pathogenicity may be found in the affected area. In many cases, although an element of infection may be strongly suspected, no organism can be found and an alternative cause may be sought. In many, loosening may be associated with particulate wear debris, and in others tissue sensitivity to the metallic elements of the components of the prosthesis has been blamed.

Infection may be introduced at the time of the initial operation and grumble on thereafter, leading to loosening, bone absorption, and distal migration of the femoral component. There may be flare-ups accompanied by more acute pain, malaise and sometimes abscess formation. In other cases, it would seem that late infections may arise as a result of infection being blood-borne from a septic focus elsewhere.

The treatment of these complications is highly specialised. In the (uncommon) case of secondary infection, investigations by blood culture and aspiration, immobilisation, and the prompt administration of the appropriate antibiotics may occasionally lead to resolution. In the case of loosening without the discovery of any organism, a revision procedure may be advised. Where there is evidence of a low-grade infection, a very thorough débridement under antibiotic cover, followed by the insertion of a fresh prosthesis of a pattern designed to accommodate any migration or loss of bone stock may be attempted (either as a one- or two-stage procedure). Additional measures to control recurrence of local infection may include the use of antibiotic-loaded cement. Where infection is well established, removal of the components and cement may be the only solution which will allow the infection to be overcome, even though limb function will obviously be seriously compromised. In some of these cases, however, once the infection has been eradicated, a further replacement procedure may sometimes be contemplated.

Hip assessment

For over 50 years attempts have been made to discover a reliable method of gauging the performance of a given hip, so that the extent and progress of any disability can be assessed, and the results of surgery evaluated. Over 80 rating systems have been devised, and the lack of standardisation has prevented the direct comparison of many reported series.

There is general agreement that certain functional parameters should be assessed. These include pain, gait and the ability to perform certain activities of daily living. A problem is that there are differences in opinion on the weight that should be placed on each of the items that is assessed. In the widely used, but often highly modified Harris System[1], a normal hip is rated as scoring 100 points, while the hip being examined is described as being so many percent of this theoretical normal. *Pain* (which is subjective and hard to assess with accuracy) is allocated 44 points. *Function*, which is highly detailed, is broken down into gait, the use of supports, and activities, and merits 47 points. *Range of movements* attracts only 5 points, and *absence of deformity* 4 points.

If a hip scoring system is being used to assess the results of a hip replacement (and this is one of the commonest indications) then it is necessary to include details of the radiographic appearances which are so important. This is a feature of many recent methods of assessment. Again, after much consultation among many interested groups, a comprehensive list of questions relating to pain, function, gait movements and radiological appearances has been produced[2]. The terminology has been described as standard and unalterable in its definition, so that without weighting results can be readily compared between series. While use of the full list (described in the reference) may have to be considered where publication is intended, the questions in the clinical assessment are of such value in assessing any case that they are appended here:

Pain

Degree
— None — no pain
— Mild — slight and occasional pain; patient has not altered patterns of activity or work
— Moderate — patient is active, but has had to modify or give up some activities or both, because of pain
— Severe — major pain and serious limitations

Occurrence
— None
— With first steps, then dissipates (start-up pain)
— Only after long (30-minute) walks
— With all walking
— At all times

Work/Level of activity

Occupation, including housewife ....

Retired:
— No
— Yes

Nursing home:
— No
— Yes (date entered....................)

Level of activity

— Bedridden or confined to a wheelchair
— Sedentary — minimum capacity for walking or other activity
— Semi-sedentary — white-collar job, bench work, light housework
— Light work — includes heavy housework, light employment, light athletic activity (e.g. walking 5 km or less)
— Moderate manual labour (e.g. work involving lifting weights of 23 kg or less), moderate athletic activity (e.g. walking or cycling more than 5 km)
— Heavy manual labour (e.g. work frequently lifting 23–45 kg), vigorous sports (e.g. tennis, squash)

Work capacity in last 3 months

— 100%
— 75%
— 50%
— 25%
— 0%

Putting on shoes and socks

— No difficulty

— Slight difficulty
— Extreme difficulty
— Unable

Ascending and descending stairs

— Normal (foot over foot)
— Foot over foot, using banister
— Two feet on each step
— Any other method
— Unable

Sitting to standing

— Can rise from chair without using arms
— Can rise from chair using arms
— Cannot rise independently

Walking capacity

Usual support needed
— None
— 1 stick for long walks
— 1 stick
— 1 crutch
— 2 sticks
— 2 crutches
— Zimmer frame or equivalent
— Unable to walk

Time walked

Without support
— Unlimited (more than an hour)
— 31–60 minutes
— 11–30 minutes
— 2–10 minutes
— Less than 2 minutes, or indoors only
— Unable to walk

With support
— Unlimited (more than an hour)
— 31–60 minutes
— 11–30 minutes
— 2–10 minutes
— Less than 2 minutes, or indoors only
— Unable to walk

References

1. Harris W H 1969 Traumatic arthritis of the hip. Journal of Bone and Joint Surgery 81-A: 737–755
2. Johnston R C et al 1990 Clinical and radiographic evaluation of total hip replacement, Journal of Bone and Joint Surgery 72-A: 161–168

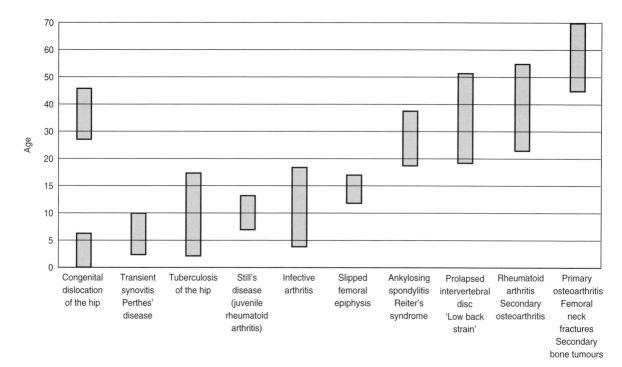

Table 10.1   Age distribution of common hip pathology.

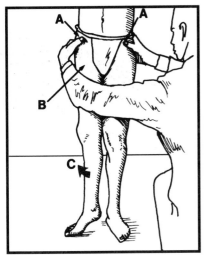

1. *Inspection* (1): Examine the standing patient from the front. Note (A) any pelvic tilting (e.g. from adduction or abduction deformity of the hip, short leg, scoliosis); (B) muscle wasting (e.g. secondary to infection, disuse, polio); (C) rotational deformity (common in osteoarthritis).

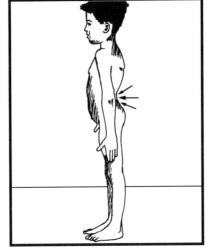

2. *Inspection* (2): Examine the patient from the side. Note any increased lumbar lordosis suggestive of fixed flexion deformity of the hip(s).

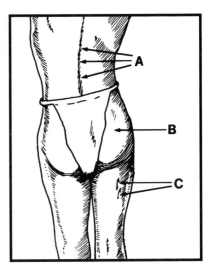

3. *Inspection* (3): Look at the patient from behind. Note (A) any scoliosis (possibly secondary to pelvic tilting, from, for example an adduction deformity of the hip); (B) gluteal muscle wasting (e.g. from disuse, infection); (C) sinus scars (e.g. secondary to tuberculosis).

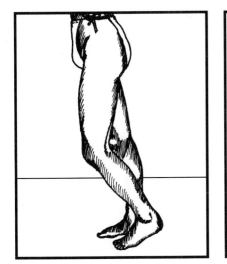

4. *Gait:* Observe the gait from the front, side and behind. Analysis is often difficult but grows from experience. In particular try to assess the stride and dwell time on each side, and the possible factors of pain, stiffness, shortening and gluteal insufficiency.

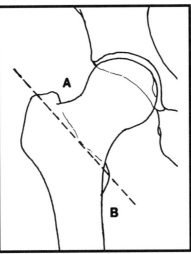

5. *Shortening* (1): It is important in the examination of the hip and the lower limb to determine the presence or absence of shortening. In *true shortening*, the affected limb is physically shorter than the other. This may be caused by pathology (A) above or proximal to the greater trochanter or (B) distal to the trochanters.

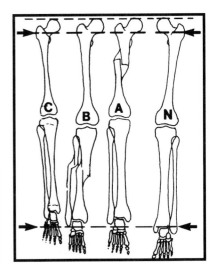

6. *True shortening* (2): True shortening from causes distal to the trochanters most frequently results from (A) old fractures of the femur or (B) of tibia, or (C) growth disturbance (e.g. from polio, bone or joint infection or epiphyseal trauma). (N) Normal side for comparison.

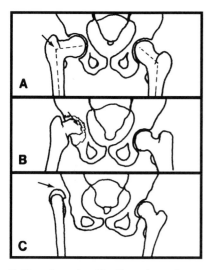

7. *True shortening* (3): Above the trochanter causes include (A) coxa vara (e.g. from femoral neck fractures, slipped upper femoral epiphysis, Perthes' disease, congenital coxa vara); (B) loss of articular cartilage (e.g. from infection, arthritis); (C) dislocation of the hip.

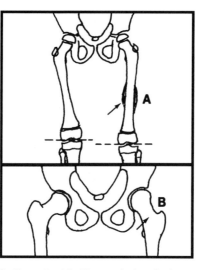

8. *Shortening* (4): Very rarely *lengthening of the other limb* gives relative true shortening. This may be due to (A) stimulation of bone growth from increased vascularity (e.g. after long bone fracture in children, or bone tumour); (B) coxa valga (e.g. following polio).

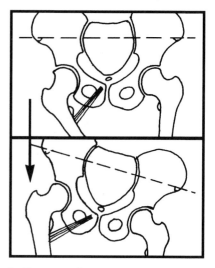

9. *Shortening* (5): In *apparent shortening* the limb is not altered in length, but appears short as a result of an adduction contracture of the hip which has to be compensated for by tilting of the pelvis.

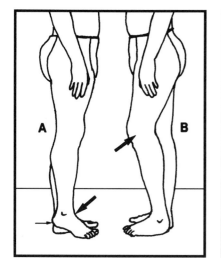

10. *Shortening* (6): Limb shortening may be compensated for by (A) plantar flexion of the foot on the affected side, by (B) flexion of the knee on the other or by (C) pelvic tilting which in turn may be compensated for by the development of a lumbar scoliosis.

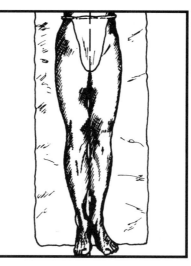

11. *Shortening: examination* (1): The patient should be adjusted to lie squarely on the couch, with the trunk and legs parallel to its edge. The position of the pelvis should be observed (by the position of the anterior superior iliac spines) and adjusted where possible.

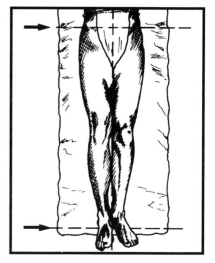

12. *Shortening: examination* (2): In the normal patient the heels should be level, and the plane of the iliac spines at right angles to the edge of the couch.

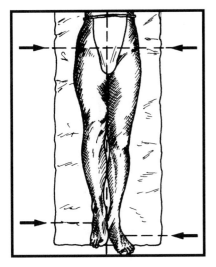

13. *Shortening: examination* (3): Where there is significant true shortening, the heels will not be level (the discrepancy is a guide to the amount of shortening) and the pelvis will not be tilted. The site and amount of shortening must now be further investigated.

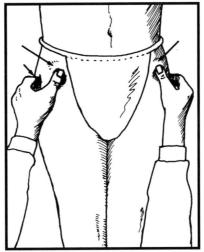

14. *Shortening: examination* (4): Begin by hooking the thumbs under the anterior spines. Feel for the greater trochanters with the fingers. If the distance between the thumb and fingers is shorter on one side, this suggests that the pathology lies above the trochanters.

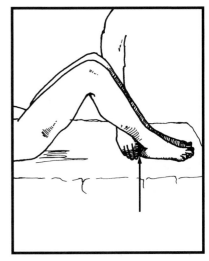

15. *Shortening: examination* (5): If in the last test there was no evidence of shortening above the trochanter, look for causes below the trochanter. Slightly flex both knees and hips, and place a hand behind the heels to check that you now have them squarely together.

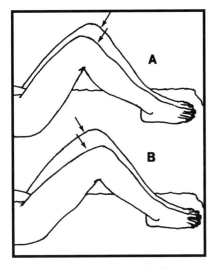

16. *Shortening: examination* (6): The position of the two knees should be compared. (A) This appearance suggests femoral shortening. (B) This appearance is suggestive of tibial shortening.

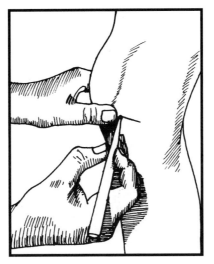

17. *Shortening: examination* (7): Further confirmation of tibial shortening may be made by direct measurement. Flex the knees and mark the line of the knee joint.

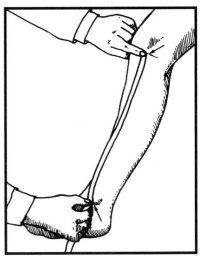

18. *Shortening: examination* (8): Now measure from the mark to the tip of the medial malleolus. Compare the two sides. Any difference indicates true tibial shortening. Note also any obvious tibial irregularity suggestive of old fracture.

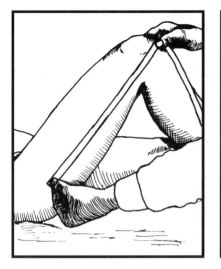

19. *Shortening: examination (9):* Measurement of femoral shaft shortening can only be attempted in the thin patient where the tip of the greater trochanter is easily palpable. Measure from the trochanter to the lateral joint line and compare the sides.

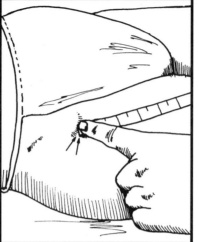

20. *Shortening: examination (10):* Measurement of total (true) leg shortening is the most valuable single assessment, although it gives itself no indication of site. Place the metal end of the tape over the anterior spine and press it backwards until it hooks under its inferior edge.

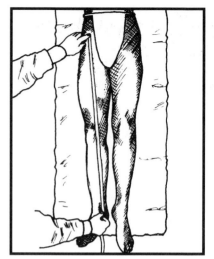

21. *Shortening: examination (11):* Now measure to the middle or inferior border of the medial malleolus. Compare the sides, and always repeat the measurements until consistency is obtained. Deformity of the pelvis (which is rare) may sometimes lead to errors in assessment.

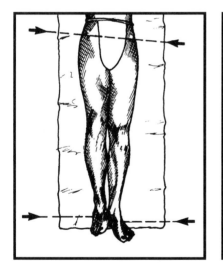

22. *Shortening: examination (12):* Pelvic tilting which is uncorrectable, with heel discrepancy, indicates apparent shortening of the limb. It may of course be accompanied by some true shortening. The discrepancy at the heels is a measure of its degree.

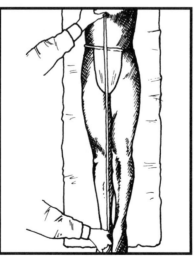

23. *Shortening: examination (13):* Apparent shortening may also be assessed by comparing the distances between the xiphisternum and each medial malleolus.

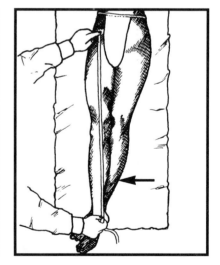

24. *Shortening: examination (14):* When there is an adduction deformity of the hip, and the leg lengths are being measured to assess any accompanying true shortening, the good leg should be adducted by the same amount before commencing measurement between the anterior spines and malleoli.

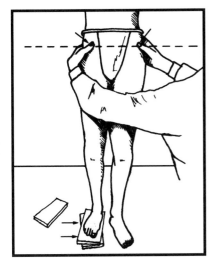

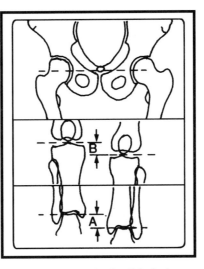

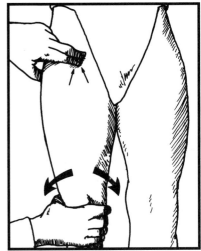

25. *Shortening: examination* (15): True leg shortening may also be measured by blocking up the short leg until both anterior superior iliac spines and the iliac crests lie horizontally, and the natal cleft is vertical; a further check of the pelvis being level is to see that the posterior iliac spines remain horizontal when the patient flexes forwards.

26. *Shortening: examination* (16): In the difficult case, sequential radiographs of the hips, knees and ankles, taken on a single plate without moving the patient, afford accurate comparison of the sides. For example, (A) indicates overall shortening; (B) indicates femoral shortening.

27. *Palpation* (1): Place the fingers over the head of the femur below the inguinal ligament, lateral to the femoral artery. Note any tenderness. Now rotate the leg medially and laterally. Crepitus arising in the hip joint may be detected in this way.

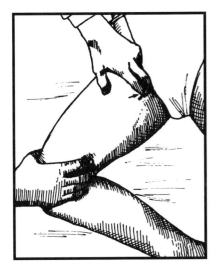

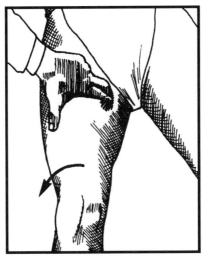

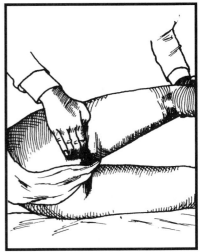

28. *Palpation* (2): Palpate the origin of adductor longus. Tenderness occurs here in sports injuries (strain of adductor longus) and in patients developing adductor contractures in osteoarthritis of the hip.

29. *Palpation* (3): Externally rotate the leg and palpate the lesser trochanter. Tenderness occurs here in strains of the ilio-psoas as a result of athletic injuries.

30. *Palpation* (4): Palpate the region of the ischial tuberosity looking for tenderness. Strain of the hamstring origin occurs as a result of athletic activities, especially in children. Less commonly athletic injuries may affect the anterior superior and inferior spines.

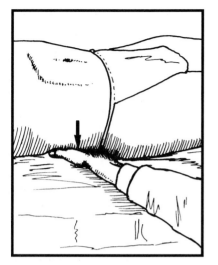

31. *Movements: extension* (1): Place a hand behind the lumbar spine so that you may assess its position.

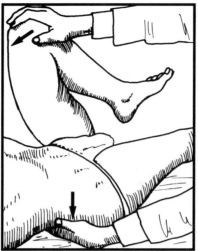

32. *Movements: extension* (2): Now flex the *good* hip fully, observing with the hand that the lumbar curvature is fully obliterated.

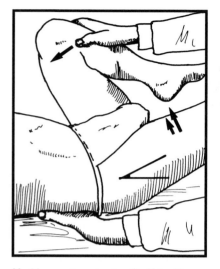

33. *Movements: extension* (3): If the hip being examined rises from the couch, this indicates *loss of extension in that hip* (also described as *fixed flexion deformity of the hip*). Any loss should be measured and recorded. This test is usually referred to as Thomas's test.

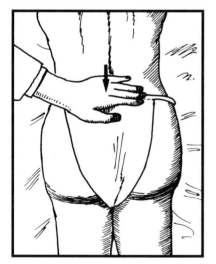

34. *Movements: extension* (4): To check smaller losses of extension, especially when the other hip is normal, turn the patient over on to his face and steady the pelvis with one hand.

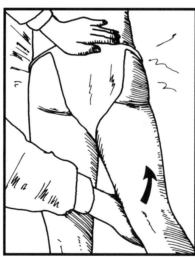

35. *Movements: extension* (5): Lift each leg and compare the range. *Normal range: 5–20°*. A loss of extension is often the first detectable sign of effusion in the hip joint.

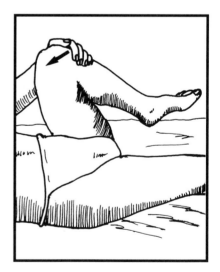

36. *Movements: flexion* (1): The good hip is first flexed to obliterate the lumbar curve and to steady the pelvis. The patient is asked to hold the leg in this position.

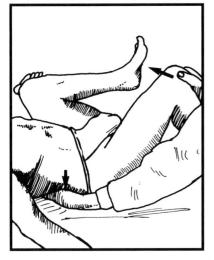

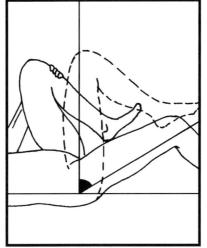

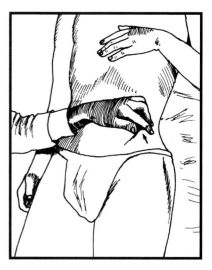

37. *Movements: flexion* (2): The hip is then flexed, using a hand to check that no further pelvic movement occurs. Note the range of movement. *Normal range: 120°*.

38. *Movements: flexion* (3): The range of flexion may be recorded in this example as 'Flexion (R) hip: 30–90°' or 'Fixed flexion deformity of 30° and hip flexes to 90°'. Flexion may also be tested with the patient lying on his side.

39. *Movements: abduction* (1): A false impression of hip movement may be gained if the pelvis tilts during the examination, so first place the left hand on the patient's left anterior superior iliac spine. Steady the other spine with the forearm.

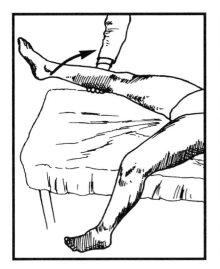

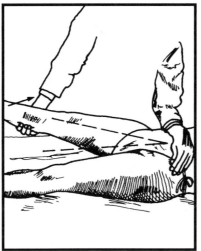

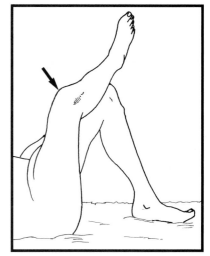

40. *Movements: abduction* (2): An alternative way of fixing the pelvis is to flex the other leg over the edge of the couch, and check movement of the pelvis by holding the anterior superior iliac spine on the side begin examined.

41. *Movements: abduction* (3): Now having fixed the pelvis, move the leg laterally and note the range achieved. *Normal range: 40°*. Abduction may also be tested from a starting position of 90° hip flexion. This is of particular value in suspected osteoarthritis of the hip or congenital dislocation (see also 10, 74).

42. *Patrick's test:* Basically this is a variation of abducting the hip from a position of 90° flexion. Pain during the manoeuvre is regarded as being the very first sign of osteoarthritis in a hip. To perform (on the right), flex both hips and knees, place the right foot on the left knee, and gently press down on the right knee. This is also known as the fabere sign (**F**lexion, **AB**duction, **E**xternal **R**otation, **E**xtension).

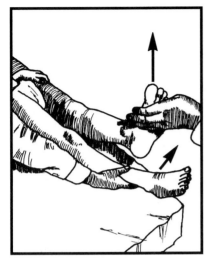

43. *Movements: adduction* (1): Ideally an assistant should lift the good leg out of the way to allow the affected leg to be adducted in full extension. *Normal range: 25°*.

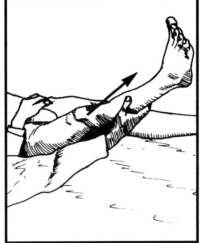

44. *Movements: adduction* (2): If an assistant is not available, cross the leg being examined over the other. This brings the leg being examined into slight flexion, but is sufficiently accurate under most circumstances. If the hip is normal, the legs should cross about mid-thigh. Adduction may also be tested from a starting position of 90° hip flexion.

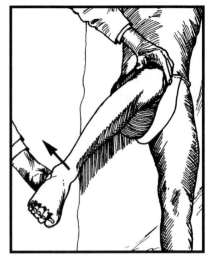

45. *Movements: internal rotation at 90° flexion* (1): Steady the flexed hip by holding the knee with one hand, and move the foot laterally to produce internal rotation of the hip. Note that this is a never-ending source of confusion; be sure that this is clear in your own mind. Although the *foot* moves *laterally* (or externally), the *hip* rotates *internally* (or medially).

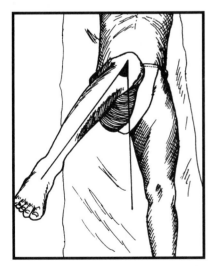

46. *Movements: internal rotation at 90° flexion* (2): Measure the range of internal rotation by comparing the position of the leg and the midline. *Normal range: 45°*. Compare the sides. Loss of internal rotation is common in most hip pathology.

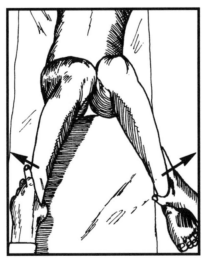

47. *Movements: internal rotation at 90° flexion* (3): A sensitive comparison of the sides may be made by asking the patient to hold the knees together while you move both feet laterally.

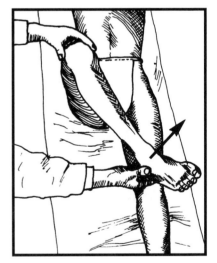

48. *Movements: external rotation at 90° flexion* (1): The position of the hip is the same as for testing internal rotation, but in this case the foot is moved medially.

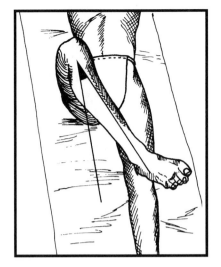

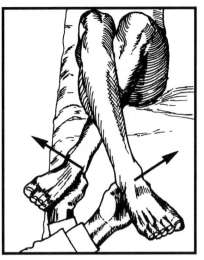

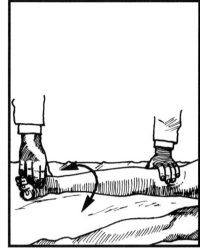

49. *Movements: external rotation at 90° flexion* (2): Measure external rotation in the same general way. *Normal range: 45°*. External rotation becomes limited in most arthritic conditions of the hip.

50. *Movements: external rotation at 90° flexion* (3): Comparison between the sides may be made by crossing one leg over the other.

51. *Movements: rotation in extension:* For a rough comparison of the sides, roll each leg medially and laterally, observing any play at the knee.

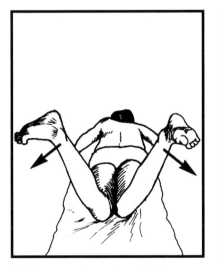

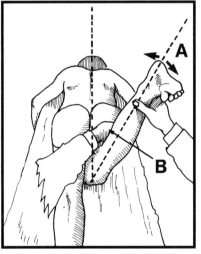

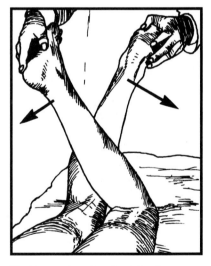

52. *Movements: internal rotation in extension:* For a more accurate assessment, the patient should be prone, with the knees flexed. The two sides can easily be compared and measurements taken. *Normal range: 35°*.

53. *Movements: anteversion of the femoral neck:* An assessment of anteversion may be made when the patient is in the same position. Hold the leg with one hand, and rock it from side to side (A) while simultaneously feeling the prominence of the greater trochanter with the other (B). When the trochanter is facing truly laterally, anteversion is equal to the angle between the leg and the vertical. This is the most accurate method of assessing anteversion.

54. *Movements: external rotation in extension:* Comparison and measurement may be made in the same way. *Normal range: 45°*.

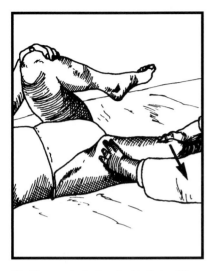

55. *Movements: testing for hip fusion* (1): When there is doubt regarding the solidity of a hip fusion, it is sometimes helpful to test for protective muscle contraction. Flex the good hip and knee. Feel for involuntary adductor contracture while suddenly abducting the leg.

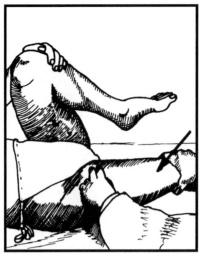

56. *Movements: testing for hip fusion* (2): Repeat the test, this time feeling for flexor (ilio-psoas) contraction while making a sudden gentle attempt to extend the hip.

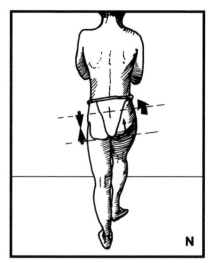

57. *Trendelenberg's test* (1): When standing on one leg, the centre of gravity (at S2) is brought over the stance foot by the hip abductors (gluteus medius and minimus). This tilts the pelvis and normally elevates the buttock of the non-stance side. The patient should be able to produce a greater pelvic tilt (by being asked to lift the side higher), and *hold* the position for 30 seconds.

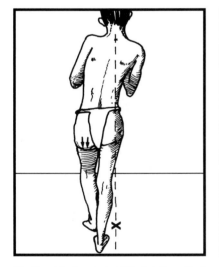

58. *Trendelenberg's test* (2): Ask the patient to stand on the affected side: any support (stick or hand) *must* be on the *same* side. Now ask him to raise the non-stance leg further. Prevent excessive trunk movements (a vertical dropped from C7 should not fall beyond the foot). If the pelvis drops below the horizontal or cannot be held steady for 30 seconds, the test is positive. It is not valid below age 4; pain, poor co-operation or bad balance may give a false positive.

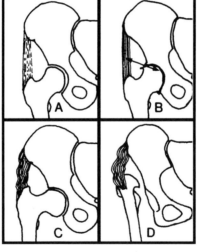

59. *Trendelenberg's test* (3): The test is positive as a result of (A) gluteal paralysis or weakness (e.g. from polio, muscle-wasting disease), (B) gluteal inhibition (e.g. from pain arising in the hip joint), (C) from gluteal inefficiency from coxa vara or (D) CDH. Nevertheless false positives have been recorded in about 10% of patients.

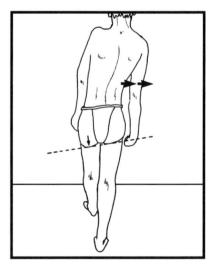

60. *Duchenne sign:* Note if the patient lurches to one side when walking. If present, this is due to the patient trying to reduce pain by shifting his body weight over the hip. This is often also somewhat confusingly referred to as an abductor or Trendelenberg lurch. It is often associated with a positive Trendelenberg sign (as shown), but not invariably.

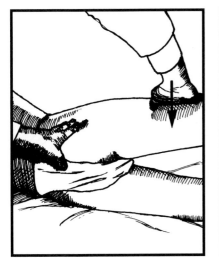

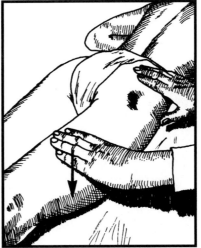

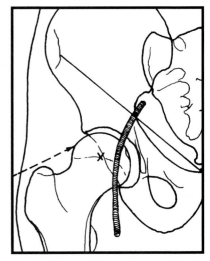

61. *Gluteal muscles* (1): Test the power of the abductors of the hip with the patient lying on the side, attempting to abduct the leg against resistance.

62. *Gluteal muscles* (2): Test the power in gluteus maximus by asking the patient to extend the hip against resistance, at the same time feeling the tone in the contracting muscle.

63. *Aspiration:* The hip may be aspirated by inserting a needle above the trochanter, allowing for femoral neck anteversion. Alternatively, a needle may be passed into the joint from in front, a little below the inguinal ligament and lateral to the femoral artery.

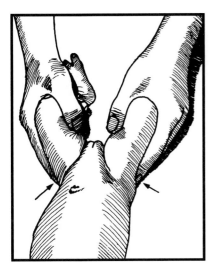

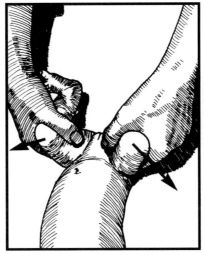

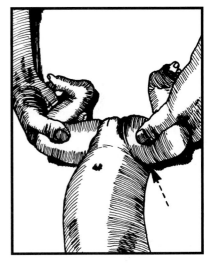

64. *Ortolani's test* (1): To be of any value the examination must be carried out on a relaxed child, preferably after feeding. Flex the knees and encircle them with the hands so that the thumbs lie along the medial sides of the thighs and the fingers over the trochanters.

65. *Ortolani's test* (2): Now flex the hips to a right angle, and starting from a position where the thumbs are touching, smoothly and gently abduct the hips.

66. *Ortolani's test* (3): If a hip is dislocated, as full abduction is approached the femoral head will be felt slipping into the acetabulum. An audible click may accompany the displacement but in no way must this be considered an essential element of the test. Note that restriction of abduction may be pathological, and represent an irreducible dislocation (see also 10, 74).

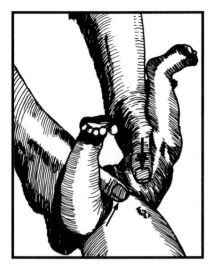

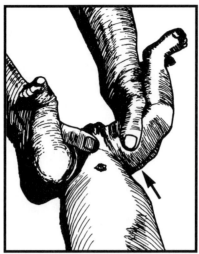

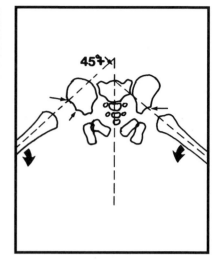

67. *Barlow's provocative test* (1): If the Ortolani test is negative the hip may nevertheless be unstable. Fix the pelvis between symphysis and sacrum with one hand. With the thumb of the other, attempt to dislocate the hip by gentle but firm backward pressure. Check both sides.

68. *Barlow's test* (2): If the head of the femur is felt to sublux backwards, its reduction should be achieved by forward finger pressure or wider abduction. The movement of reduction should also be appreciated with the fingers. If Barlow's test is positive (and Ortolani's negative), recheck at weekly intervals. Instability persisting for more than 3 weeks is an indication for splintage, or for further investigation with ultrasound and X-ray.

69. *Radiographic examination of the neonate:* Because of a degree of unreliability and the risks of unnecessary radiation, reserve this for the suspicious but uncertain case only. (A) *van Rosen method:* An antero-posterior (AP) view should be taken with the hips in at least 45° abduction and full internal rotation. On the films, a line projected along the line of the femur in the normal hip should strike the acetabulum, and in a case of dislocation, the region of the anterior superior spine.

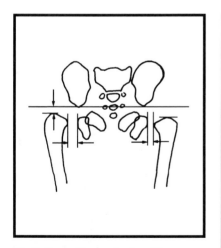

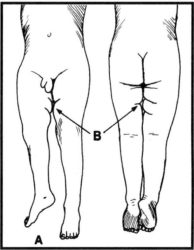

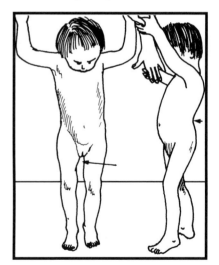

70. *Radiographic examination:* (B) *Edinburgh method:* An AP film is taken with the child's legs held parallel, with slight traction and no external rotation. Centre the beam at a standard distance of 100 cm. Measure the gap between the most medial part of the femur and the lateral edge of the ischium. This is normally 4 mm; over 5 mm is suspicious; 6 mm is regarded as diagnostic of CDH. Proximal migration can also be measured in the same film.

71. *CDH: the older child* (1): *appearance:* (A) The affected leg in a case of unilateral congenital dislocation of the hip may appear slightly shorter, and lie in external rotation. (B) There may be asymmetry of the skin folds in the thigh, although this sign is of limited reliability.

72. *CDH: the older child* (2): If both hips are involved, there is usually widening of the perineum due to the hip displacement. If the child has been walking, there will be a compensatory increase in lumbar lordosis.

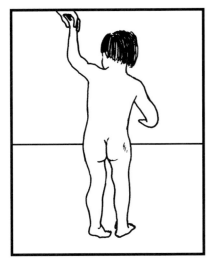

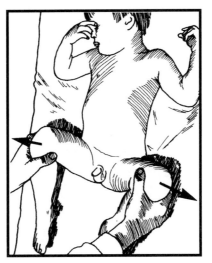

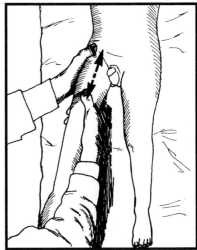

73. *CDH: the older child* (3): Trendelenberg's test will be positive (see 10, 57) and the gait will be abnormal with excessive shoulder sway. In unilateral cases, the child will dip on the affected side; in bilateral cases the child will have a waddling gait.

74. *CDH: the older child* (4): Test the range of abduction from a position of 90° flexion of the hip. Abduction is restricted in CDH in this position, and of course is most obvious in the unilateral case. Less than 60° of abduction is regarded as being of particular significance.

75. *CDH: the older child* (5): Attempt to elicit telescoping in the affected limb. Steady the pelvis with one hand, and push and pull along the axis of the femur with the other. Abnormal excursion of the limb is suggestive of CDH. Always compare the sides. For interpretation of radiographs, see 10, 69.

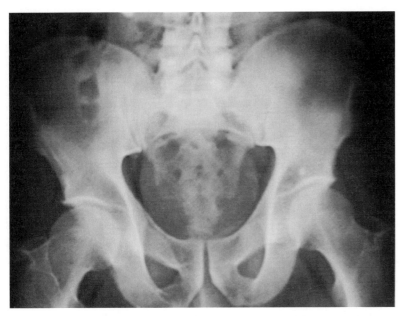

76. *Radiographs* (1): Normal antero-posterior projection of the pelvis.

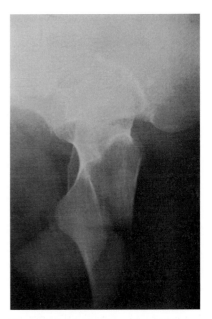

77. *Radiographs* (2): Normal lateral hip.

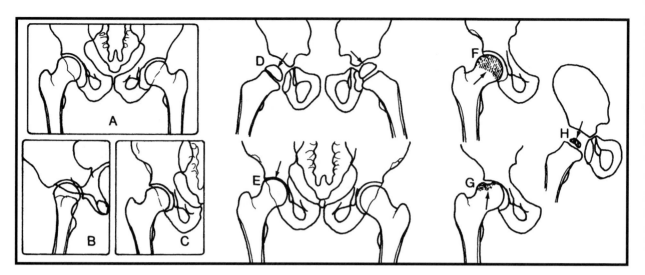

78. *Radiographs* (3): An antero-posterior view showing both hips (A) is the most useful single screening film as it allows both sides to be compared. If the joint is strongly suspect, an additional lateral projection (B) and an antero-posterior centred on the hip (C) are essential. Note first in the films any *disturbance of bone texture* (e.g. Paget's disease, osteoporosis, tumour). Now note the *joint space* (which indicates the depth of articular cartilage and interposing fluid) which may be (D) increased in Perthes' disease, synovitis and infection and (E) decreased in the later stages of infection and arthritis. Note the relative *density* of the femoral head which may be decreased. e.g. in rheumatoid arthritis, infection and osteoporosis, and increased in (F) avascular necrosis, (G) segmental avascular necrosis and (H) Perthes' disease.

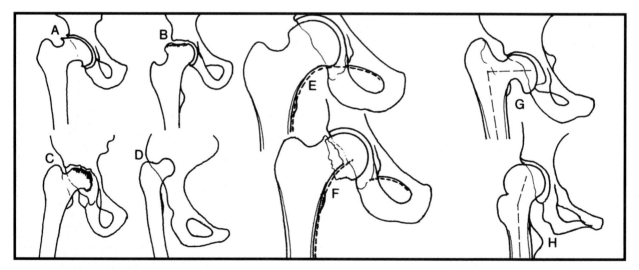

79. *Radiographs* (4): Now note the *shape* of the femoral head which may, for example, be (A) buffer-shaped after Perthes' disease, (B) flattened after avascular necrosis (total or segmental), (C) irregular or destroyed after infection, (D) atrophic in persistent congenital hip dislocation. Note *Shenton's line* which normally forms a smooth curve flowing from the superior pubic ramus to the femoral neck (E). Compare the sides if possible. Distortion occurs in many conditions involving the femoral neck and head, particularly fractures (F) and subluxations. Note the *neck/shaft angle*. This is decreased in (G) congenital coxa vara, and coxa vara secondary to rickets, Paget's disease, osteomalacia, fracture etc. It is increased in coxa valga secondary to polio (H) and other neurological disturbances.

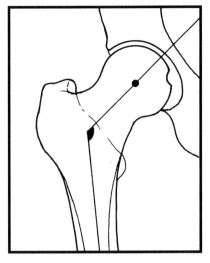

80. *The neck/shaft angle:* may be measured from lines drawn through the shaft and along the neck into the centre of the head. *Normal: Males 128°; Female 127°.* The centre of the head may be easily found with the aid of an orthopaedic rule or similar transparent drawing template inscribed with concentric circles of different radii.

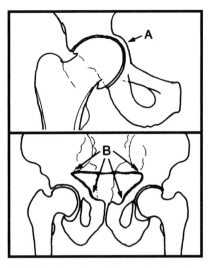

81. *Pelvic distortion:* This may be found in (A) protrusio acetabuli (often hereditary, and with associated osteoarthritis); (B) osteomalacia (and other diseases accompanied by bone softening, e.g. rickets, Paget's disease).

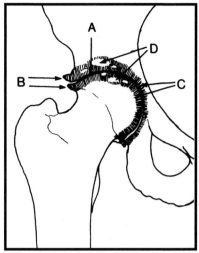

82. *Osteoarthritis:* Note the presence of any of the changes commonly seen in osteoarthritis, such as (A) joint space narrowing; (B) marginal osteophytes; (C) marginal sclerosis; (D) cystic changes in the head and acetabulum.

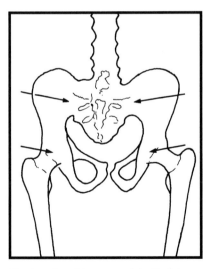

83. *Complete obliteration of the hip joint (bony ankylosis):* This is seen in ankylosing spondylitis (where there is invariably involvement of the sacro-iliac joints). It is also seen as a late result of tuberculous and other infections, and after surgical fusion.

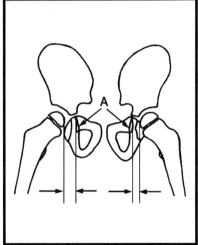

84. *Perthes' disease* (1): The earliest radiographic sign is an increase in joint space (also seen in synovitis of the hip and in infective arthritis). Minor degrees of joint widening may be detected by measuring the distance between (A) the 'tear drop' and the head on both sides.

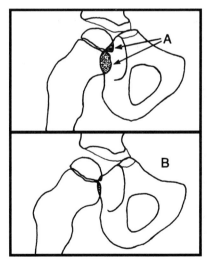

85. *Perthes' disease* (2): If the 'tear drop' (formed by the anterior acetabular floor) is not clear, note (A) the overlap shadows of the head and neck on the acetabulum, comparing one hip with the other. Alteration (B) occurs in Perthes' disease, synovitis and infection.

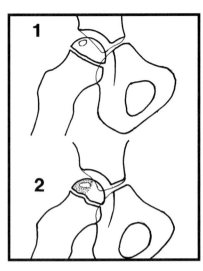

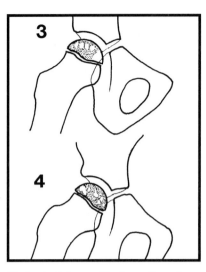

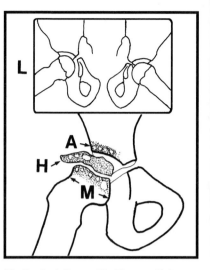

86. *Perthes' disease* (3): *Catterall grading:* This is the commonest method of assessing the severity of bone changes when they appear. *Grade 1:* Cyst formation occurs in the antero-lateral aspect of the capital epiphysis. Revascularisation may be completed without bone collapse, and the prognosis without treatment is good. *Grade 2:* A little more of the head is involved, and bony collapse is inevitable.

87. *Perthes' disease* (4): *Catterall grading ctd: Grade 3:* Most of the head is involved. *Grade 4:* The whole head is affected. Bony collapse is inevitable in grades 3 and 4, and the prognosis is poorer.

88. *Perthes' disease* (5): The so-called 'frog' lateral (Loewenstein projection (L)) is routine in assessing these cases. Apart from in the capital epiphysis, cystic changes may also appear in the acetabulum (A) and the metaphysis which may widen (M). The femoral head may flatten and extrude laterally (H).

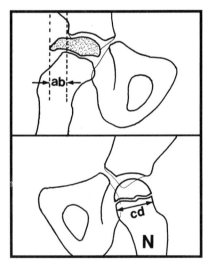

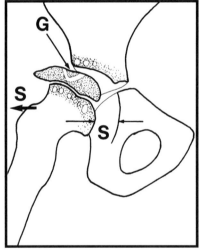

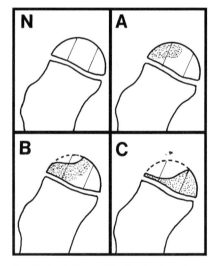

89. *Perthes' disease* (6): Lateral extrusion may be expressed as a percentage of the diameter of the metaphysis on the normal side (N): if ab/cd × 100 >20% then the prognosis is poor. An accurate assessment of the amount of avascular bone may be made by radionuclide bone scanning. Prognosis is mainly dependent on the mass and degree of epiphyseal involvement (assessed for example by Catterall grading).

90. *Perthes' disease* (7): Other adverse factors placing the case in the 'head-at-risk' category include (a) presentation above the age of 4; (b) calcification seen lateral to the epiphysis or other evidence of major extrusion; (c) lateral subluxation (S); (d) a positive Gage sign (a sequestrum surrounded by a 'V' of viable epiphysis (G)).

91. *Perthes' disease* (8): *Herring lateral pillar classification:* Divide the head into three columns during the fragmentation stage; then if the lateral is of normal height (Herring A) the prognosis is excellent. If the lateral is depressed up to 50% (even with the central column involved), Herring B, the results are generally good under age 9. In Herring C the lateral pillar is less than 50%, and all develop permanent deformity.

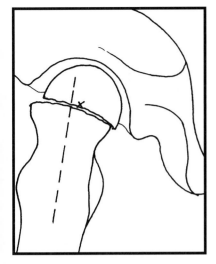

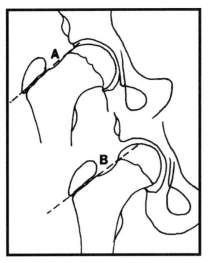

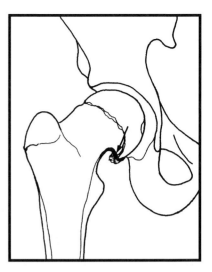

92. *Slipped femoral epiphysis* (1): The earliest changes are seen in the lateral projection. A line drawn up through the centre of the neck fails to meet the midpoint of the base of the epiphysis.

93. *Slipped femoral epiphysis* (2): Later, in the antero-posterior view, the first sign is that a tangential line drawn on the upper femoral neck fails to strike the epiphysis (A), while in a normal well-centred view, such a tangent (B) includes part of the epiphysis.

94. *Slipped femoral epiphysis* (3): In the later stages, some weeks after the initial slip (now the so-called 'chronic slip' stage), there is distortion of the inferior part of the femoral neck with new bone formation ('buttressing').

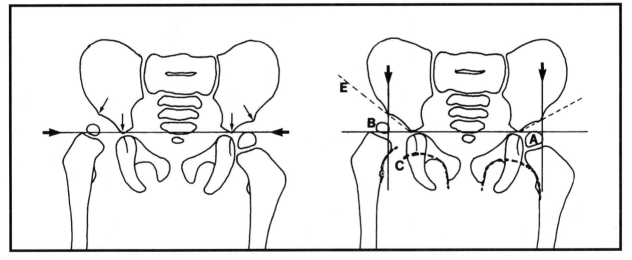

95. *Radiographs:* Interpretation of hip radiographs in the older child is dependent on the presence of ossification in the epiphysis of the femoral head. This normally appears between 2 and 8 months, but is often delayed in CDH. The position of the capital epiphysis in relation to the other pelvic elements must be determined. First draw a horizontal line (Hilgenreimer line) across the pelvis. On each side this should touch the downward-pointing apex of the acetabular element of the ilium. Vertical lines (Perkins lines) should then be drawn from the lateral limit of the acetabulum. These lines divide the region of each hip into four areas. The epiphysis of the femoral head should normally lie within the lower and inner quadrant (A), but in CDH the head moves upwards and outwards (as at B). Shenton's line (C) may be disturbed. Dysplasia of the acetabulum alters its slope (E) which decreases with growth (it usually does not exceed 30° at 6 months). There are a number of other measurements of a specialised nature which may be made (and compared with tables detailing average values relating to age and sex) when a more detailed assessment of suspected acetabular dysplasia is required. Additional information regarding the head, acetabulum and limbus may be obtained by MRI scans or contrast arthrography. The techniques and interpretation are specialised.

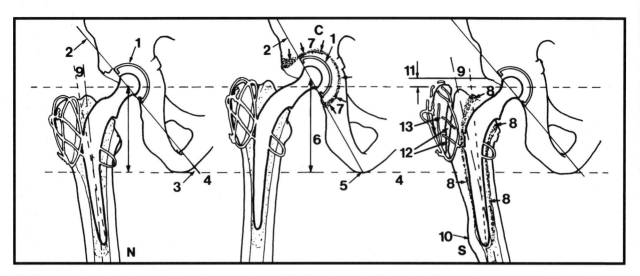

96. *Component loosening after total hip replacement: the cup* (C): The wire marker (1) sunk within the radiolucent cup aids the analysis of any radiographic series. The plane (2) of the socket lies at an angle (3) to the plane of the pelvis (4), shown by a line drawn between the ischial tuberosities. This angle may be altered (5) by rotation of the cup if it loosens. The cup may also migrate proximally: look for any disturbance in the relationship between the wire marker and the fixed landmarks of the pelvis. An increase in the distance (6) between the centre of the cup and the ischium may be suggestive of migration, although errors of positioning and tube/film distances make this a little unreliable. Development of a radiolucent zone (7) (between cement and bone) exceeding 1 mm and extending right round the cup is a strong indicator of loosening. (Note that the appearance of a radiolucent line *between the cement and a component* is diagnostic of loosening.)
The stem (S): Look for a radiolucent zone of more than 1 mm between cement and bone (8) or between the stem and the cement. Note any *change* in the angle between the axes of the femur and prosthetic stem (9), or any local bone disturbance (10). Check for sinking of the prothesis, by noting the distance between the upper edge of the acetabulum and the greater trochanter (11). Non-union of the greater trochanter (12) and wire fracture and fragmentation (13) should also recorded.

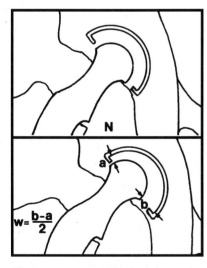

97. *Component wear:* This is posing much less of a problem than was originally anticipated by both surgeon and patient. Wear involves the softer acetabular component; head wear is negligible. To determine this, measure the gap between the prosthetic head and the wire marker at their upper and lower limits. *Half* the difference between these is a measure of wear in the wall of the cup. 3 mm or more suggests an appreciable amount.

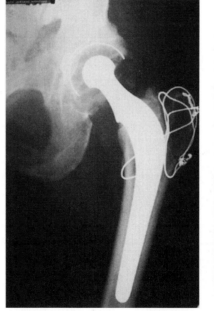

98. *Radiographs:* In this (normal) Charnley total hip replacement, the stem of the prosthesis is well placed. The greater trochanter is uniting in good position, and the wires are intact. The head of the femoral component is concentric with the acetabular wire marker.

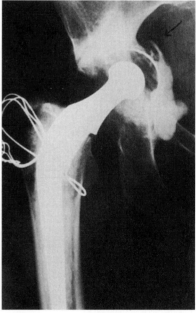

99. *Hip radiographs: examples of pathology* (1): After a total hip replacement the floor of the acetabulum has given way, and the cup is becoming centrally displaced.

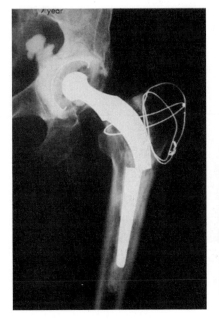

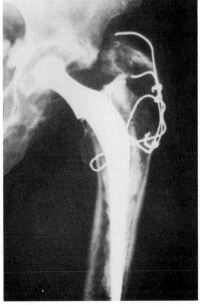

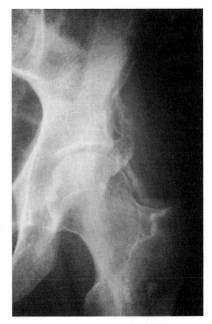

100. *Pathology* (2): After a total hip replacement the prosthetic stem has fractured with loss of the ability to weight-bear. Note the cement which has extruded into the pelvis during the insertion of the device. There is some evidence of loosening of both the cup and the stem.

101. *Pathology* (3): In this case of total hip replacement, the trochanteric wires have broken; the trochanter has displaced proximally and failed to unite. The stem has loosened, and its distal end is in danger of broaching the femoral cortex. Note the extensive translucency at the bone–cement interface.

102. *Pathology* (4): Following a dislocation of the hip which was successfully reduced, this patient complained of great stiffness in the hip. Note the extensive new bone formation round the joint typical of myositis ossificans.

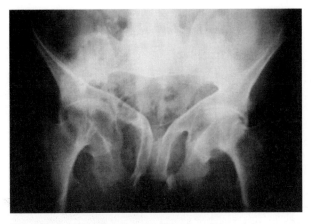

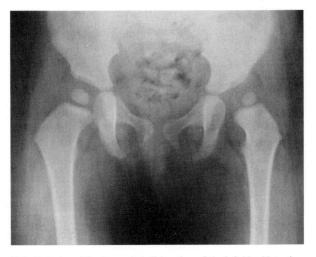

103. *Pathology* (5): There is gross distortion of the pelvis, secondary to osteomalacia.

104. *Pathology* (6): Congenital dislocation of the left hip. Note the lateral and proximal displacement of the upper femoral epiphysis; compare this with the other (normal) side.

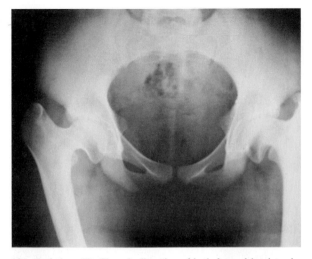

105. *Pathology* (7): There is distortion of both femoral heads and necks due to congenital coxa vara.

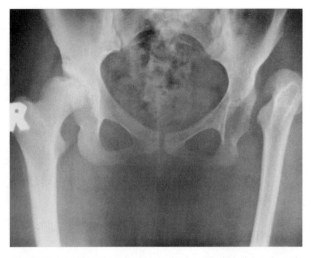

106. *Pathology* (8): There is an untreated congenital dislocation of the left hip. The right hip is dysplastic, and poorly contained by a shallow, sloping acetabulum. The joint space is already narrowed due to early osteoarthritis.

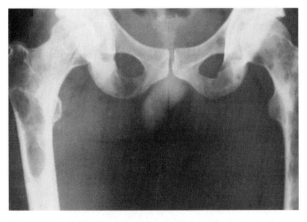

107. *Pathology* (9): There is widespread cystic change in both femora and the pelvis due to hyperparathyroidism.

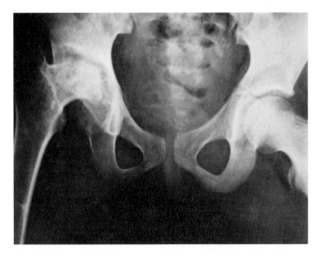

108. *Pathology* (10): There is gross destruction of the right hip joint secondary to infection; in this adolescent boy, the cause was tuberculosis.

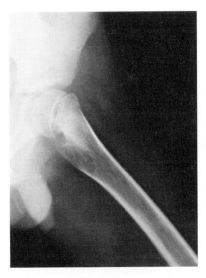

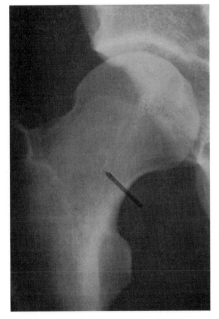

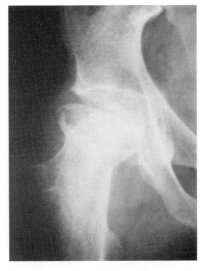

109. *Pathology* (11): This lateral projection of the hip shows displacement of the proximal femoral epiphysis on the femoral neck due to slipped femoral epiphysis.

110. *Pathology* (12). The pointer marks a ringed area of bone in the femoral neck with a central nidus, typical of osteoid osteoma, and the source of niggling bone pain.

111. *Pathology* (13): Following a previous hip fracture there has been collapse of the femoral head due to avascular necrosis. There are secondary osteoarthritic changes in the hip.

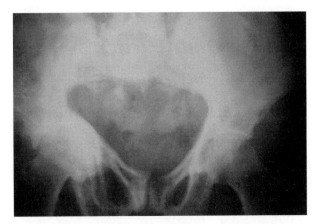

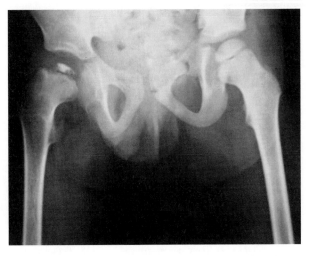

112. *Pathology* (14): There is gross disturbance of the bony architecture of the right hemipelvis typical of Paget's disease.

113. *Pathology* (15): The epiphysis of the right femoral head is small and of increased density. There is some broadening of the metaphysis. The appearances are those of Perthes' disease.

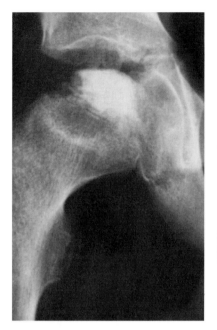

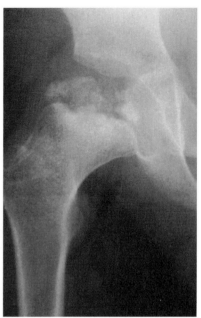

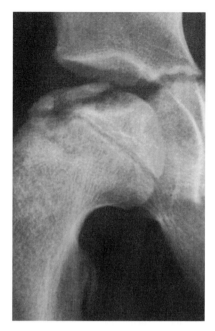

114. *Pathology (16): Perthes' disease:* There is increased density of the epiphysis, and some cystic change in the metaphysis. The area of sclerosis along the inferior margin of the cyst is sometimes referred to as the 'sagging rope' sign.

115. *Pathology (17): Perthes' disease:* There is fragmentation of the capital epiphysis.

116. *Pathology (18): healing Perthes' disease:* Fragmentation of the epiphysis is obvious, but the bone density is returning to normal.

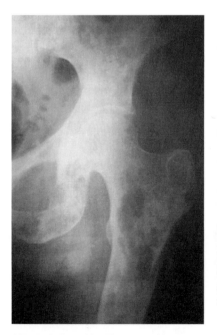

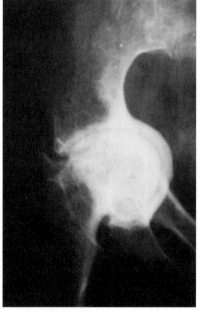

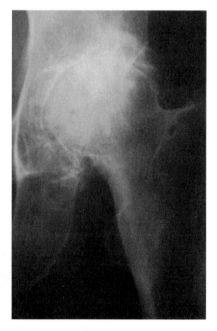

117. *Pathology (19):* There are widespread changes in the femur and pelvis due to metastatic bone disease.

118. *Pathology (20):* There is distortion of the acetabulum which is projecting into the pelvis (protrusio acetabuli), associated with osteoarthritis.

119. *Pathology (21):* There is loss of joint space typical of osteoarthritis of the hip.

11. The knee

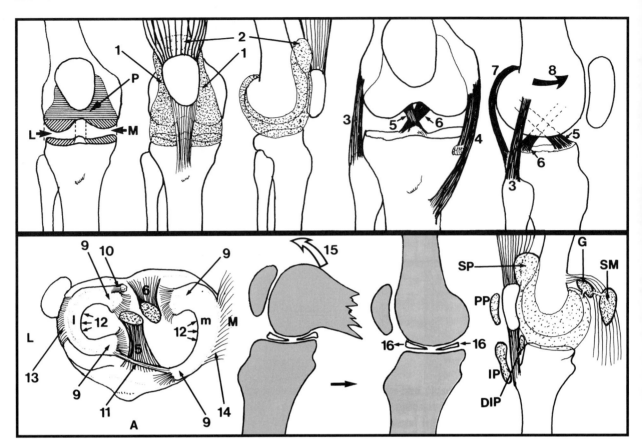

Fig. 11.A

Anatomical features

The knee joint combines three articulations (medial tibio-femoral (M), lateral tibio-femoral (L) and patello-femoral (P)) which share a common synovial sheath; anteriorly, this extends a little to either side (1) of the patella and an appreciable amount proximal to its upper pole (2). This portion lies deep to the quadriceps muscle and is known as the suprapatellar pouch.

There is little congruency between the articular surfaces of the tibia and femur; as a result, there is a well-developed system of ligaments to give the knee stability, and an arrangement of intra-articular menisci to reduce the contact loadings between femur and tibia.

Ligaments

(a) *The lateral ligament* (3) extends between the lateral epicondyle and the head of the fibula.

(b) *The medial ligament* (4), consisting of superficial and deep parts, is attached above to the medial epicondyle of the femur, and below to the medial surface of the tibia on either side of the semimembranosus groove.

(c) *The anterior cruciate ligament* (5) runs between the tibial plateau anteriorly and the lateral femoral condyle posteriorly.

(d) *The posterior cruciate ligament* (6) runs between the tibial plateau posteriorly and the medial femoral condyle anteriorly.

Both cruciate ligaments lie within the confines of the intercondylar notch of the femur, thereby avoiding being trapped between the articular surfaces during movement of the joint.

(e) *The posterior ligament* (7) is attached to posterior aspects of the femur and the tibia just outside their articular margins.

During the last 10° or so of knee extension the ligaments of the joint are twisted taut as a result of medial rotation (8) of the femur on the tibia; at the start of flexion, this tightening is undone by lateral rotation of the femur, aided by contraction of the popliteus muscle.

Menisci

In plan view the *medial* (m) and *lateral* (l) menisci are C-shaped; they are triangular in cross section, and formed from dense avascular fibrous tissue. Their extremities (horns) (9) are attached to the upper surface of the tibia on which they lie; the posterior horn of the lateral meniscus has an additional attachment (10) to the femur, while both anterior horns are loosely connected (11). The concave margin (12) of each meniscus is unattached; the convex margin of the lateral meniscus is anchored to the tibia by coronary ligaments (13), while the corresponding part of the medial meniscus is attached to the joint capsule (14), and thereby loosely united to both femur and tibia.

During extension of the knee (15) the menisci slide forwards (16) on the tibial plateau and become progressively more compressed, adapting in shape to the altering contours of the particular portions of the femur and tibia between which they come to lie.

Only the peripheral edges of the menisci have an appreciable blood supply, so that meniscal tears have little potential for healing.

Bursae

Numerous bursae have been described round the knee, but from the practical point of view only a few are of any real significance.

At the front.

(a) *The suprapatellar pouch* (SP) or *bursa* is a normal extension of the synovial compartment of the knee; it may become prominent as a result of a joint effusion, but treatment is always directed at the underlying cause rather than this local effect.

(b) *A pre-patellar bursa* (PP) may form between the patella and the overlying skin as a result of repeated local friction, e.g. from kneeling.

(c) *An infrapatellar bursa* (IP) may form between the skin and the tibial tubercle or patellar ligament, again usually as a result of local friction from kneeling. Bursae forming deep to the patellar ligament (DIP) also occur, but are rather uncommon.

At the back. Bursal enlargements may be encountered in the popliteal fossa, and these are generally referred to as *Baker's cysts* or enlarged *semimembranosus bursae*. Some are found to communicate with the knee joint (sometimes with a valve-like mechanism), and tend to keep pace in terms of distension with any effusion in the knee.

Others are quite unconnected with the joint. The anatomical explanation is that while the semimembranosus bursa (SM) itself never communicates with the knee, it is often connected to the bursa (G) under the medial head of gastrocnemius (which does).

Swelling of the knee

The knee may become swollen as a result of the accumulation within the joint cavity of excess synovial fluid, blood or pus (synovitis, haemarthrosis, pyarthrosis). Much less commonly the knee swells beyond the limits of the synovial membrane. This is seen in soft tissue injuries of the knee when haematoma formation and oedema may be extensive. It is also a feature of fractures, infections and tumours of the distal femur, where confusion may result either from the proximity of the lesion to the joint or because it involves the joint cavity directly. Although primary tumours of the knee are rare, in malignant synovioma there is striking swelling of the joint, and this often extends beyond the limits of the synovial cavity.

Synovitis, effusion

The synovial membrane secretes the synovial fluid of the joint; excess synovial fluid indicates some affection of the membrane. Joint injuries cause synovitis by tearing or stretching the synovial membrane. Infections act directly by eliciting an inflammatory response which causes the synovial membrane to secrete more fluid. The membrane itself becomes thickened and its function disturbed in rheumatoid arthritis and villo-nodular synovitis; both conditions are usually accompanied by large effusions. In long-standing meniscus lesions and in osteoarthritis of the knee, the synovial membrane may not be directly affected, and consequently no effusion may be present in either of these conditions. Minor injuries of the knee which do not materially damage any of the main structural elements are in some cases followed by rather persistent effusions (traumatic synovitis). In spite of these exceptions, the recognition of fluid in the joint is of great importance. Effusion indicates damage to the joint, and the presence of a major lesion must always be eliminated. A tense synovitis may be aspirated to relieve discomfort.

Haemarthrosis

Blood in the knee is seen most commonly following acute injuries where there is tearing of structures which are vascular. The menisci are avascular, and there may be no haemarthrosis when a meniscus is torn. Bleeding into the joint will take place, however, if the meniscus has been detached at its periphery or if there is accompanying damage to other structures within the knee (e.g. the cruciate ligaments). In injuries of the medial ligament, a haematoma may track distally without involvement of the joint cavity. Nevertheless the presence of a haemarthrosis generally indicates a substantial injury to the joint and is a serious finding. Its physical presence alone may give rise to great discomfort and make diagnosis of its underlying cause rather difficult. In view of this a tense, painful haemarthrosis should be aspirated.

Pyarthrosis

Infections of the knee joint are rather uncommon, and usually blood-borne. Sometimes the joint is involved by direct spread from an osteitis of the femur or tibia; rarely the joint becomes infected following surgery or penetrating wounds.

In acute pyogenic infections the onset is usually rapid and the knee very painful; swelling is tense, tenderness is widespread, and movement resisted. There is pyrexia and general malaise. Pyogenic infections occurring in patients suffering from rheumatoid arthritis have often a much slower onset. Although the joint is invariably swollen, other inflammatory changes are often suppressed, especially if the patient is receiving steroids.

Tuberculous infections of the knee, now uncommon in the UK, have a slow onset spread over weeks. The knee appears small and globular, with the associated profound quadriceps wasting contributing to this appearance.

In gonococcal arthritis, great pain and tenderness, often apparently out of proportion to the local swelling and other signs, are the striking features of this condition.

When pus is suspected in a joint, aspiration should always be carried out to empty it and obtain specimens for bacteriological examination. If tuberculosis is suspected, synovial biopsy to obtain specimens for culture and histology is required. All knee infections are treated by splintage and an appropriate antibiotic regime.

The extensor mechanism of the knee

Extension of the knee is produced by the quadriceps muscle acting through the quadriceps ligament, patella, patellar ligament and tibial tubercle. *Weakness of extension* leads to instability, repeated joint trauma and effusion. There is often a vicious circle of pain → quadriceps inhibition → quadriceps wasting → knee instability → ligament stretching and further injury → pain. *Loss of full extension* also leads to instability, as there is failure of the screw-home mechanism which tightens the ligaments of the joint at terminal extension.

Rapid wasting of the quadriceps is seen in all painful and inflammatory conditions of the knee. Weakness of the quadriceps is also sometimes found in lesions of the upper lumbar intervertebral discs, as a sequel to poliomyelitis, in multiple sclerosis and other neurological disorders, and in the myopathies. Difficulty in diagnosis is common when wasting is the presenting feature of a diabetic neuropathy or secondary to femoral nerve palsy from an iliacus haematoma. Maintenance of good quadriceps tone and breaking the quadriceps vicious circle is an essential part of the treatment of virtually all conditions affecting the knee joint.

Disruption of the extensor mechanism of the knee is seen in a number of conditions. *Fractures of the patella* seldom give difficulty in diagnosis provided the appropriate radiographs are taken. *Ruptures of the quadriceps tendon or patellar ligament* result from sudden, violent contraction of the quadriceps and are seen in the middle-aged when there has been some accompanying degenerative change in the structures involved. *Avulsion of the tibial tuberosity* may also be seen as a result of a sudden muscle contraction. All these acute lesions are generally treated surgically.

There are a number of conditions short of disruption which may affect the patellar ligament and its extremities, with the generic title of jumper's knee. In the *Sinding-Larsen-Johansson* syndrome, seen in children in the 10–14 age group, there is aching pain in the knee, associated with X-ray changes in the distal pole of the patella. *Osgood-Schlatter's disease* (which is often thought due to a partial avulsion of the tuberosity) occurs in the 10–16 age group. There is recurrent pain over the tibial tuberosity which becomes tender and prominent. Radiographs may show partial detachment or fragmentation of the tuberosity. Pain usually ceases with closure of the epiphysis, and the management is usually conservative. In an older age group (16–30) the patellar ligament itself may become painful and tender. This almost invariably occurs in athletes, and there may be a history of giving-way of the knee. CT scans may show changes in the patellar ligament which becomes expanded centrally. Exploration and incision of the patellar ligament are usually advised.

The ligaments of the knee

The cruciate, collateral, posterior and capsular ligaments, and the menisci, form an integrated stabilising system which prevents the tibia from shifting or tilting under the femur in an abnormal fashion. The pathological movements which may occur after ligamentous injury are (a) tilting of the knee into varus or valgus, (b) shifting of the tibia directly forwards or backwards, and (c) rotation of the tibia under the femur so that the medial or lateral tibial condyle subluxes forwards or backwards.

Ligament injuries are important to detect as they may account for appreciable disability in the form of incidents of giving-way of the joint, recurrent effusion, lack of confidence in the knee, difficulty in undertaking strenuous or athletic activities, and sometimes trouble in using stairs or walking on uneven ground.

The diagnosis and interpretation of instability in the knee is difficult and somewhat controversial for the following reasons:

1. Several structures may be simultaneously damaged.

2. Each of the main ligamentous structures round the knee has primary and secondary supportive functions: if a ligament whose primary role in preventing a certain abnormal movement is torn, that movement may be prevented by other structures which have a secondary supporting function. Later, however, the secondary structures may stretch, giving rise to increasing disability. As a result, the symptoms and the clinical signs may be masked during the intial stages, and only become obvious later.

3. A plethora of terms describing these instabilities makes the interpretation of the literature somewhat difficult. The present trend both in examination and management is to analyse and treat the instability; less emphasis is placed on the diagnosis of the precise anatomical disturbance. Nevertheless, the main supportive structures have certain distinctive features which should be noted.

The medial ligament and capsule

The medial ligament stretches between the femur and tibia, and has superficial and deep layers. Considerable violence (usually in the form of a valgus strain or a blow on the lateral side of the knee) is required to damage the medial ligament. When the forces are moderately severe, a few fibres only may be torn, usually near the upper attachment (sprain of the medial ligament). Then, when the knee is examined clinically, no instability will be demonstrated, but stretching the ligament will cause pain. Minor tears of the medial ligament may be followed eventually by calcification in the accompanying haematoma, and this may give rise to sharply localised pain at the upper attachment (Pellegrini-Stieda disease).

With greater violence, the whole of the deep part of the ligament ruptures, followed in order by the superficial part, the medial capsule, the posterior ligament, the posterior cruciate ligament and sometimes finally the anterior cruciate ligament. Acute complete tears give rise to serious instability in the knee which can move or be moved into valgus. They are usually dealt with by immediate surgical repair. Partial tears do well by immobilization for 6 weeks in a pipe-stem plaster. Chronic lesions may be accompanied by tibial condylar subluxation (see later), although there is some doubt as to whether this is indeed possible without there being some additional damage to the anterior cruciate ligament. Surgical treatment may be indicated for such instability. Medial ligament tears may accompany fractures of the lateral tibial table, which will require additional attention.

The lateral ligament and capsule

This ligament may be damaged by blows on the medial side of the knee, throwing it into varus. It most frequently tears at its fibular attachment. As in the case of the medial ligament, increasing violence will lead to tearing of the posterior capsular ligament and the cruciates. In addition, the common peroneal nerve may be stretched and sometimes irreversibly damaged. These injuries are usually treated by operative repair, and where applicable, exploration of the common peroneal nerve. Again, any associated fracture of the medial tibial table may require attention. Chronic lesions may be associated with tibial condylar subluxations.

The anterior cruciate ligament

Impaired anterior cruciate ligament function is seen most frequently in association with tears of the medial meniscus. In some cases this is due to progressive stretching and attrition rupture. (This may occur as an attempt is made to obtain full extension in a knee blocked by a meniscal fragment.) In others, the anterior cruciate ligament tears at the same time as the meniscus, and in the most severe injuries the medial ligament may also be affected (O'Donoghue's triad).

Isolated ruptures of the anterior cruciate ligament are uncommon and are not usually treated surgically unless accompanied by avulsion of bone at the anterior tibial attachment or if there is a so-called positive pivot shift test.

When the tear is acute and accompanies a meniscal lesion, the meniscus is preserved if at all possible to reduce the risks of tibial subluxation and secondary osteoarthritic change, although the damage may be such that excision cannot be avoided. After attention to the meniscus, many would then advocate direct repair of the anterior cruciate ligament, supplemented by a ligament reinforcement (e.g. using a woven synthetic), or a reconstruction procedure (e.g. using part of the patellar ligament and its bony attachments). When an acute anterior cruciate tear is associated with damage to the medial or less commonly the lateral collateral ligament, a similar approach may be employed.

Chronic anterior cruciate ligament laxity generally results from old injuries, and may cause problems from acute, chronic or recurrent tibial subluxations. There may be a history of giving-way of the knee, episodic pain, and functional impairment. There is often quadriceps wasting and effusion, and secondary osteoarthritis may develop. Intense quadriceps and hamstring muscle building is usually advised as a first measure. In resistant cases, a ligament reconstruction may be advocated. There is no doubt that procedures of this nature are often intially very successful, but as yet the long-term results tend to be disappointing.

The posterior cruciate ligament

Posterior cruciate ligament tears are produced when in a flexed knee the tibia is forcibly pushed backwards (as for example in a car accident, when the upper part of the shin strikes the dashboard). Most advise immediate surgical repair if the injury is seen at the acute stage, as persisting instability and osteoarthritis are common sequelae in the untreated case.

Rotatory instability in the knee: tibial condylar subluxations

In this group of conditions, when the knee is stressed, the tibia may sublux forwards or backwards on either the medial or lateral side, giving rise to pain and a feeling of instability in the joint. The main forms are as follows:

1. *The medial tibial condyle subluxes anteriorly* (antero-medial rotatory instability): In the most severe cases, this occurs as a result of tears of both the anterior cruciate ligament and the medial structures (medial ligament and capsule). The medial meniscus may also be damaged and contribute to the instability. In the less severe cases there is some controversy regarding which structures may be spared. Clinically, the condition should be suspected on the evidence of the anterior drawer and Lachman tests, and the demonstration of instability on applying a valgus stress to the joint.

2. *The lateral tibial condyle subluxes anteriorly* (antero-lateral rotatory instability): In the more severe cases, the anterior cruciate ligament and the lateral structures are torn, and there may be an associated lesion of the anterior horn of the lateral meniscus. It may be diagnosed from the results of the anterior drawer and Lachman tests, and by demonstrating instability on applying a varus stress to the knee, although a number of specific tests may afford additional confirmation.

3. *The lateral tibial condyle subluxes posteriorly* (postero-lateral rotatory instability): This may follow rupture of the lateral and posterior cruciate ligaments, and be recognised by the presence of instability in the knee on applying varus stress, in combination with eliciting an abnormal posterior drawer test. There are also specific tests for this instability.

4. *Combinations of these lesions* (particularly 1 and 2, and 2 and 3) may be found, especially where there is major ligamentous disruption of the knee.

Where symptoms are demanding, and when a firm diagnosis has been established, the stability of the joint may be restored by an appropriate ligamentous re-attachment or reinforcement procedure.

Lesions of the menisci

Congenital discoid meniscus. This abnormality, most frequently involving the lateral meniscus, commonly gives rise to presenting symptoms in childhood. The meniscus does not have its usual semilunar form, but is rather more D-shaped, with its central edge extending in towards the tibial spines. It may produce a very pronounced clicking from the lateral compartment, a block to extension of the joint, and other derangement signs. It is usually treated by excision.

Meniscus tears in the young adult. The commonest cause is a sporting injury, when a twisting strain is applied to the flexed, weight-bearing leg. The entrapped meniscus commonly splits longitudinally, and its free edge may displace inwards towards the centre of the joint (bucket-handle tear). This prevents full extension (with physiological locking of the joint), and if an attempt is made to straighten the knee, a painful elastic resistance is felt ('springy block to full extension'). In the case of the medial meniscus, prolonged loss of full extension may lead to stretching and eventual rupture of the anterior cruciate ligament.

The aim in treating meniscal tears is to correct the mechanical problems that they have created within the joint, while preserving as much of each meniscus as is possible; this, it is thought, will reduce the risks of instability and the onset of secondary osteoarthritis. In many cases the torn part of the meniscus (e.g. the handle of a bucket-handle tear) only is excised, but some major meniscal tears may require total meniscectomy. In certain lesions, particularly those involving the periphery of the meniscus, repair by direct suture is sometimes attempted. Most surgical procedures are performed arthroscopically, thereby facilitating early recovery.

Degenerative meniscus lesions in the middle-aged. Loss of elasticity in the menisci through degenerative changes associated with the ageing process may give rise to horizontal cleavage tears within the substance of the meniscus. These tears may not be associated with any remembered traumatic incident, and sharply localised tenderness in the joint line is a common feature. In an appreciable number of cases symptoms may resolve without surgery, although excision may sometimes be required.

Cysts of the menisci. Ganglion-like cysts occur in both menisci, but are much more common in the lateral. Medial meniscus cysts must be carefully distinguished from ganglions arising from the pes anserinus (the insertion of sartorius, gracilis and semitendinosus). In true cysts there is often a history of a blow on the side of the knee over the meniscus. They are tender, and as they restrict the mobility of the menisci, they render them more susceptible to tears. They are generally treated by excision, and sometimes simultaneous meniscectomy may be required, especially if there are problems with recurrence. Some workers believe that all meniscal cysts have an associated tear, and prefer to deal with the problem by arthroscopic resection of the tear and simultaneous decompression of the cyst through the substance of the meniscus.

Patello-femoral instability

The patella always has a tendency to lateral dislocation, as the tibial tuberosity lies lateral to the dynamic axis of the quadriceps (Fig. 11.B); any tightness in the extensor mechanism (e.g. from quadriceps contraction or fibrosis) generates a lateral component of force which tends to displace the patella laterally. Normally, at the beginning of knee flexion, the patella engages in the groove separating the two femoral condyles (the trochlea), and this keeps it in place as flexion continues. This system may be disturbed in a number of ways. The side thrusts which tend to cause the patella to sublux laterally may be increased by an abnormal lateral insertion of the quadriceps, tight lateral structures, or by increases in the angle between the axis of the quadriceps and the line of the patellar ligament (e.g. as a result of knock-knee deformity or by a broad pelvis). The lateral condyle which supports and guides the patella may be deficient, or the patella itself may be small and poorly formed (hypoplasia). If the patella is highly placed (patella alta) it may fail to engage in the condylar groove (trochlea) at the beginning of flexion. This condition is often associated with genu recurvatum. Medial to the patella the soft tissues which would normally help prevent an abnormal lateral excursion of the patella may be deficient, sometimes as a result of stretching from previous dislocations.

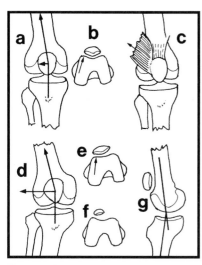

Fig. 11.B Some factors relating to patellar instability. Because the quadriceps and the patellar ligament meet at an angle (Q angle), there is a lateral component of force when the quadriceps contracts, and this tends to dislocate the patella laterally (a). This is resisted by the femoral sulcus in which the patella lies, and the prominence of the lateral femoral condyle (b). This mechanism may be interfered with by an abnormal lateral insertion of the quadriceps (c), or an increase in the Q (quadriceps) angle (e.g. in knock knee) (d). The lateral femoral condyle may be hypoplastic and the condylar sulcus shallow (e); or the patella itself may be hypoplastic (f). The patella may be highly placed, especially in genu recurvatum (g), so that it fails to engage in the condylar gutter.

There are a number of conditions characterised by loss of normal patellar alignment:

Acute traumatic dislocation of the patella. This injury occurs most frequently in adolescent females during athletic activity (e.g. playing hockey). There may be a history of a direct blow on the inside of the knee. The patella dislocates laterally, and causes a striking deformity which has often reduced by the time that the patient is first seen. If, however, it is still displaced when the patient reaches hospital, it is reduced by manipulation; thereafter a period of fixation in a cylinder plaster is usually advised in all cases. Some advocate exploration, with reefing of the medial structures and release of those on the lateral side.

Recurrent lateral dislocation. Further painful dislocations of the patella may occur, often with increasing frequency and ease. Surgical stabilisation is usually advised in the well-established case, to reduce the risks of secondary patello-femoral osteoarthritis and prevent the danger that the patient might be exposed to should the dislocation occur in a hazardous situation. The type of procedure carried out is aimed at correcting the underlying defect, which should be established by investigation.

Congenital dislocation of the patella. The patella may be dislocated at birth in association with congenital abnormalities. The dislocation is irreducible. Surgical correction is difficult, and the results often poor.

Habitual dislocation of the patella. The patella dislocates every time the knee flexes, and this is pain-free. It often arises in childhood and may be due to an abnormal attachment of the ilio-tibial tract. In a number of cases in the neonatal period it results from fibrosis in a quadriceps muscle which has been used for intra-muscular injections. The condition also occurs in joint laxity syndromes. In the established case there is usually a severe associated deficiency in the trochlea. It may be treated by extensive lateral releases, medial reefing, and sometimes transposition of the tibial tubercle.

Permanent dislocation of the patella. This is uncommon, and may result from an untreated childhood or adolescent dislocation. The patella is permanently displaced, and the power of the quadriceps and the strength of the knee are greatly reduced.

Retro-patellar pain syndromes/chondromalacia patellae

These are characterised by chronic ill-localised pain at the front of the knee, often made worse by prolonged sitting, walking on slopes or stairs. It is commonest in females in the 15–35 age group, and the pathology is often uncertain. In some there is softening or fibrillation of the articular cartilage lining the patella (chondromalacia patellae), and some of these cases progress to develop patello-femoral osteoarthritis.

Cases suffering from retro-patellar knee pain may be divided into two groups: in one, no significant cause can be found, while in the other there is evidence of patellar malalignment. In this latter group some of the factors responsible for recurrent dislocation may be found to be present (even although there may be no history of frank dislocation). While symptoms are often prolonged, they are not usually severe, and may be dealt with by restriction of the activities which are known to aggravate the symptoms, and by physiotherapy. In some cases, where symptoms are particularly severe and unresponsive, and where there is evidence of malalignment, lateral release and patellar débridement procedures are often practised. Where the articular surface of the patella is seriously involved, patellectomy is sometimes advocated.

Osteochondritis dissecans

This occurs most frequently in males in the second decade of life, and most commonly involves the medial femoral condyle. Possibly as a result of impingement against the tibial spines or the cruciate ligaments, a segment of bone undergoes avascular necrosis, and a line of demarcation becomes established between this area and the underlying healthy bone. Complete separation may occur so that a loose body is formed. The symptoms are initially of aching pain and recurring effusion, with perhaps locking of the joint if a loose body is present. Good results generally follow conservative treatment with quadriceps exercises and continued weight-bearing if the condition is found before epiphyseal closure. If the fragment becomes loose, it should be fixed surgically (e.g. with the use of Smillie pins). If the lesion is long-standing, with a fragment smaller than its crater, it should be excised. The cavity may be drilled in an attempt to encourage vascularisation of its base. In all cases, the damaging effects of a loose body must be prevented.

Fat pad injuries

The infrapatellar fat pads may become tender and swollen and give rise to pain on extension of the knee, especially if they are nipped between the articulating surfaces of femur and tibia. This may occur as a complication of osteoarthritis, but is seen more frequently in young women when the fat pads swell in association with premenstrual fluid retention. Excision of the pads may be required to relieve the symptoms.

Loose bodies

Loose bodies are seen most frequently as a sequel to osteoarthritis or osteochondritis dissecans. Much less commonly, numerous loose bodies are formed by an abnormal synovial membrane in the condition of synovial chondromatosis. Loose bodies are treated by excision, but synovectomy may be required in synovial chondromatosis if massive recurrence is to be avoided.

Affections of the articular surfaces

Osteoarthritis (osteoarthrosis). The stresses of weight-bearing mainly involve the medial compartment of the knee, and it is in this area that primary osteoarthritis usually first occurs. This is an exceedingly common condition, arising without any obvious previous pathology in the joint. Overweight, the degenerative changes accompanying old age, and overwork are common factors. Secondary osteoarthritis may follow ligament and meniscus injuries, recurrent dislocation of the patella, osteochondritis dissecans, joint infections and other previous pathology. It is seen in association with knock-knee and bow-leg deformities which throw additional mechanical stresses on the joint.

In osteoarthritis, the articular cartilage undergoes progressive change, flaking off into the joint and thereby producing the narrowing that is a striking feature of radiographs of this condition. The subarticular bone may become eburnated, and often small marginal osteophytes and cysts are formed. Exposure of bone and free nerve endings gives rise to pain and crepitus on movement. Distortion of the joint surfaces is one cause of progressive loss of movement and fixed flexion deformities. Treatment is generally conservative, by quadriceps exercises, short-wave diathermy, analgesics and weight reduction. Surgery may be considered in severe cases. The procedures available include joint replacement, osteotomy (especially in cases of genu varum and valgum), and arthrodesis.

Rheumatoid arthritis. Characteristically the knee is warm to the touch, there is effusion, limitation of movements, muscle wasting, synovial thickening, tenderness and pain. Fixed flexion, valgus and (less commonly) varus deformities are quite common. Generally other joints are also involved, although the mono-articular form is occasionally seen. Active cases are often treated by synovectomy in an attempt to avoid or delay the progress of the condition. An acute flare-up of symptoms may be treated by temporary splintage. Either joint replacement, osteotomy or arthrodesis may be considered in the well-selected case.

Reiter's syndrome. This usually presents as a chronic effusion accompanied by discomfort in the joint. It is often bilateral, with an associated conjunctivitis. There is often a history of urethritis or colitis.

Ankylosing spondylitis. The first symptoms of ankylosing spondylitis are generally in the spine, but occasionally the condition presents at the periphery, with swelling and discomfort in the knee joint. Stiffness of the spine and radiographic changes in the sacro-iliac joints are nevertheless almost invariably present.

Disturbances of alignment

Genu varum (bow leg). This commonly occurs as a growth abnormality of early childhood, and usually resolves spontaneously. Rarely genu varum is caused by a growth disturbance involving both the tibial epiphysis and proximal tibial shaft (tibia vara), and treatment by osteotomy may be required. In adults this deformity most frequently results from osteoarthritis, where there is narrowing of the medial joint compartment. It also occurs in Paget's disease and rickets. It is less common in rheumatoid arthritis unless secondary osteoarthritic changes supervene in that condition.

Genu valgum (knock knee). This is seen most often in young children where it is usually associated with flat foot. Nearly all cases resolve spontaneously by the age of 6. It is also seen in the plump adolescent girl, and it may be a contributory factor in recurrent dislocation of the patella. In adults it most frequently occurs as a result of the bone softening and ligamentous stretching accompanying rheumatoid arthritis. It occurs after uncorrected fractures of the lateral tibial table with depression, and as a sequel to a number of paralytic neurological disorders where there is ligament stretching and altered epiphyseal growth. Selected cases may be treated by corrective osteotomy.

Genu recurvatum. Hyperextension at the knee is seen after ruptures of the anterior cruciate ligament and in girls where the growth of the upper tibial epiphysis may be retarded from much point work in ballet classes or from the wearing of high-heeled shoes in early adolescence. In the latter cases there is corresponding elevation of the patella (patella alta), contributing to a tendency to recurrent dislocation. More rarely, the deformity is seen in congenital joint laxity, poliomyelitis and Charcot's disease.

Bursitis

Cystic swelling occurring in the popliteal region in both sexes is usually referred to as enlargement of the semimembranosus bursa. In fact, several of the bursae known to the anatomist may be involved — singly or together. The swelling sometimes communicates with the knee joint and may fluctuate in size. Rupture may lead to the appearance of bruising on the dorsum of the foot, and this may help to distinguish it from deep venous thrombosis or cellulitis. If there is any doubt about the diagnosis, or if the swelling is persistent and producing symptoms, excision is advised.

Fluctuant bursal swellings may also occur over the patella (pre-patellar bursitis or housemaid's knee) or the patellar ligament (infrapatellar bursitis or clergyman's knee). Chronic pre-patellar bursitis, with or without local infection, is common in miners where it is referred to as 'beat knee'; it is also associated with other occupations where prolonged kneeling is unavoidable (e.g. it is common in plumbers and carpet layers). If the swelling is bulky or tense it is aspirated; recurrent swellings, if troublesome, are excised.

How to diagnose a knee complaint

1. Note the patient's age and sex, bearing in mind the following important distribution of the common knee conditions:

Age group	Males	Females
0–12	Discoid lateral meniscus	Discoid lateral meniscus
12–18	Osteochondritis dissecans Osgood-Schlatter's disease	First incidents of recurrent dislocation of the patella Osgood-Schlatter's disease
18–30	Longitudinal meniscus tears	Recurrent dislocation of the patella Chondromalacia patellae Fat pad injury
30–50	Rheumatoid arthritis	Rheumatoid arthritis

Age group	Males	Females
40–55	Degenerative meniscus lesions	Degenerative meniscus lesions
45+	Osteoarthrosis	Osteoarthritis

Table 11.1

Infections are comparatively uncommon and occur in both sexes in all age groups.

Reiter's syndrome occurs in adults of both sexes; ankylosing spondylitis nearly always occurs in male adults. Both are comparatively rare.

Ligamentous and extensor apparatus injuries occur in both sexes, but are rare in children.

2. Find out if the knee swells. An effusion indicates the presence of pathology which must be determined. (Note however that the absence of effusion does not necessarily eliminate significant pathology.)

3. Try to establish whether there is a mechanical problem (internal derangement) accounting for the patient's symptoms. Do this by:

(a) *Obtaining a convincing history of an initiating injury*. Note the degree of violence, and its direction. The initial incapacity is important. For example, a footballer is unlikely to be able to finish a game with a freshly torn meniscus. Note whether there was bruising or swelling after the injury, and whether the patient was able to weight-bear.

(b) *Asking if the knee 'gives way'*. 'Giving-way' of the knee on going down stairs or jumping from a height follows cruciate ligament tears, loss of full extension in the knee, and quadriceps wasting. 'Giving-way' on twisting movements or walking on uneven ground follows many meniscus injuries.

(c) *Asking if the knee 'locks'*. Patients often confuse stiffness and true locking. Ask the patient to show the position the knee is in if it locks. *Remember that the knee never locks in full extension.* Locking due to a torn meniscus generally allows the joint to be flexed fully or nearly fully, but the last 10–40° of extension are impossible. Attempts to obtain full extension are accompanied by pain. Ask what produces any locking. With long-standing meniscus lesions, a slight rotational force, such as the foot catching on the edge of a carpet, may be quite sufficient. In chronic lesions, weight-bearing is not an essential factor, locking not infrequently occurring during sleep. If the knee is not locked at the time of the patient's attendance, ask how it became free. Unlocking with a click is suggestive of a meniscus lesion. Locking from a loose body may occur at varying positions of flexion. Locking from a dislocating patella may be noted to be accompanied by deformity.

(d) *Asking about pain*. Find out the circumstances in which it is present and ask the patient if he can localise it by pointing to the site with one finger.

In a high proportion of cases the likely diagnosis will have been established by this stage, requiring only confirmation by clinical examination.

Additional investigations. Occasionally a firm diagnosis cannot be made on the basis of the history and clinical examination alone. The following additional investigations are often helpful:

Suspected internal derangement.

(a) *Arthroscopy.* This may give much useful information, and in conjunction with the clinical examination will permit a firm, accurate diagnosis to be made in the majority of cases. Incorrect diagnoses are most common in lesions involving the menisci in their posterior thirds. An increasing number of conditions are amenable to arthroscopic surgery, which can often follow diagnostic arthroscopy in the same session.

(b) *MRI scans.* These can be useful in diagnosing lesion of the menisci and ligaments, but it has been suggested that they should only be used if there is diagnostic uncertainty. An accuracy of 90% is claimed. However, there is often an increase in signal intensity in the region of the posterior third of the medial mensicus (from the myxoid degeneration which may occur in the ageing process, or after previous surgery), and this can lead to false interpretations.

(c) *Arthrography.* This may be helpful, although the interpretation of the radiographs is specialised and often difficult.

(d) *Examination under anaesthesia.* If pain prevents full examination (e.g. by preventing flexion), anaesthesia may be helpful. This is frequently followed by arthroscopy.

(e) *Provocative exercises.* These are carried out under the supervision of a trained physiotherapist. They aim to throw considerable stress on the menisci by applying torsional stresses to the weight-bearing knee. If the meniscus has been damaged, the exercises are likely to be followed by localised pain, swelling and sometimes even locking, so that any doubtful meniscus lesion is likely to declare itself.

Suspected acute infections.

(a) Aspiration and culture of the synovial fluid.
(b) Blood culture.
(c) Full blood count, including differential white count, and estimation of the sedimentation rate and C-reactive protein.

Suspected tuberculosis of the knee.

(a) Chest radiograph.
(b) Synovial biopsy, with specimens of synovial membrane being sent for both histological and bacteriological examination. At the same time, synovial fluid specimens are also sent for bacteriology and sensitivities.
(c) Mantoux test.

Suspected rheumatoid arthritis.

(a) Examination of other joints.
(b) Estimations of rheumatoid factor.

(c) Full blood count and sedimentation rate.
(d) Serum uric acid.

Further investigation of poor mineralisation, bone erosions etc.

(a) Estimation of serum calcium, phosphate and alkaline phosphatase.
(b) Estimation of rheumatoid factor.
(c) Serum uric acid.
(d) Full blood count and differential count.
(e) Skeletal survey and chest radiograph.
(f) Radio-isotope scan.
(g) Bone biopsy.

Further investigation of chronic effusion, aspirate negative.

(a) Tests as for suspected rheumatoid arthritis.
(b) Brucellosis agglutination tests.
(c) Radiography of the chest and sacro-iliac joints.
(d) Exploration and synovial biopsy.

Further investigation of severe undiagnosed pain.

(a) Radiography of the chest, pelvis and hips.
(b) Exploration.

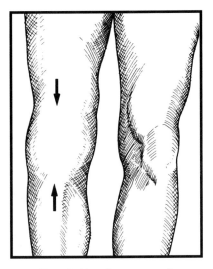

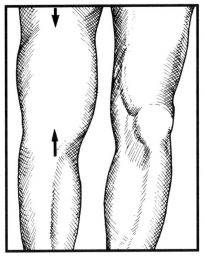

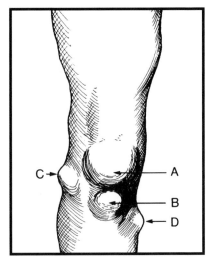

1. *Swelling* (1): Note the presence of swelling confined to the limits of the synovial cavity and suprapatellar pouch — suggesting effusion, haemarthrosis, pyarthrosis or a space-occupying lesion in the joint.

2. *Swelling* (2): Note if the swelling extends beyond the limits of the joint cavity, suggesting infection (of the joint, femur or tibia), tumour or major injury.

3. *Lumps:* Note presence of localised swellings, e.g. (A) pre-patellar bursitis (housemaid's knee); (B) infra-patellar bursitis (clergyman's knee); (C) meniscus cyst (in joint line); (D) diaphyseal aclasis (exostosis, often multiple and sometimes familial) (see also 11, 31). In beat knee there is chronic anterior bursal enlargement, often with thickening of the overlying skin.

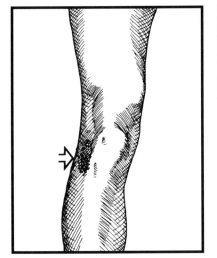

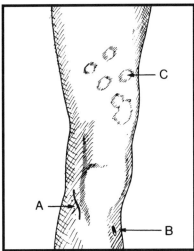

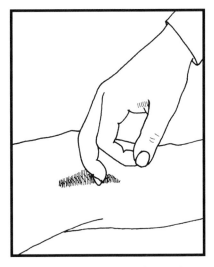

4. *Discoloration:* Note any bruising which suggests trauma to the superficial tissues, or knee ligaments. Note that bruising is not usually seen in meniscus injuries. Note any redness suggesting inflammation.

5. *Skin marks:* Note (A) scars of previous injury or surgery — the relevant history must be obtained. (B) Sinus scars are indicative of previous infections, often of bone, and with the potential for reactivation. (C) Evidence of psoriasis, with the possibility of psoriatic arthritis.

6. *Temperature* (1): Note any increased local heat and its extent, suggesting in particular rheumatoid arthritis or infection. There may also be increased local heat as part of the inflammatory response to injury, and in the presence of rapidly growing tumours. Always compare the two sides.

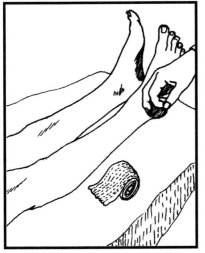

7. *Temperature* (2): A warm knee and cold foot suggest a popliteal artery block. Always make allowance for any warm bandage the patient may have been wearing just prior to the examination, and check the peripheral pulses.

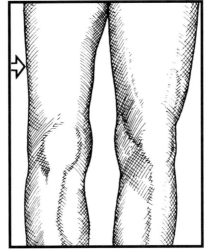

8. *The quadriceps* (1): Inspect the relaxed quadriceps muscle. Slight wasting and loss of bulk are normally apparent on careful inspection.

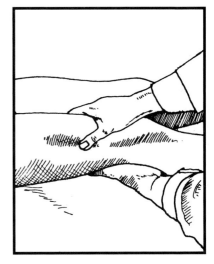

9. *The quadriceps* (2): Examine the contracted quadriceps. Place a hand behind the knee and ask the patient to press the leg against the hand. Feel the muscle tone with the free hand.

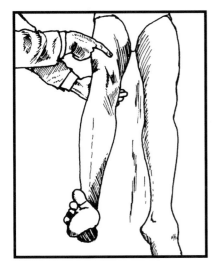

10. *The quadriceps* (3): Repeat the last test, this time asking the patient to dorsiflex the inverted foot. This demonstrates the important vastus medialis portion of the quadriceps, which may be involved in recurrent dislocation of the patella.

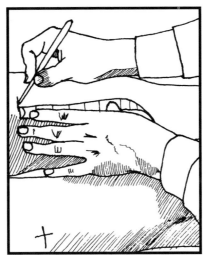

11. *The quadriceps* (4): Substantial wasting, especially in the fat leg, may be confirmed by measurement, assuming the other limb is normal. This test, being objective, may be valuable for repeat assessments and in medico-legal cases. Begin by locating the knee joint (see 11, 28) and mark it with a ball point pen. Make a second mark on the skin 18 cm above this. Repeat on the other leg.

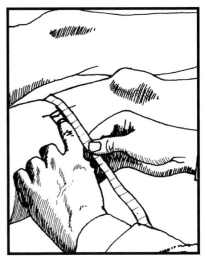

12. *The quadriceps* (5): Compare the circumference of the legs at the marked levels. Wasting of the quadriceps occurs most frequently as the result of disuse, generally from a painful or unstable lesion of the knee, or from infection or rheumatoid arthritis.

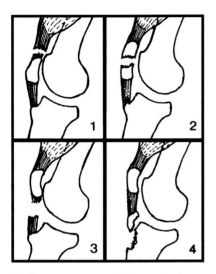

13. *Extensor apparatus* (1): Loss of active extension of the knee (excluding paralytic conditions) follows (1) rupture of the quadriceps tendon, (2) many patellar fractures, (3) rupture of the patellar ligament or (4) avulsion of the tibial tubercle.

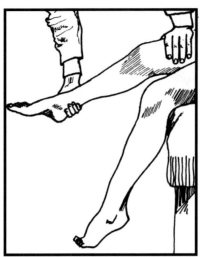

14. *Extensor apparatus* (2): With the patient sitting with his legs over the end of the examination couch, ask him to straighten the leg while you support the ankle with one hand. Feel for quadriceps contraction, and look for active extension of the limb.

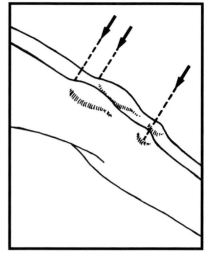

15. *Extensor apparatus* (3): Note the position of the patella in relation to the joint line and the tibial tuberosity. If its upper border is high, this suggests that it is proximally displaced, and that you should suspect lesion 2, 3 or 4.

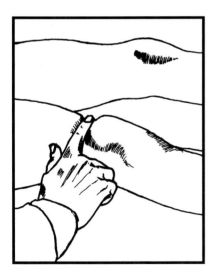

16. *Extensor apparatus* (4): If the patella is normally placed, lay a finger along its upper border. Loss of normal soft tissue resistance is suggestive of a rupture of the quadriceps tendon (1).

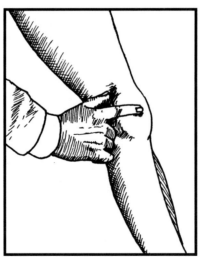

17. *Extensor apparatus* (5): Look for gaps and tenderness at the other levels to help differentiate between lesions 2, 3 and 4. Radiographs of the knee are essential.

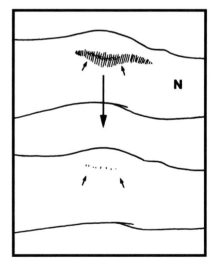

18. *Effusion* (1): Small effusions are detected most easily by inspection. The first signs are bulging at the sides of the patellar ligament and obliteration of the hollows at the medial and lateral edges of the patella.

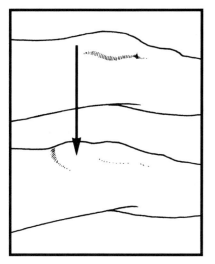

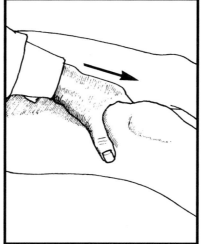

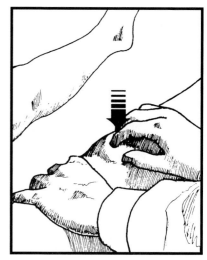

19. *Effusion* (2): With greater effusion into the knee the suprapatellar pouch becomes distended. Effusion indicates synovial irritation from trauma or inflammation.

20. *Effusion* (3): *patellar tap:* Squeeze any excess fluid out of the suprapatellar pouch with the index and thumb, slid firmly distally from a point about 15 cm above the knee to the level of the upper border of the patella.

21. *Effusion* (4): *patellar tap:* Place the tips of the thumb and three fingers of the free hand squarely on the patella, and jerk it quickly downwards. A click indicates the presence of effusion. If, however, the effusion is slight or tense, the tap test will be negative.

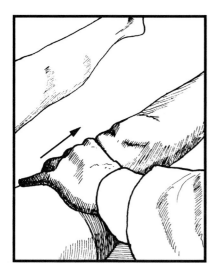

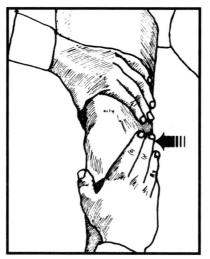

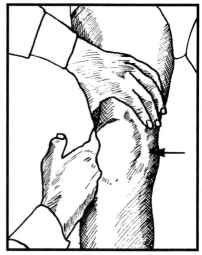

22. *Effusion* (5): *fluid displacement test* (1): Small effusions may be detected by this manoeuvre. Evacuate the suprapatellar pouch as before in the patellar tap test.

23. *Effusion* (6): *fluid displacement test* (2): Stroke the medial side of the joint to displace any excess fluid in the main joint cavity to the lateral side of the joint.

24. *Effusion* (7): *fluid displacement test* (3): Now stroke the lateral side of the joint while watching the medial closely. Any excess fluid present will be seen to move across the joint and distend the medial side. This test will be negative if the effusion is gross and tense.

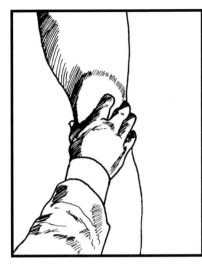

25. *Haemarthrosis:* A haemarthrosis is a sign of major joint pathology, is usually obvious within half an hour of injury, and gives a doughy feel in the suprapatellar region. A tense haemarthrosis should be aspirated to relieve pain and permit a more thorough clinical (and usually) arthroscopic examination.

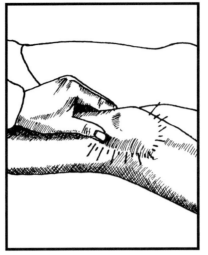

26. *Pyarthrosis:* Tenderness in pyarthrosis is usually widespread. There is generally a severe systemic upset and quadriceps wasting. If pyarthrosis is suspected, the knee should always be aspirated.

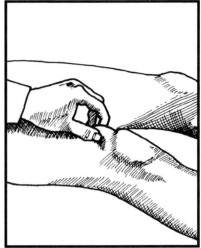

27. *Synovial membrane:* Pick up the skin and the relaxed quadriceps tendon to assess the thickness of the synovial membrane in the suprapatellar pouch. The synovial membrane is thickened in inflammatory conditions, e.g. rheumatoid arthritis, and in villo-nodular synovitis.

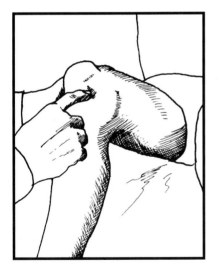

28. *Tenderness* (1): It is the first essential to identify the joint line quite clearly. Begin by flexing the knee, and looking for the hollows at the sides of the patellar ligament; these lie over the joint line. Then confirm by feeling with the fingers or thumb for the soft hollow of the joint, with the firm prominences of the femur above and the tibia below.

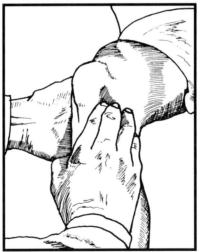

29. *Tenderness* (2): *joint line structures:* Begin by palpating carefully from the front of the joint backwards along the joint line on each side. Localised tenderness here is commonest in meniscus, collateral ligament and fat pad injuries.

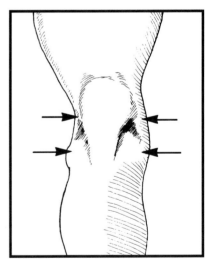

30. *Tenderness* (3): *collateral ligaments:* Now systematically examine the upper and lower attachments of the collateral ligaments. Associated bruising and oedema are features of acute injuries.

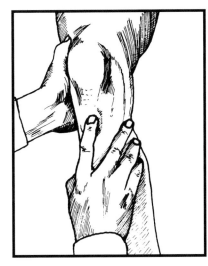

31. *Tenderness* (4): *tibial tubercle:* In children and adolescents, tenderness is found over the tibial tubercle (which may be prominent) in Osgood-Schlatter's disease and after acute avulsion injuries of the patellar ligament and its tibial attachment. Tenderness over the lower pole of the patella is found in Sinding-Larsen-Johansson disease.

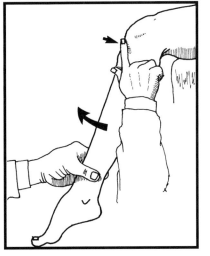

32. *Tenderness* (5): *patellar ligament:* Where in an athletic patient a problem with the patellar ligament is suspected, look for patellar ligament tenderness while the patient is attempting to extend the leg against resistance. This test is best performed with the leg over the end of the examination couch.

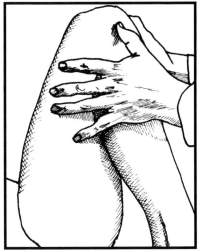

33. *Tenderness* (6): *femoral condyles:* In suspected osteochondritis dissecans, flex the knee fully and look for tenderness over the femoral condyle. Osteochondritis dissecans most frequently involves the medial femoral condyles, and particular attention should therefore be paid to the medial side.

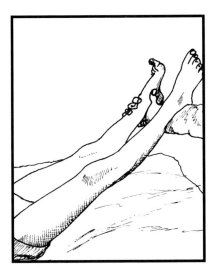

34. *Movements* (1): *extension:* First make sure that the knee can be fully extended. If in doubt, lift both legs and sight along the good and affected leg. Full extension is recorded as 0°. Loss of full extension may be recorded as 'The knee lacks X° of extension.'

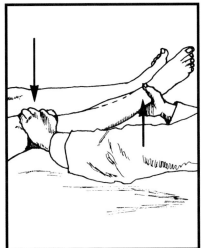

35. *Movements* (2): *extension:* Try to obtain full extension if this is not obviously present. A springy block to full extension is very suggestive of a bucket-handle meniscus tear. A rigid block to full extension (commonly described as a fixed flexion deformity) is often present in arthritic conditions affecting the knee.

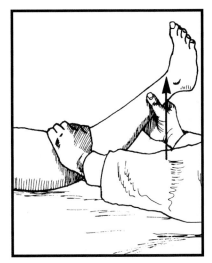

36. *Movements* (3): *hyperextension (genu recurvatum):* This is present if the knee extends beyond the point when the tibia and femur are in line. Attempt to demonstrate this by lifting the leg while at the same time pressing back on the patella. If severe, look for other signs of joint laxity, particularly in the elbow, wrist and fingers, keeping in mind the rare Ehlers-Danlos syndrome.

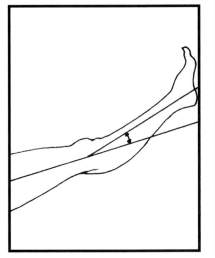

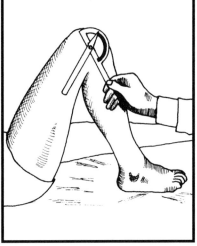

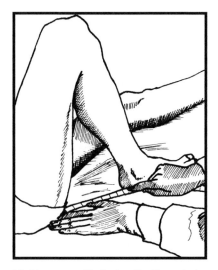

37. *Movements* (4): *hyperextension:* If present, record as 'X° hyperextension'. It is seen most frequently in girls, and is often associated with a high patella, chondromalacia patellae, recurrent dislocation of the patella, and sometimes tears of the anterior cruciate, medial ligament or medial meniscus.

38. *Movements* (5): *flexion* (1): Measure the range of flexion in degrees, starting from the zero position of normal full extension. Flexion of 135° and over is regarded as normal, but compare the two sides. There are many causes of loss of flexion, the commonest of which are effusion and arthritic conditions.

39. *Movements* (6): *flexion* (2): Alternatively, measure the heel-to-buttock distance with the leg fully flexed. This can be a very accurate way of detecting small alterations in the range (1 cm = 1.5° approximately) and is useful for checking daily or weekly progress.

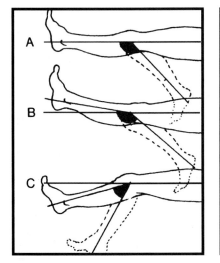

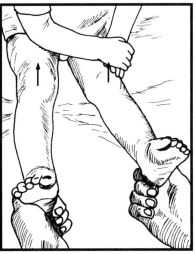

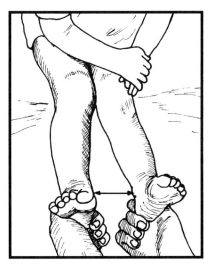

40. *Movements* (7): *recording:* The range of movements in the examples would be recorded as follows: (A) 0–135° (normal range); (B) 5° hyperextension — 140° flexion; (C) 10–60° (or 10° fixed flexion deformity with a further 50° flexion).

41. *Genu valgum (knock knee) in children* (1): Note whether unilateral or bilateral; the latter is more common. The severity of the deformity is recorded by measuring the intermalleolar gap. Grasp the child by the ankles, and rotate the legs until the patellae are vertical.

42. *Genu valgum in children* (2): Now bring the legs together to touch *lightly* at the knees, and measure the gap between the malleoli. (Normally the knees *and* malleoli should touch.) Serial measurements, often every 6 months, are used to check progress. Note that with growth, a static measurement is an angular improvement. In the 10–16 age group, < 8 cm in females and < 4 cm in males is regarded as normal.

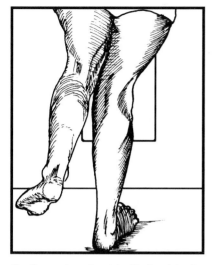

43. *Genu valgum in adults* (1): In adults the deformity is seen most often in association with rheumatoid arthritis. It is also common in teenage girls. It is best measured by X-ray, and the films should be taken with the patient taking all his weight on the affected side.

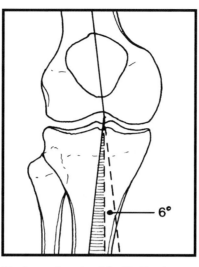

44. *Genu valgum in adults* (2): The degree of valgus may be roughly assessed by measuring the angle formed by the tibial and femoral shafts. Allow for the 'normal' angle, which is approximately 6° in the adult. The shaded area represents genu valgum. (Note that the tibio-femoral angle is virtually the same as the Q angle used in the assessment of patellar instability.)

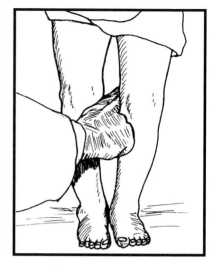

45. *Genu varum (bow leg)* (1): Measure the distance between the knees, using the fingers as a gauge. Ideally the patient should be weight-bearing, and it is essential that both patellae should be facing forwards to counter any effect of hip rotation. In the 10–16 age group, < 4 cm in females and < 5 cm in males is regarded as being within normal limits.

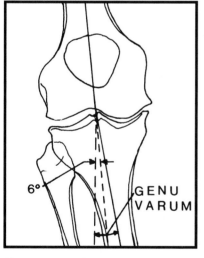

46. *Genu varum* (2): An assessment of the deformity may also be carried out radiographically as in genu valgum, with the patient weight-bearing during the exposure of the films. The deformity is seen most commonly in osteoarthritis and Paget's disease. It may occur in rheumatoid arthritis, although genu valgum is commoner in that condition.

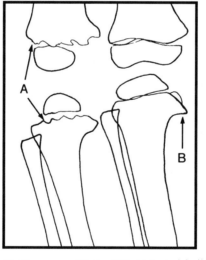

47. *Genu varum* (3): In children, radiography may be helpful. In (A) *rickets*, note the wide and irregular epiphyseal plates. In (B) *tibia vara*, note the sharply downturned medial metaphyseal border. Note that radiological varus is normal till a child is 18 months old.

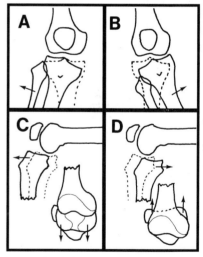

48. *Instability* (1): The following *potential* deformities may be looked for: (A) *valgus* (when the medial ligament is torn: severe when the posterior cruciate is also damaged); (B) *varus* (when the lateral ligament is torn: severe when the posterior cruciate is also torn); (C) *anterior displacement of the tibia* (anterior cruciate tears: worse if medial and/or lateral structures torn); (D) *posterior displacement of the tibia* (posterior cruciate ligament tears).

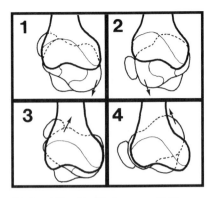

49. *Instability* (2): (E) *Rotatory:* (1) *The medial tibial condyle subluxes anteriorly* (antero-medial instability): this is usually due to combined tears of the anterior cruciate and medial structures; (2) *the lateral condyle subluxes anteriorly* (antero-lateral instability): this is usually due to tears of the anterior cruciate plus the lateral structures; (3) *the lateral tibial condyle subluxes posteriorly* (postero-lateral instability) or (4) the *medial tibial condyle subluxes posteriorly* (postero-medial instability). 3 and 4 are mainly due to tears of the posterior cruciate and lateral or medial structures. (5) Combinations of these instabilities (not shown).

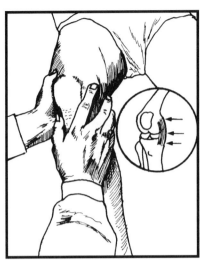

50. *Valgus stress instability* (1): Begin by examining the medial side of the joint, and the medial ligament in particular. *Tenderness* in injuries of the medial ligament is commonest at the upper (femoral) attachment and in the medial joint line. *Bruising* may be present after recent trauma, but haemarthrosis may be absent.

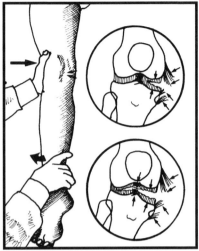

51. *Valgus stress instability* (2): Extend the knee fully. Use one hand as a fulcrum, and with the other attempt to abduct the leg. Look for the joint opening up, and the leg going into valgus. *Moderate* valgus is suggestive of a major medial and posterior ligament rupture. *Severe* valgus may indicate additional cruciate (particularly posterior cruciate) rupture.

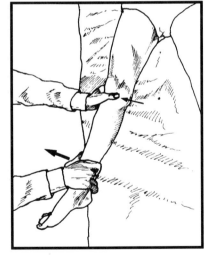

52. *Valgus stress instability* (3): If in doubt, use the heel of the hand as a fulcrum, and use the thumb or index, placed in the joint line, to detect any opening up of the joint as it is stressed. If there is still some uncertainty, compare the two sides.

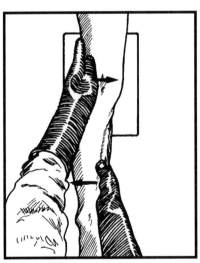

53. *Valgus stress instability* (4): *stress films* (1): If there is still some doubt, then radiographs of both knees should be taken while applying a valgus stress to each joint.

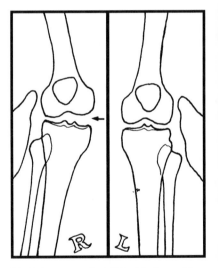

54. *Valgus stress instability* (5): *Stress films* (2): The films of both sides are then compared. Any instability should be obvious.

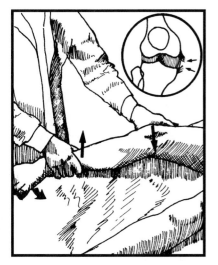

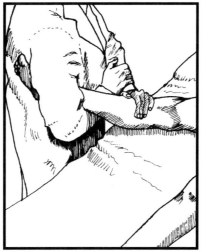

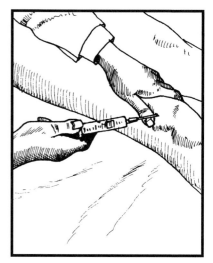

55. *Valgus stress instability* (6): If no instability has been demonstrated with the knee fully extended, repeat the tests with the knee flexed to 30° and the foot internally rotated. Some opening up of the joint is normal, and *it is essential to compare sides*. Demonstration of an abnormal amount of valgus suggests less extensive involvement of the medial structures (e.g. partial medial ligament tear).

56. *Valgus stress instability* (7): If the knee is very tender, and will not permit the pressure of a hand as a fulcrum, attempt to stress the ligament with this cross-over arm grip, with one hand placed over the proximal part of the tibia *distal* to the knee joint.

57. *Valgus stress instability* (8): If a haemarthrosis is present (and this is not always the case) preliminary aspiration of the joint may allow a more meaningful examination of the joint.

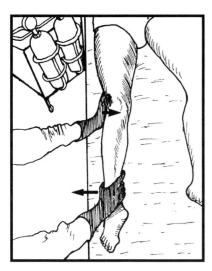

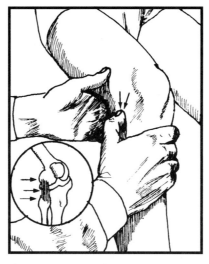

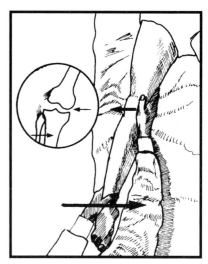

58. *Valgus stress instability* (9): If the knee remains too painful to permit examination, the joint should be fully tested under anaesthesia; there should be provision to carry on with a surgical repair should major instability be demonstrated (i.e. where there is the involvement of several major structures), or with an arthroscopy.

59. *Varus stress instability* (1): Begin by examining the lateral side of the joint. Tenderness is most common over the head of the fibula or in the lateral joint line in acute injuries of the lateral joint complex (lateral ligament and capsule).

60. *Varus stress instability* (2): Attempt to produce a varus deformity by placing one hand on the medial side of the joint and forcing the ankle medially. Carry out the test as in the case of valgus stress instability, first in full extension and then in 30° flexion, and compare one side with the other.

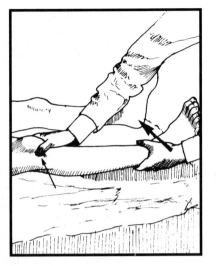

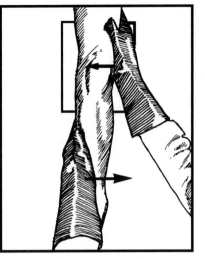

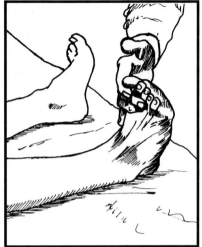

61. *Varus stress instability* (3): Again, for a more sensitive assessment of 'give', the thumb can be placed in the joint line. If there is varus instability in extension as well as flexion, it suggests tearing of the posterior cruciate ligament as well as the lateral ligament complex.

62. *Varus stress instability* (4): As in the case of valgus stress instability, stress films may be taken, and if examination is not possible even after aspiration, arrange to examine the knee under general anaesthesia.

63. *Varus stress instability* (5): Always check that the patient is able to dorsiflex the foot, to ensure that the motor fibres in the common peroneal nerve (lateral popliteal) have escaped damage.

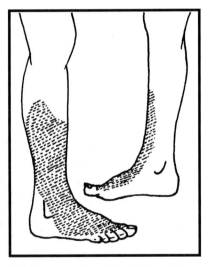

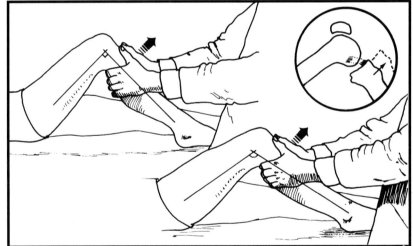

64. *Varus stress instability* (6): In addition, test for sensory disturbance in the distribution of the common peroneal nerve.

65. *The anterior drawer test* (1): Flex the knee to 90°, with the foot pointing straight forwards, and steady it by sitting close to it. Grasp the leg firmly with the thumbs on the tibial tubercle. Check that the hamstrings are relaxed, and jerk the leg towards you. Repeat with the knee flexed to 70°, and compare the sides. *Note:* significant displacement (i.e. the affected side more than the other) confirms anterior instability of the knee. When the displacement is marked (say 1.5 cm or more), then the anterior cruciate is almost certainly torn, and there is a strong possibility of associated damage to the medial complex (medial ligament and medial capsule) and even the lateral complex. If the displacement is less marked, and one tibial condyle moves further forward than the other, then the diagnosis is less clear: it may suggest an isolated anterior cruciate ligament laxity or a tibial condylar subluxation (rotatory instability).

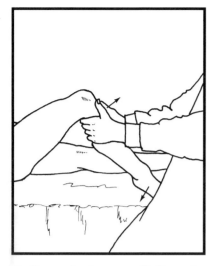

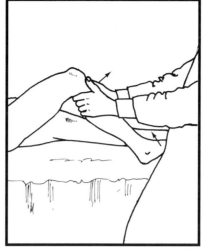

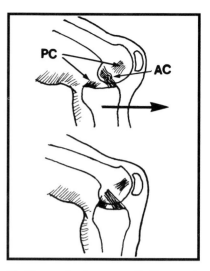

66. *The anterior drawer test* (2): Repeat the test with the foot in 15° of external rotation. Excess excursion of the medial tibial condyle suggests a degree of antero-medial (rotatory) instability, with possible involvement of the medial ligament as well as the anterior cruciate ligament.

67. *The anterior drawer test* (3): Now turn the foot into 30° of internal rotation, and repeat the test. Anterior subluxation of the lateral tibial condyle suggests some antero-lateral rotational instability, with possible damage to the posterior cruciate and the posterior ligament as well as the anterior cruciate ligament.

68. *The anterior drawer test* (4): Beware of the following fallacy: a tibia already displaced backwards as a result of a *posterior* cruciate ligament tear may give a false positive in this test. This also applies to the Lachman tests described in the following figures. Check by inspection of the contours of the knee prior to testing.

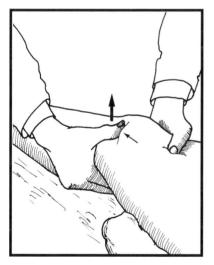

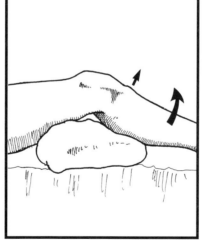

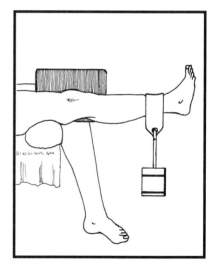

69. *The Lachman tests* (1): The Lachman tests are also used to detect anterior tibial instability. In the *manipulative Lachman test*, the knee should be relaxed and in about 15° flexion. One hand stabilises the femur, while the other tries to lift the tibia forwards. The test is positive if there is anterior tibial movement (detected with the thumb in the joint), with a spongy end point. Some claim that the test is easier to perform with the patient prone.

70. *The Lachman tests* (2): In the *active Lachman test* the relaxed knee is supported at 30° and the patient asked to extend it. If the test is positive, there will be anterior subluxation of the lateral tibial plateau as the quadriceps contracts, and posterior subluxation when the muscle relaxes. It is considered that this is best seen from the medial side. Repeat, resisting extension by applying pressure to the ankle.

71. *Radiological analysis of anterior cruciate function* (1): Anterior subluxation of the tibia in extension may also be demonstrated radiologically. The lower thigh is supported by a sandbag, and the leg extended against the resistance of a 7-kg weight. The limb should be in the neutral position, with the patella pointing upwards, and the X-ray film cassette placed between the legs.

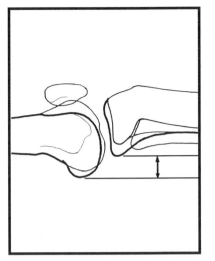

72. *Radiological analysis* (2): On the films, draw two lines parallel to the posterior cortex of the tibia, tangential to the medial tibial plateau and the medial femoral condyle. Measure the distance between them. *Normal: 3.5 mm, plus or minus 2 mm.* Ruptured anterior cruciate = 10.2 mm, plus or minus 2.7 mm. The latter figure is slightly increased if the medial meniscus is also torn. The diagnostic reliability is high.

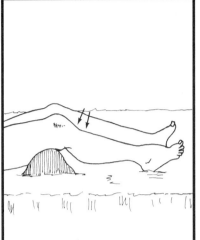

73. *Posterior tibial instability: testing the posterior cruciate ligament* (1): *the gravity test:* Rupture, detachment or stretching of the posterior cruciate ligament may permit the tibia to sublux backwards, frequently giving rise to a striking deformity of the knee which allows the diagnosis to be made on inspection alone. The knee should be flexed 20°, with a sandbag under the thigh.

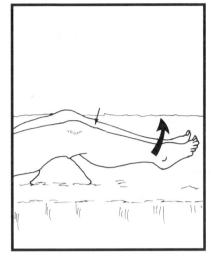

74. *Posterior cruciate ligament* (2): With the leg still in 20° flexion, ask the patient to lift the heel from the couch, while observing the knee from the lateral side. Any posterior subluxation should normally correct during this extension of the knee, confirming the diagnosis.

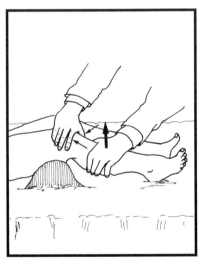

75. *Posterior cruciate ligament* (3): Place the thumb on one side of the joint line and the index on the other to help you assess any tibial movement. Try to pull the tibia forwards with the other hand. If the posterior cruciate ligament is torn, and the tibia subluxed posteriorly, the forward movement as the tibia reduces will be easily felt.

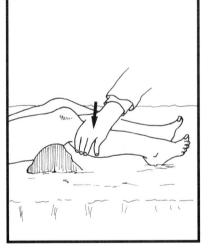

76. *Posterior cruciate ligament* (4): If the posterior cruciate is lax or torn, but subluxation has not yet occurred (uncommon), then backward pressure on the tibia will normally produce a detectable, excessive posterior excursion of the tibia.

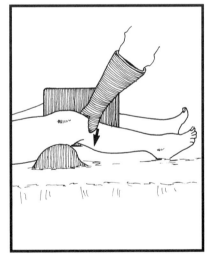

77. *Radiological examination of posterior cruciate ligament function* (1): A sandbag is placed behind the thigh, and the proximal tibia forcibly pressed backwards (with an equivalent force of 25 kg). This is repeated, and after the second pre-loading cycle, radiographs are taken while the same force is maintained.

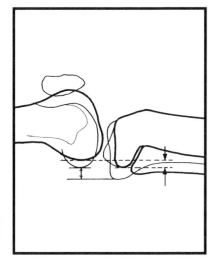

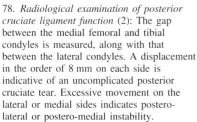

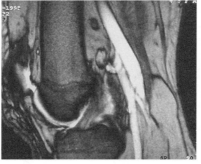

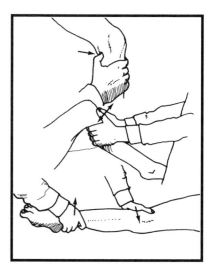

78. *Radiological examination of posterior cruciate ligament function* (2): The gap between the medial femoral and tibial condyles is measured, along with that between the lateral condyles. A displacement in the order of 8 mm on each side is indicative of an uncomplicated posterior cruciate tear. Excessive movement on the lateral or medial sides indicates postero-lateral or postero-medial instability.

79. *Visualisation of the cruciate ligaments:* MRI scans allow an accurate assessment of the state of the cruciate ligaments in 80% of cases. (Note that this is inferior to clinical assessment.) (Illustration: intact anterior cruciate ligament.) The cruciates may also be inspected by arthroscopy. The ability of the cruciate ligaments to prevent abnormal tibial movements can be assessed mechanically using dynamic testing rigs.

80. *Assessing tibial subluxations (rotatory or torsional instabilities):* (1) Look for medial or lateral tenderness or oedema. (2) Perform the drawer tests noting variations. (3) Test for laxity on valgus stress (often positive in anterior subluxations of the medial tibial condyle). (4) Test for laxity on varus stress (usually positive when the lateral tibial condyle subluxes forwards or backwards). (5) Carry out tests 81–84.

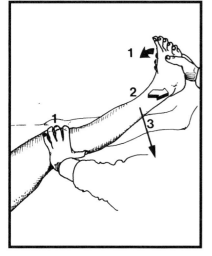

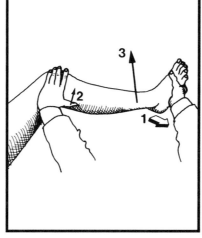

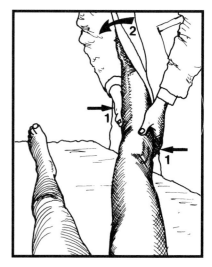

81. *MacIntosh test for anterior subluxation of the lateral tibial condyle (the pivot shift test):* Fully extend the knee while holding the foot in internal rotation (1). Apply a valgus stress (2). In this position, if instability is present, the tibia will be in the subluxed position. Now flex the knee (3): reduction should occur at about 30° with an obvious jerk. A positive test indicates an anterior cruciate abnormality, with or without other pathology.

82. *Losee pivot shift test for anterior subluxation of the lateral tibial condyle:* The patient should be completely relaxed, with no tension in the hamstrings. Apply a valgus force to the knee (1), at the same time pushing the fibular head anteriorly (2). The knee should be partly flexed. Now extend the joint (3). As full extension is reached, a dramatic clunk will occur as the lateral tibial condyle subluxes forwards (if rotatory instability is present). *Note:* the patient should relate this to the sensations experienced in activity.

83. *Modified pivot shift or jerk test for anterior subluxation of the lateral tibial condyle:* Grasp the foot between the arm and the chest, and apply a valgus stress (1); lean over to rotate the foot internally (2). Now flex the knee. If the test is positive, and because the tibia is firmly held, the lateral *femoral* condyle will appear to jerk anteriorly. Now extend the knee, and as the tibia subluxes, the femoral condyle will appear to jerk backwards.

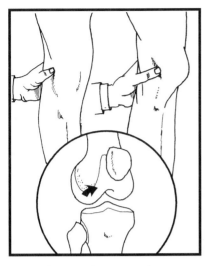

84. *Standing apprehension test for postero-lateral instability:* The patient should be taking his weight through the slightly flexed knee. Grasp the knee and with the thumb at the joint line press the anterior part of the lateral femoral condyle medially. The test is positive if movement of the condyle occurs (allowing the tibia to slip posteriorly under it), and if this is accompanied by a feeling of giving way.

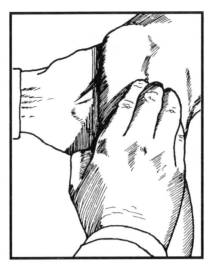

85. *The menisci* (1): Look for tenderness in the joint line, and test for a springy block to full extension. These two signs in association with evidence of quadriceps wasting are the most *consistent and reliable signs* of a torn meniscus.

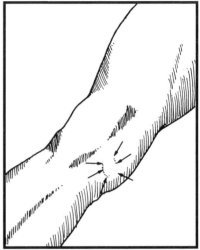

86. *The menisci* (2): In recent injuries, look for tell-tale oedema in the joint line. Bruising is *not* a feature of meniscal injuries.

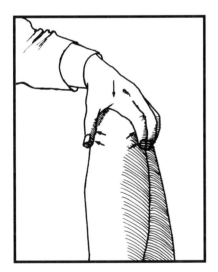

87. *The menisci* (3): *posterior lesions* (1): Fully flex the knee and place the thumb and index along the joint line. The palm of the hand should rest on the patella. You are now in a position to be able to locate any clicks emanating from the joint.

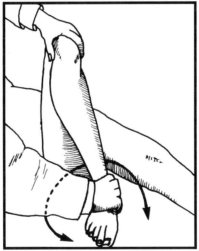

88. *The menisci* (4): *posterior lesions* (2): Sweep the heel round in a U-shaped arc, looking and feeling for clicks from the joint accompanied by pain. Watch the patient's face, not the knee, while carrying out this test.

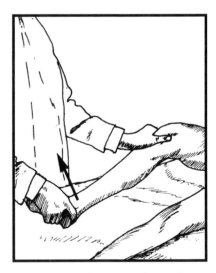

90. *The menisci* (5): *anterior lesions:* Press the thumb firmly into the joint line at the medial side of the patellar ligament. Now extend the joint. Repeat on the other side of the ligament. A click, accompanied by pain, is often found in anterior meniscus lesions.

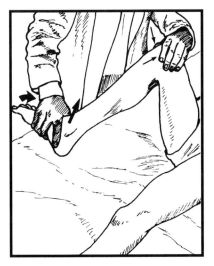

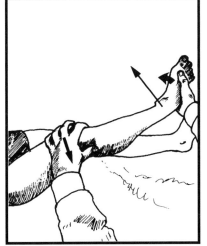

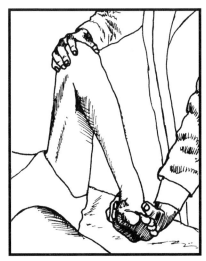

90. *The menisci (6): McMurray manoeuvre for the medial meniscus:* Place the thumb and index along the joint line to detect any clicks. *Flex* the leg fully; *externally rotate* the foot, *abduct* the lower leg, and *extend* the joint smoothly. A click arising in the medial joint line, accompanied by complaint of pain, is indicative of a medial meniscus tear.

91. *The menisci (7): McMurray manoeuvre for the lateral meniscus:* Repeat the last test with the foot internally rotated and the leg *adducted.* Use the hand to pick up the source of any clicks which are accompanied by pain. A grating sensation may be felt in degenerative lesions of the meniscus.

92. *The menisci (8):* If any clicks are detected, the normal limb should be examined to help eliminate symptomless, non-pathological clicks which may be arising from tendons or other soft tissues snapping over bony prominences (e.g. the biceps tendon over the femoral condyle), or from the patella clicking against a femoral condyle.

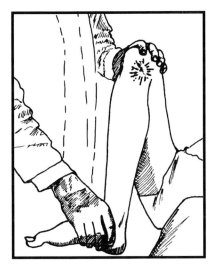

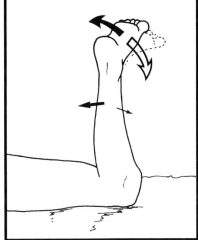

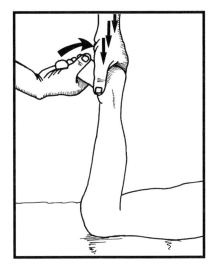

93. *The menisci (9):* If a unilateral painful click is obtained, repeat the test with the sensing finger or thumb removed. The cause of the click, whether meniscus or tendon, may be visible on close inspection of the joint line.

94. *The menisci (10): Apley's grinding tests* (1): In the tests, the suspect meniscus is subjected to compression and shearing stresses; sharp pain is suggestive of a tear. The patient is prone. The foot is externally rotated and the knee flexed fully; then the foot is internally rotated and the leg extended. The sides are compared. This demonstrates any limitation of rotation, or where any pain occurs.

95. *The menisci (11): grinding tests* (2): While standing on a stool the examiner throws his weight along the axis of the limb, and externally rotates the foot. Severe sharp pain is indicative of a medial meniscus tear. Repeat in a greater degree of flexion to test the posterior horn. To test the lateral meniscus, repeat the tests with the foot forcibly rotated internally.

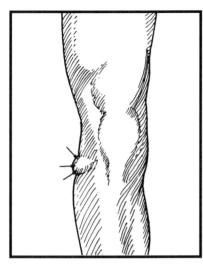

96. *The menisci* (12): Meniscal cysts lie in the joint line, feel firm on palpation, and are tender on deep pressure. Cysts of the menisci may be associated with tears. Lateral meniscus cysts are by far the commonest. Cystic swellings on the medial side are sometimes due to ganglions arising from the pes anserinus (insertion of sartorius, gracilis and semitendinosus).

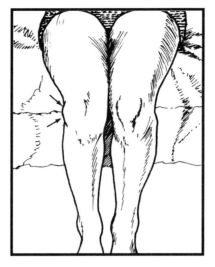

97. *The patella* (1): Examine both knees flexed over the end of the couch. This may show a torsional deformity of the femur or tibia, and a laterally placed patella (which will be predisposed to instability (e.g. recurrent dislocation) or chondromalacia patellae).

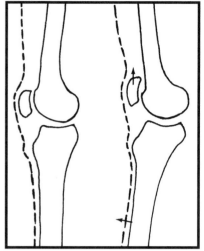

98. *The patella* (2): Look for genu recurvatum and the position of the patella relative to the femoral condyles. A high patella (patella alta) is a predisposing factor in recurrent lateral dislocation of the patella.

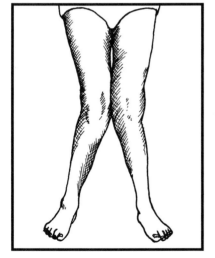

99. *The patella* (3): Is there any knock-knee deformity? Because this leads to an increase in the Q angle (quadriceps angle), it predisposes the knee to recurrent dislocation, anterior knee pain and chondromalacia patellae. The deformity is particularly common in adolescent girls. The intermalleolar distance may be measured, or the Q angle (which is similar to the tibio-femoral angle) may be determined.

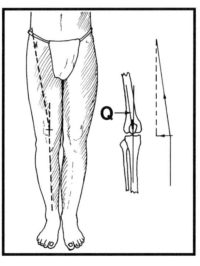

100. *The patella* (4): *finding the Q angle:* This is the angle (normally about 6°) between (a) a line joining the anterior superior iliac spine with the centre of the patella, and (b) the line of the patellar ligament. (To assess, ask the patient (who must be standing) to hold the end of a tape measure on his anterior spine while you centre the other over the patella. Then align a goniometer with the tape and the patellar ligament.)

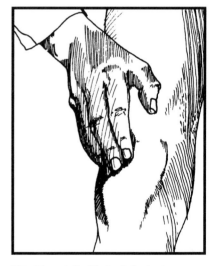

101. *The patella* (5): Look for tenderness over the anterior surface of the patella, and note if a tender, bipartite ridge is present. Lower pole tenderness occurs in Sinding-Larsen-Johannson disease. (Tenderness may also occur over the patellar ligament, quadriceps tendon and tibial tuberosity in other extensor apparatus traction injuries and variants of 'jumper's knee'.)

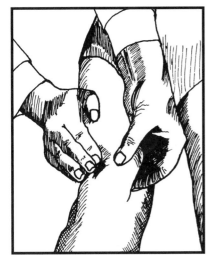

102. *The patella* (6): Displace the patella medially and palpate its articular surface. Tenderness is found when the articular surface is diseased, e.g. in chondromalacia patellae. Repeat the test, displacing the patella laterally. Two-thirds of the articular surface is thus normally accessible.

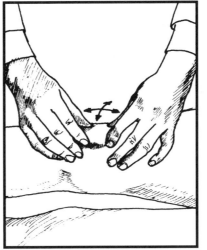

103. *The patella* (7): Test the mobility of the patella by moving it up and down and from side to side. Reduced mobility is found in retro-patellar arthritis. The quadriceps must be relaxed for adequate performance of this test. Decreased patellar mobility will obviously impair the performance of the previous test.

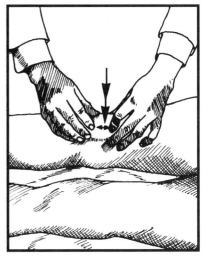

104. *The patella* (8): Move the patella proximally and distally, at the same time pressing it down hard against the femoral condyles. Pain is produced in chondromalacia patellae and retro-patellar osteoarthritis.

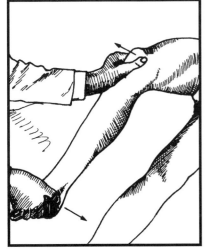

105. *The patella* (9): *the apprehension test:* Try to displace the patella laterally while flexing the knee from the fully extended position. If there is a tendency to recurrent dislocation, the patient will be apprehensive and try to stop the test, generally by pushing the examiner's hand away.

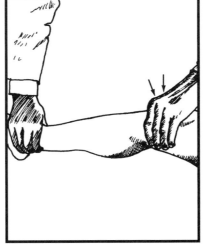

106. *Articular surfaces* (1): Place the palm of the hand over the patella, and the thumb and index along the joint line. Flex and extend the joint. The source of crepitus from damaged articular surfaces can then be detected. Compare one side with the other. If in doubt, auscultate the joint. Ignore single patellar clicks.

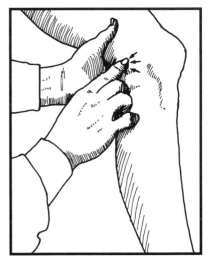

107. *Articular surfaces* (2): Apparent broadening of the joint and palpable exostoses occur commonly in osteoarthritis. (Both sides of the joint are affected in the later stages of tibio-femoral osteoarthritis, but in the early stages of this condition the *medial* side of the joint is often affected first, leading to a bow-leg deformity and frequently laxity of the medial ligament.)

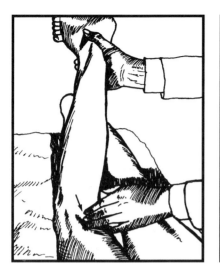

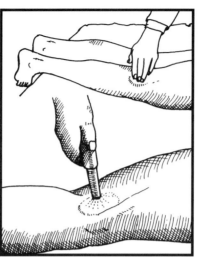

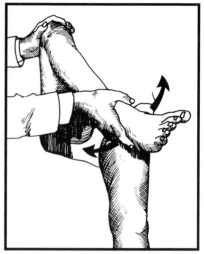

108. *Popliteal region* (1): All the previous tests have involved examination of the joint *from the front*. Do not forget to examine the *back* of the joint both by inspection and palpation. If the knee is flexed the roof of the fossa is relaxed, and deep palpation becomes possible.

109. *Popliteal region* (2): Semimembranosus bursae become obvious when the knee is extended. Compare the sides. A bursa may be small at the time of examination, and transillumination is worth trying although not always positive. Note that semimembranosus bursae may be secondary to rheumatoid arthritis or other pathology in the joint.

110. *The hip:* Always examine the hip, especially in the presence of severe, undiagnosed pain, as hip pain is often referred to the knee joint. The hip may be screened by testing rotation at 90° flexion, noting pain or restriction of movements.

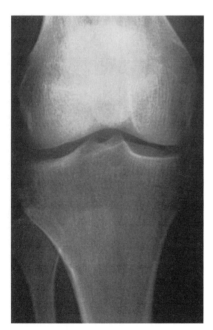

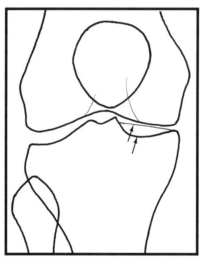

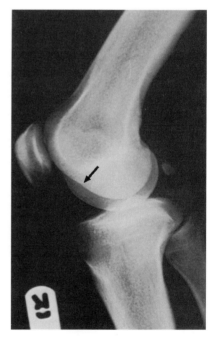

111. *Radiographs* (1): Normal antero-posterior radiograph of the knee.

112. *Radiographs* (2): The contours of the femur, tibia and fibula are obvious. The patellar shadow is usually rather faint and difficult to make out. Note on the medial side the two tibial shadows formed by the anterior and posterior rims of the concave medial tibial plateau. (The lateral tibial plateau is convex and has a single shadow.)

113. *Radiographs* (3): Normal lateral radiograph of the knee. The arrow points to the condylo-patellar sulcus; this helps identify the lateral femoral condyle, which is larger and flatter.

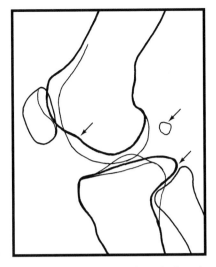

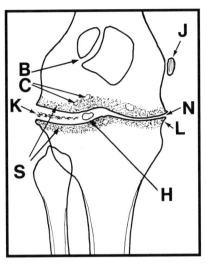

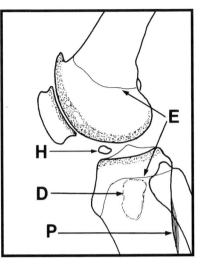

114. *Radiographs* (4): Note here the *lateral condyles* of the femur and of the tibia are drawn with a heavy line. The *lateral tibial condyle* may often be identified by the fibular articulation. The outline of the *medial tibial condyle* tends to blend with the shadow of the tibial spines. Note the fabella, an inconstant sesamoid bone lying in the lateral head of gastrocnemius; do not mistake it for a loose body.

115. *Radiographs* (5): Note any joint space narrowing (indicating cartilage loss) (N), lipping (L), marginal sclerosis (S), cysts (C), loose bodies (H), varus or valgus (these are all common in osteoarthritis). Do not mistake a bipartite patella (B) for fracture (this anomaly affects the *outer* quadrant). Note any abnormal calcification as in Pellegrini-Stieda disease (J), calcified meniscus and pseudo-gout (K).

116. *Radiographs* (6): Look for alterations in bone texture (e.g. in Paget's disease, rheumatoid arthritis, osteomalacia, infections). Note any bone defects (D) suggestive of tumour or infection, or areas of periosteal reaction (P), perhaps indicative of tumour or infection. Do not mistake epiphyseal lines (E) for hairline or other fractures. H = loose body.

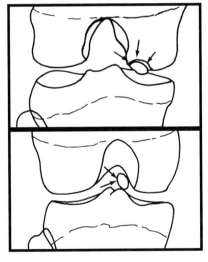

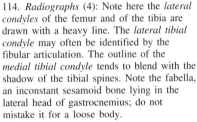

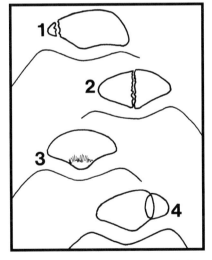

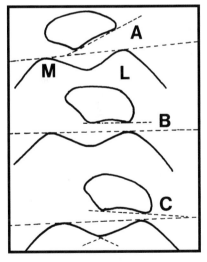

117. *Radiographs* (7): Intercondylar radiographs are often of help in confirming the diagnosis of osteochondritis dissecans, as they show the common sites more clearly, especially in the medial femoral condyle. They are also of value in locating loose bodies.

118. *Radiographs* (8): Where the patella is suspect, a tangential (skyline) view should be obtained. This may show (1) a marginal (medial) osteochondral fracture, common in recurrent dislocation of the patella; (2) other fractures; (3) occasionally, evidence of chondromalacia patellae; (4) bipartite patella.

119. *Radiographs* (9): A 20° projection may help in assessing patellar instability. Draw tangents to show the *lateral patello-femoral angle*. The angle is positive in 97% of normal subjects (A). In those suffering from recurrent dislocation of the patella it is zero in 80% (B), or negative in 20% (C). This angle may also be defined by CAT scans. Note also if the sulcus is shallow (> 170°).

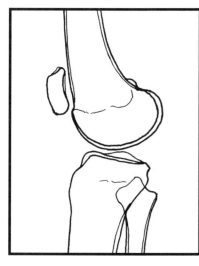

120. *Radiographs* (10): Again, in suspected recurrent dislocation of the patella the lateral projection should be taken with the knee weight-bearing and held in full extension. This may confirm the presence of a highly placed and susceptible patella (patella alta).

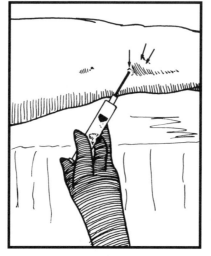

121. *Aspiration* (1): Aspirate the knee (a) in the presence of a tense haemarthrosis or (b) to obtain specimens for bacteriology in suspected infections. Begin with full aseptic precautions by raising a skin weal with local anaesthetic just above and lateral to the patella.

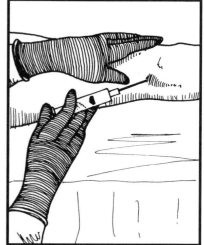

122. *Aspiration* (2): Infiltrate the tissues more deeply down to the level of the synovial membrane of the suprapatellar pouch.

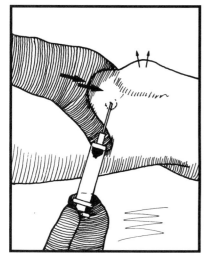

123. *Aspiration* (3): Unless the knee is very tense, squeeze fluid from the upper limits of the suprapatellar pouch to float the patella forwards before inserting the aspiration needle.

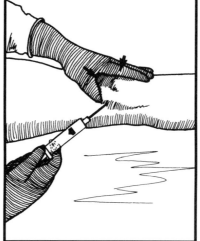

124. *Aspiration* (4): Squeeze the superior aspect and sides of the joint during the terminal stages of aspiration to empty the joint. After withdrawal of the needle, apply a sterile dressing over the aspiration site.

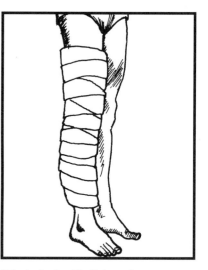

125. *Aspiration* (5): Unless other treatment is contemplated, apply a Jones compression bandage. This consists of several layers (2–4) of wool in the form of wool roll, gamgee, or cotton-wool sheets, each held in place with firmly, but not tightly, applied calico, domette or crepe bandaging.

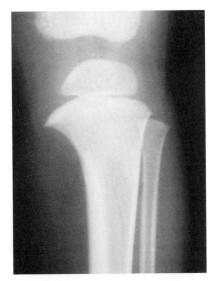

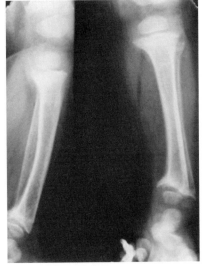

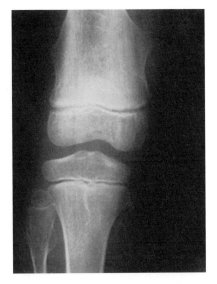

126. *Radiographs of the knee: examples of pathology* (1): Tibia vara: note the beaking of the proximal part of the tibial metaphysis. Bowing of the legs is the outstanding clinical feature.

127. *Pathology* (2): Rickets associated with bow-leg deformity: note the widening of the metaphyses of the tibia, with their characteristic irregularity and cupping.

128. *Pathology* (3): Diaphyseal aclasis (sometimes also referred to as metaphyseal aclasis): note the prominent femoral exostoses (the main clinical feature) and the deformity of the proximal end of the fibula.

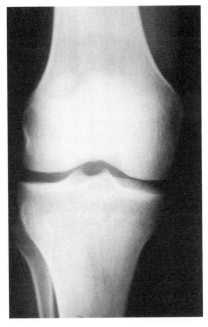

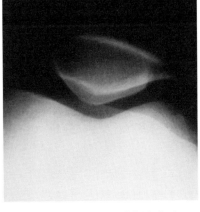

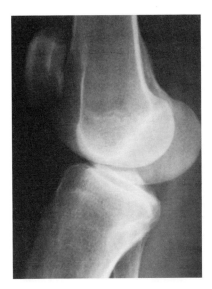

130. *Pathology* (5): Tangential (skyline) projection of the previous case showing the lateral irregularity (to the right of the figure).

131. *Pathology* (6): This weight-bearing lateral in an adolescent girl confirms the presence of genu recurvatum; note how the patella is in contact with the femur proximal to its articular surface (patella alta).

129. *Pathology* (4): Bipartite patella: note the separate centre of ossification involving the supero-lateral quadrant of the patella. The constancy of the site may often help differentiate it from fracture.

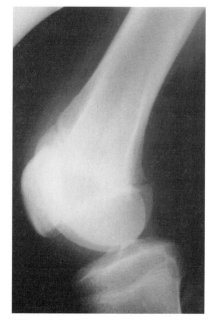

132. *Pathology* (7): Lateral dislocation of the patella. This radiograph is of an acute injury.

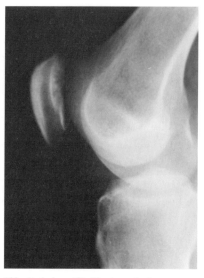

133. *Pathology* (8): The irregularity involving the proximal two-thirds of the articular surface of the patella in a young woman is secondary to a severe degree of chondromalacia patellae.

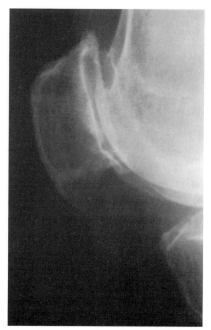

134. *Pathology* (9): This localised view shows a severe degree of retro-patellar osteoarthritis; note the narrowing of the joint space and the arthritic lipping of the patella.

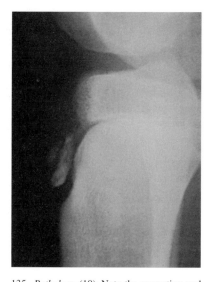

135. *Pathology* (10): Note the separation and fragmentation of the tongue-like downward projecting proximal tibial epiphysis: Osgood-Schlatter's disease.

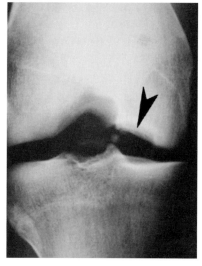

136. *Pathology* (11): Antero-posterior view of the knee positioned to show the intercondylar notch (tunnel projection). Note the punched-out area in the medial femoral condyle due to osteochondritis dissecans.

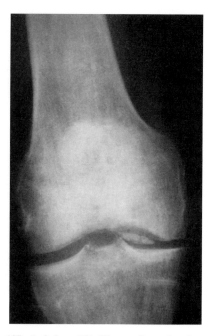

137. *Pathology* (12): These radiographs of a young man (note the degree of epiphyseal fusion) show separation of a large fragment from the medial femoral condyle due to long-standing osteochondritis dissecans.

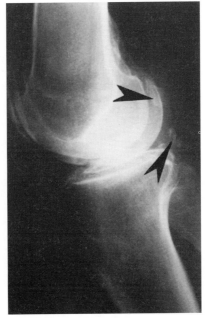

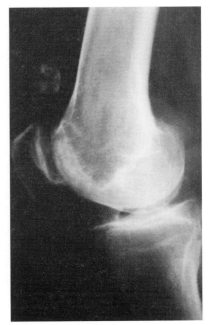

138. *Pathology* (13): The arrow points to a small spherical loose body in the lateral compartment, associated with osteoarthritis: note the irregularity of the articular surface of the lateral femoral condyle.

139. *Pathology* (14): The *upper* arrow points to a normal fabella. The *lower* arrow indicates two loose bodies, lying in the posterior part of the joint. These are secondary to osteoarthritis.

140. *Pathology* (15): There is a large loose body in the suprapatellar pouch; note the osteoarthritic changes involving the patella.

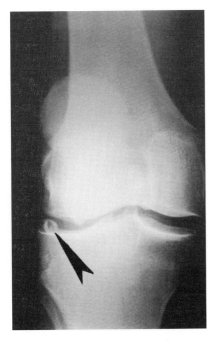

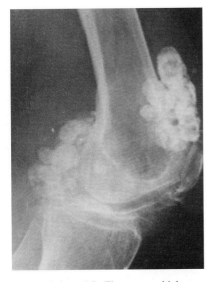

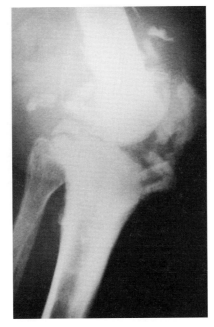

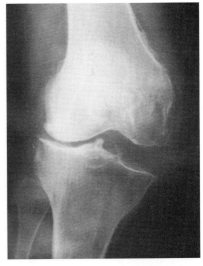

141. *Pathology* (16): There are multiple loose bodies in the knee joint due to synovial chondromatosis.

142. *Pathology* (17): There is gross disorganisation of the knee due to Charcot's disease.

143. *Pathology* (18): This radiograph, taken following acute trauma, shows widening of the medial joint line secondary to rupture of the medial ligament. It is uncommon to see such a degree of deformity without stress being applied to the joint while the films are being exposed.

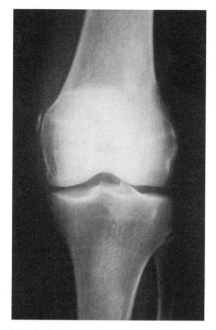

144. *Pathology* (19): There is calcification at the upper pole of the medial ligament characteristic of Pellegrini-Stieda disease.

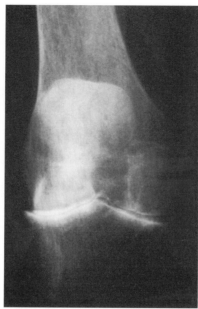

145. *Pathology* (20): There is gross narrowing of the joint space with a degree of osteoporosis typical of rheumatoid arthritis.

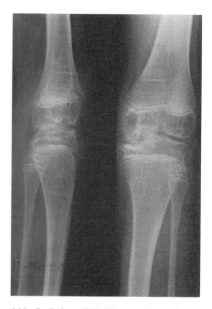

146. *Pathology* (21): There is destruction of the medial joint compartment secondary to chronic infection (tuberculosis). Note the horizontal striations (Looser's zones) in the femur, indicative of repeated incidents of temporary growth arrest.

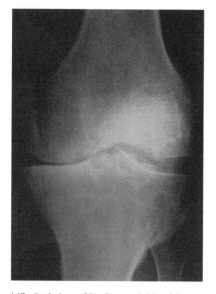

147. *Pathology* (22): Osteoarthritis of the knee: note in particular the narrowing of the medial joint compartment. There has been an old injury to the lateral tibial plateau.

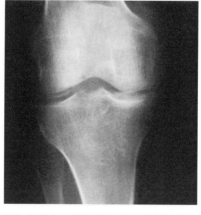

148. *Pathology* (23): There is calcification in the lateral meniscus; this is a common finding in pseudo-gout.

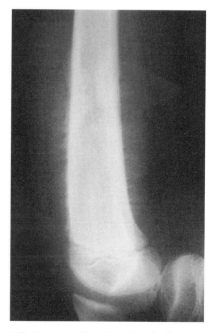

149. *Pathology* (24): There is a fusiform swelling of the femoral shaft encroaching the knee joint. Note the radial spiculation typical of osteogenic sarcoma.

12. The tibia

Common causes of pain in the anterior aspect of the lower leg

Note: Knock-knee and bow-leg deformities are included with the knee joint.

Osteitis of the tibia. Osteitis of the tibia occurs predominantly in children, with or without a history of previous trauma or sore throat. Pain is intense, tenderness is acute and initially well localised over the metaphyseal area, and there is inability to weight-bear. There is systemic upset with fever and tachycardia, and often but not always a polymorph leucocytosis. Admission and investigation with repeated blood cultures are essential. Radiographs of the tibia are initially normal. When this condition is suspected, it is customary to administer a broad-spectrum antibiotic, effective against the penicillin-resistant *Staphylococcus*, and in large doses to achieve adequate bone levels, prior to the results of blood culture. Splintage of the affected area is often helpful, and in proven cases antibiotics are administered for 4 weeks. Surgical drainage is seldom necessary and is avoided unless failure of response to antibiotics, profound toxicity and spread of the infection make it essential.

Cellulitis from insect stings, small wounds and abrasions, and hair follicle infections may sometimes cause difficulty in diagnosis.

Low-grade osteitis of the tibia (Brodie's abscess) may give rise to chronic upper tibial pain.

Bone tumours. The tibia is a common site for many primary bone tumours, so that radiographic examination of the tibia is essential in any case of undiagnosed leg pain.

Anterior tibial compartment syndrome. In this condition pain in the front of the leg is usually preceded by intense (usually athletic) activity. Oedema and swelling within the confines of the anterior compartment produce ischaemia, and eventually necrosis of muscle. The leg is diffusely swollen and tender, and the skin has a glossy appearance. Tibialis anterior and extensor hallucis longus are first affected, with weakness and later inability to extend the ankle and great toe. The dorsalis pedis pulse may be absent, and there may be sensory loss in the first web space from ischaemic changes in the deep peroneal nerve. Immediate surgical decompression of the anterior tibial compartment is essential if muscle necrosis is to be avoided.

Stress fracture of the tibia. In this condition, the onset of leg pain may be sudden or less acute. There is sharply localised bone tenderness and overlying oedema. Radiographic demonstration of the hairline fracture may be difficult, and with persistent pain repeated examination is essential. A radio-isotope bone scan may be helpful in diagnosing a local 'hot spot'. In many cases the diagnosis may not be firmly established until a small area of tell-tale callus is showing. The condition is also common in Paget's disease where, of course, there is an easily identifiable radiological abnormality.

Medial tibial syndrome. Pain on the medial side of the shin in sportsmen and sportswomen (shin splints) may be severe, and gives rise to tenderness along the postero-medial border of the lower part of the shin. In a number of cases the symptoms may arise from stress fractures of the tibia, but in others the pathology is less clear. (Other causes include compartment syndromes, fascial hernias, interosseous membrane tears, periosteal avulsions, tendinitis, muscle sprains and periostitis.) Where symptoms are of a chronic nature, and fracture has been excluded, division of the attachments of the crural fascia may give relief.

Tabes dorsalis. Severe pain in the shins (lightning pains) is common in tabes dorsalis. Usually other criteria are present (e.g. Argyll-Robertson pupils) and serological tests will confirm the diagnosis.

Common causes of pain in the posterior aspect of the lower leg

1. 'Ruptured plantaris tendon'. Sudden pain in the calf during activity, with diffuse tenderness in the upper and outer part of the calf, is now regarded as being due to tearing of muscle fibres of soleus or gastrocnemius rather than injury to the plantaris muscle. Pain often persists for several months and a period of plaster immobilisation is often helpful in relieving pain in the acute initial stages.

2. Thrombo-phlebitis. Thrombosis in the superficial veins of the calf with local inflammatory changes is a common cause of recurrent calf pain and the presence of tenderness and other inflammatory signs along the course of a calf vein makes diagnosis easy. Thrombosis in the deep veins is often silent, and its importance in the post-operative situation is well known.

3. Other causes of posterior leg pain. Pain in the calf is common in patients suffering from prolapsed intervertebral discs. Claudication pain is a feature of vascular insufficiency and spinal stenosis. Lesions of the foot and ankle which lead to protective muscle spasm on standing and walking frequently give rise to marked calf and leg pain.

Deformities of the tibia

Alteration in the normal curvature of the tibia is not uncommon and may be a cause for complaint. The bone may curve convex laterally (tibial bowing), convex anteriorly (tibial kyphosis) or undergo a rotational deformity (tibial torsion). Deformities of these types are particularly likely to occur in infants and young children when the immature bone may yield under the weight of a relatively heavy child. In the majority of cases no other cause is apparent and spontaneous correction by the time the child reaches the age of 6 is the rule. Nevertheless rickets and other osteodystrophies must be excluded and continuous observation is essential.

Pseudarthrosis of the tibia is a rare congenital abnormality of the tibia which leads to progressive tibial kyphosis. The tibia becomes progressively thinner and undergoes spontaneous fracture which proceeds to non-union. It is particularly resistant to treatment. The diagnosis is made on the radiographic findings.

In the adult, deformity of the tibia may be seen following rickets in childhood, malunited fractures, Paget's disease and syphilis.

Guide to commoner causes of leg pain

In children	Osteitis or other infections
	Bone tumour
Adolescents and young adults	Stress fracture tibia
	Bone tumours (especially osteoid osteoma, osteoclastoma, osteosarcoma)
	Brodie's abscess
	Anterior compartment syndrome
	Shin splints
Adults	PID and spinal stenosis
	Vascular insufficiency
	Thrombo-phlebitis
	Paget's disease
	'Ruptured plantaris tendon'
	Painful conditions of the foot
	Syphilis
	Bone tumours

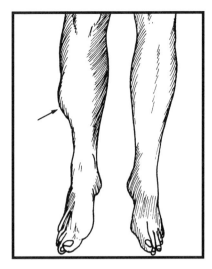

1. *Inspection* (1): *soft tissue swelling:* Note the site and extent of any swelling. In the case of oedema, note particularly if bilateral (suggesting a general rather than a local cause). Unilateral leg oedema in women over 40 is a common sign of intra-pelvic neoplasm.

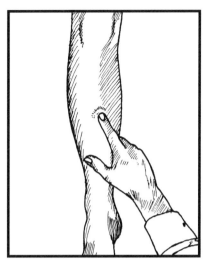

2. *Inspection* (2): *localised oedema:* Localised oedema is common over inflammatory lesions and stress fractures.

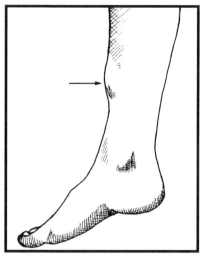

3. *Inspection* (3): *local bone swelling:* This is suggestive of neoplasm (e.g. osteoid osteoma) or old fracture. Multiple or single exostoses commonly occur in the tibia in diaphyseal aclasis. Thickening of the ends of the tibia is seen in rickets and osteoarthritis.

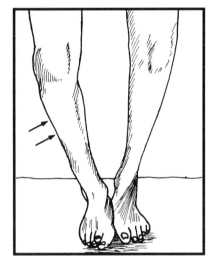

4. *Inspection* (4): *general bone thickening:* Extensive thickening of bone is characteristic of Paget's disease and long-standing osteitis. In the latter case there are usually other signs such as scarring or sinuses.

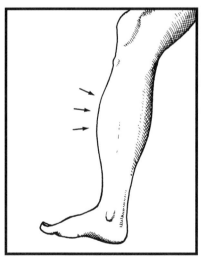

5. *Inspection* (5): *tibial shape:* Note any abnormal anterior curvature, possibly secondary to Paget's disease, malunited fracture, syphilis or rickets. Rickets affects the distal half of both tibia and fibula, and there are associated lateral and torsional deformities.

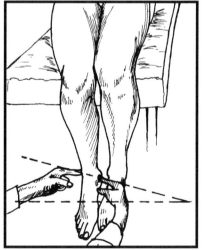

6. *Tibial torsion* (1): Flex the legs over the edge of the examination couch. The tibial tubercles must face directly forwards. Place the index fingers over the malleoli. The medial malleolus normally lies in front of the lateral 20° to the coronal plane.

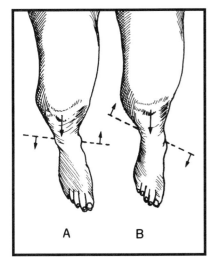

7. *Tibial torsion* (2): (A) *Medial* torsional deformity (a decrease in the angle) is associated with flat foot and intoeing. (B) *Lateral* torsional deformity (an increase in the angle) is seen in pes cavus.

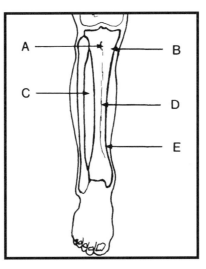

8. *Tenderness* (1): At the front, tenderness is characteristically situated in the following: (A) Osgood-Schlatter's disease; (B) Brodie's abscess, osteitis; (C) anterior tibial compartment syndrome; (D) stress fracture; (E) shin splints.

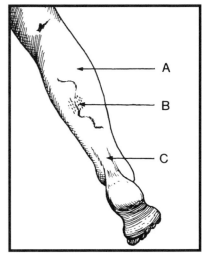

9. *Tenderness* (2): At the back of the leg, tenderness is characteristically situated in the following: (A) 'ruptured plantaris tendon' syndrome; (B) over varicosities in superficial thrombo-phlebitis; (C) over the tendo calcaneus in partial tears and complete ruptures.

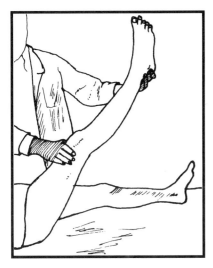

10. *Screening tests* (1): The following tests should be carried out in the investigation of any case of leg pain. The straight-leg-raising test (see 8, 31) should be carried out. In many cases pain in the leg below the knee is referred from the spine.

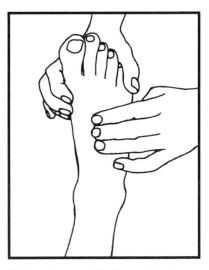

11. *Screening tests* (2): The lower limb reflexes should be elicited, and if indicated, test the pupils for reaction to light and accommodation. Lower leg pain is a common symptom of late syphilis.

12. *Screening tests* (3): The peripheral pulses should be sought (see also 14, 59). Ischaemia is an extremely common cause of leg pain.

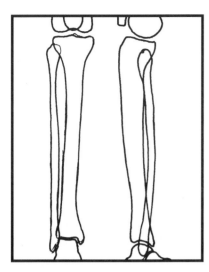

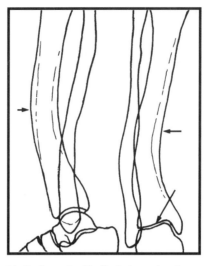

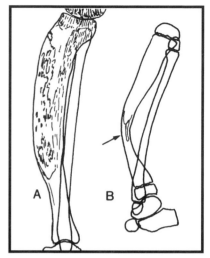

13. *Radiographs* (1): The standard films are an antero-posterior and lateral which include both ends of tibia and fibula. For better visualisation of a suspect area, localised views are required. CAT and MRI scans are often of value, especially in evaluating cystic defects, and radio-isotope scans may be helpful in assessing local vascularity.

14. *Radiographs* (2): Begin by noting the general shape of the bones, their texture and their mineralisation. For example, in *rickets* during the phase of bone softening, deformity follows weight-bearing. Note angulation of the plane of the ankle (which may theoretically predispose to osteoarthritis).

15. *Radiographs* (3): Deformity is common in *Paget's disease* (A) where there is disturbance of form and texture, and sometimes sarcomatous change. In *pseudarthrosis of the tibia* (B) there is local thinning and angulation of the bone which progresses to tibial dissolution, the fibula remaining normal.

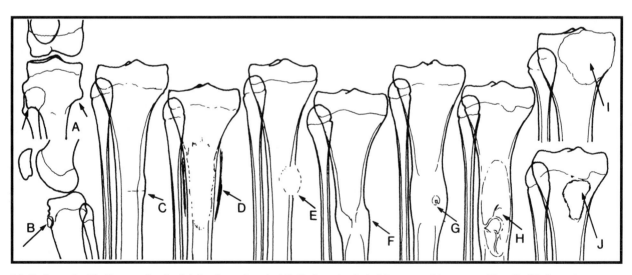

16. *Radiographs* (4): Note any localised deformity such as in (A) diaphyseal aclasis (often several bones are affected); (B) Osgood-Schlatter's disease; (C) localised periosteal reaction in the region of a stress fracture; (D) more extensive subperiosteal new bone formation in the later stages of osteitis, or at the site of a bone tumour. Note (E) cortical bone destruction suggesting a lytic neoplasm or infection. Localised thickening of bone is seen after a healed fracture (F) or again at a tumour site (e.g. in osteoid osteoma where there is often a central nidus (G)). Examine the cavity and ends of the bone for space-occupying lesions such as (H), a unicameral bone cyst occurring in the shaft, (I) an osteoclastoma occurring in the epiphysis and (J) a Brodie's abscess in the metaphysis.

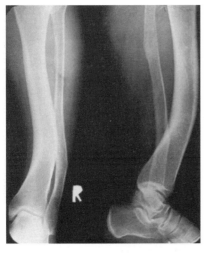

17. *Radiographs of the tibia: examples of pathology* (1): Persisting deformity of the tibia in two planes following rickets in childhood.

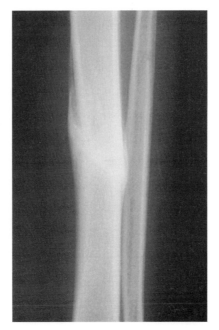

18. *Pathology* (2): Old fracture of the mid-shaft of the tibia, responsible for persisting local bone thickening.

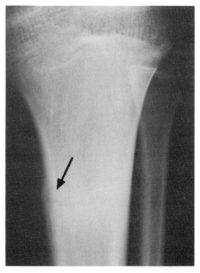

19. *Pathology* (3): The arrow points to a stress fracture of the tibia. Note the periosteal reaction with the slight increase in bone density at the same level.

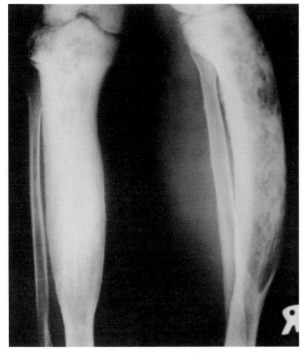

20. *Pathology* (4): Paget's disease of the tibia: note the striking alteration in bone texture, the bone thickening showing in the antero-posterior view, and the marked curvature apparent in the lateral. In this case there was no malignant change.

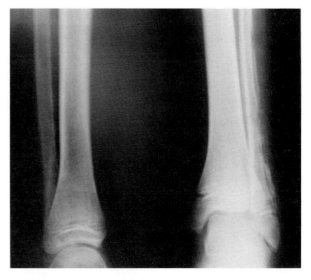

21. *Pathology* (5): In the left fibula (on the right of the figure) there is extensive bone destruction and subperiosteal new bone formation, characteristic of osteitis some weeks after the onset — which was heralded with fever, malaise and severe local pain.

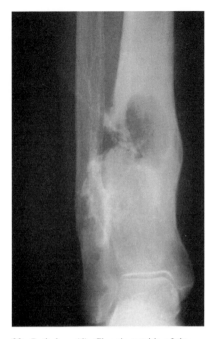

22. *Pathology* (6): Chronic osteitis of the tibia. Note the cavity in the bone and the sinus (which leads to the skin). No sequestra are apparent.

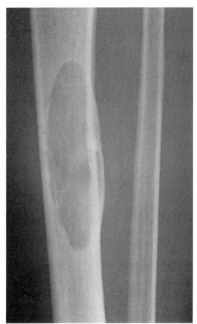

23. *Pathology* (7): Unicameral (simple) bone cyst involving the medullary canal of the tibia.

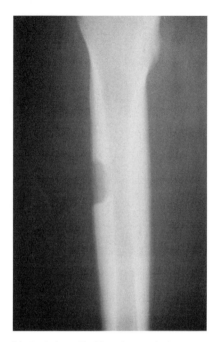

24. *Pathology* (8): Note the punched-out appearance of the defect in this femur, characteristic of the highly malignant Ewing's tumour. Lesions in the tibia are not uncommon, and have a similar appearance.

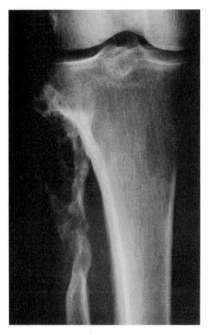

25. *Pathology* (9): There is destruction and deformity of the proximal fibula typical of osteoclastoma. The tumour in this case was only locally malignant, but was associated with a common peroneal nerve palsy and drop foot.

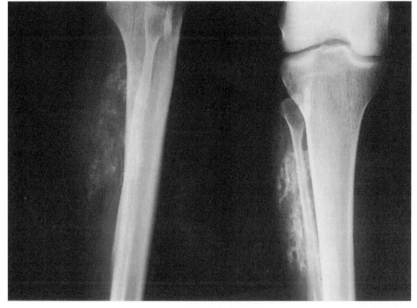

26. *Pathology* (10): There is an extensive area of new bone formation in a haematoma which has formed on the lateral aspect of the leg following a crack fracture of the fibula. The appearances are typical of myositis ossificans; here the only complaint was of local swelling.

13. The ankle

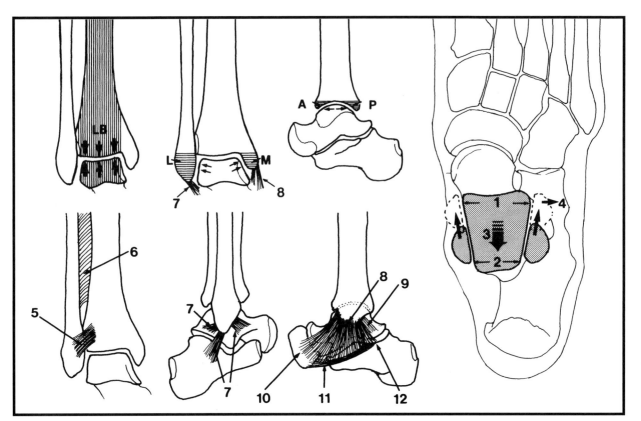

Fig. 13.A

Anatomical features

The ankle joint is basically a simple hinge joint, normally permitting movement in one plane (dorsiflexion and plantar flexion); but in addition, up to 18° of axial rotation of the talus in the tibial mortice may occur. Load-bearing stresses (LB) are taken by the upper articular surface of the talus and the tibia; the fibula plays no part in this.

Medial displacement of the talus is prevented by the medial malleolus (M), and *lateral* displacement by the lateral malleolus (L). *Posterior talar shift* is blocked by the downward-projecting curved articular surface of the tibia (P) behind, while the corresponding surface in front (A) prevents *anterior subluxation*. Any of these bony prominences may be fractured, resulting in potential instability.

When viewed from above, the articular surface of the talus may be seen to be wider anteriorly (1) than posteriorly (2). This means that as the ankle is dorsiflexed (3), the talus is gripped more firmly between the malleoli, and pushes the fibula laterally (4). When the ankle is plantar-flexed, there is a greater degree of freedom (and instability) of the talus in the ankle mortice.

The natural congruency of the bony components of the ankle accounts for its inherent stability, and this is reinforced by the disposition and strength of the associated ligaments. These include the following:

(a) The inferior tibio-fibular ligaments (anterior and posterior) (5), which bind the tibia to the fibula. They are assisted by the weak interosseous membrane (6).

(b) The lateral (external) ligament (7) has three parts which arise from the fibula; distally the anterior and posterior fasciculi are attached to the talus, while the central slip is attached to the calcaneus.

(c) The medial ligament (8), immensely strong, is triangular in shape (hence the alternative term deltoid ligament), and is attached proximally to the medial malleolus. Its deep fibres (9) pass to the medial surface of the talus, while its superficial part is attached to the navicular (10), the spring ligament (11) and the calcaneus (12).

Note that a careful examination of the foot is often also required in the investigation of many ankle complaints.

Soft tissue injuries of the ankle

Soft tissue injuries of the ankle are extremely common and in the severer cases difficult to differentiate from undisplaced fractures. Radiographic examination is essential in all but the most minor lesions, and is also necessary where symptoms are persistent. When fracture has been excluded after a significant injury a diagnosis has still to be made, as this manifestly affects treatment.

Injuries of the lateral ligament

The lateral ligament is damaged in inversion injuries. In an incomplete tear, some fibres only are ruptured (ankle sprain). Treatment is then symptomatic and a full early recovery can be expected. When the ligament is completely torn or detached from the fibula, the talus is free to tilt in the mortice of the tibia and fibula. If the lateral ligament fails to heal, chronic instability of the ankle results. If this injury is diagnosed in the acute stages, it should be treated by prolonged immobilisation in plaster or operative repair. In late-diagnosed cases, good results generally follow lateral ligament reconstruction procedures.

In *functional instability of the ankle* the patient complains of frequent sensations of the ankle giving way, and pain, stiffness and swelling related to activity, but no evidence of ligament instability can be found. It is thought that in many of these cases there is a degree of motor incoordination arising from some disorder of proprioception. Most respond to specialised physiotherapy (using tilt boards and other measures to improve muscular coordination).

Inferior tibio-fibular ligaments

When the foot is dorsiflexed the distal end of the fibula moves laterally (and proximally), as it is engaged by the wedge-shaped upper articular surface of the talus. This movement is restricted by the inferior tibio-fibular ligaments, and to a lesser extent the interosseous membrane. Damage to these structures may lead to lateral displacement of the fibula and lateral drift of the talus (diastasis). In treatment, the talus must be re-aligned with the tibia, and any fibular displacement reduced. This reduction may be held by cross screwing of the fibula to the tibia, or by plaster fixation.

Medial ligament

The medial ligament is immensely strong and if stressed in ankle joint injuries generally avulses the medial malleolus rather than itself tearing. Nevertheless tears do occur, and are seen particularly in conjunction with lateral malleolar fractures. Meticulous reduction of any associated fracture is essential, and operative repair may sometimes be undertaken.

Achilles tendon (tendo calcaneus)

Sudden plantar flexion of the foot may rupture the Achilles tendon, especially when it is weakened as a result of the degenerative changes seen in middle age. Surgical repair may be carried out, although in most cases excellent results may be achieved by conservative management in plaster.

Other common conditions seen round the ankle

Tenosynovitis. Inflammatory changes in the tendon sheaths behind the malleoli may give rise to pain at the sides of the ankle joint. Tenosynovitis may follow unusual excessive activity or be associated with degenerative changes, flat foot or rheumatoid arthritis. There is puffy swelling in the line of the tendons, with tenderness extending often for several centimetres along their length. Tibialis posterior and peroneus longus are most frequently involved, and stretching these structures by forced inversion and eversion of the foot gives rise to pain. Spontaneous rupture is not uncommon. Symptoms generally respond to immobilisation for short periods in a below-knee walking plaster.

Footballer's ankle. Ill-localised pain in the front of the ankle may follow repeated incidents of forced plantar flexion of the foot which result in tearing of the anterior capsule of the ankle joint. This is found to occur frequently in footballers where this form of stress is common. Calcification in the resulting areas of avulsion and haemorrhage leads to the appearance of characteristic exostoses in lateral radiographic projections of the ankle. These may lead to mechanical restriction of dorsiflexion.

Osteochondritis of the talus. Although rather uncommon, this condition, which is seen most frequently in adolescents and young men, may give disabling pain in the ankle. It is now generally agreed that the condition starts as an osteochondral fracture. It is the frequent source of complaints of chronic disability following a so-called simple sprain of the ankle. The diagnosis is made on the radiological findings, although the site of the pain and local tenderness over the upper articular surface of the talus may lead one to suspect it. CAT and MRI scans are invaluable in doubtful cases. If loose bodies are produced, they must be excised. The treatment of the local lesion in principle follows that of osteochondritis dissecans of the knee.

Snapping peroneal tendons. This is an uncommon cause of ankle pain and is due to tearing of the superior peroneal retinaculum. The patient complains of a clicking sensation in the ankle and is usually able to demonstrate the peroneal tendons riding over the lateral malleolus. The treatment is by surgical reconstruction of the retinaculum.

Osteoarthritis. Primary osteoarthritis of the ankle is rare. Secondary osteoarthritis is sometimes seen after ankle fractures, avascular necrosis of the talus, or osteochondritis of the talus.

Rheumatoid arthritis. Rheumatoid arthritis of the ankle is not uncommon, but is seldom seen as a primary manifestation of the disease, so that diagnosis seldom presents difficulty.

Tuberculosis. Tuberculous infections of the ankle joint are now rare in the UK. When they occur there is swelling of the joint, wasting of the calf, and the usual signs of inflammation. The patient develops a painful limp, and as the joint is comparatively superficial, sinus formation is common at a comparatively early stage.

Shortening of the Achilles tendon (tendo calcaneus). Shortening of the Achilles tendon results in plantar flexion of the foot and clumsiness of gait as the heel fails to reach the ground. The more severe degrees of Achilles tendon shortening are accompanied by a tendency to flat foot. In many cases flexion of the knee, by taking the tension off the gastrocnemius, will permit dorsiflexion of the foot. Shortening of the Achilles tendon may occur as an apparently isolated condition with no obvious predisposing cause, but in a great many cases it is associated with congenital deformities of the foot or neurological disorders of which subclinical poliomyelitis is one of the commonest (for talipes deformities see Chapter 14). Occasionally it may result from ischaemic contracture of the calf muscles.

Guide to painful conditions round the ankle

History of recent injury	Sprain of lateral ligament
	Complete tear of lateral ligament
	(Ankle fracture, fracture of the fifth metatarsal base)
	Tibio-fibular diastasis
	Ruptured Achilles tendon (tendo calcaneus)
History of past injury	Complete tear of lateral ligament
	Secondary osteoarthritis (e.g. previous ankle fracture)
No history of injury	Osteochondritis tali
	Rheumatoid arthritis
	Primary osteoarthritis
	Footballer's ankle
	Secondary osteoarthritis (e.g. osteochondritis tali)
	Tenosynovitis
	Snapping peroneal tendons

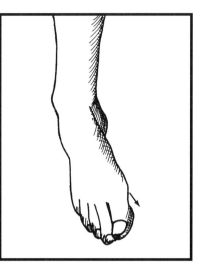

1. *Inspection* (1): Look for (A) deformity of shape, suggesting recent or old fracture; (B) sinus scars, suggesting old infection, particularly tuberculosis.

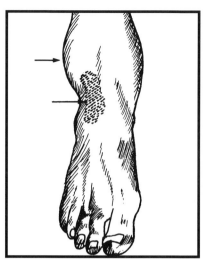

2. *Inspection* (2): Look for deformity of posture (e.g. plantar flexion from short tendo calcaneus, talipes deformity (see 14, 1), ruptured tendo calcaneus or drop foot).

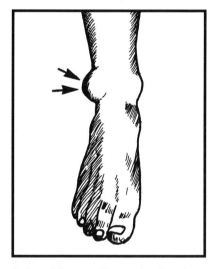

3. *Inspection* (3): Look for bruising, swelling or oedema. If there is any swelling, note if diffuse or localised. Note also if oedema is bilateral, suggesting a systemic rather than a local cause.

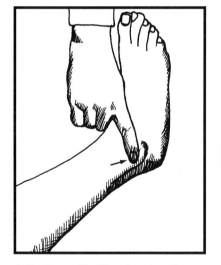

4. *Tenderness* (1): When there is tenderness localised over the malleoli following injury, radiographic examination is necessary to exclude fracture.

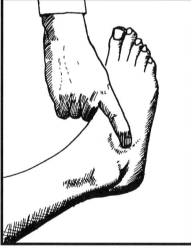

5. *Tenderness* (2): After inversion sprains, tenderness is often diffuse. Swelling, to begin with, lies in the line of the fasciculi of the lateral ligament.

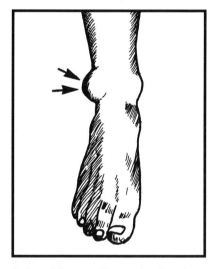

6. *Lateral ligament* (1): *complete lateral ligament tear:* Swelling is rapid, and if seen within 2 hours of injury, is egg-shaped and placed *over the lateral malleolus* (McKenzies' sign).

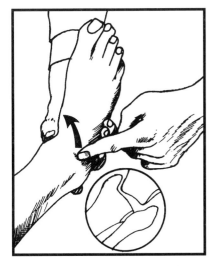

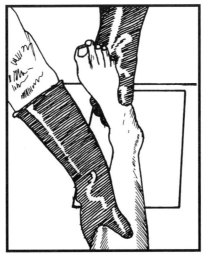

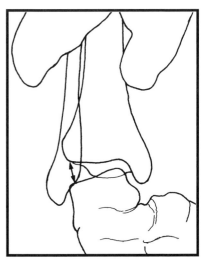

7. *Lateral ligament* (2): *stress testing for complete lateral ligament tears* (1): Grasp the heel and forcibly invert the foot, feeling for any opening-up of the lateral side of the ankle between tibia and talus.

8. *Lateral ligament* (3): *stress testing for complete lateral ligament tears* (2): If in doubt, have a radiograph taken while the foot is forcibly inverted.

9. *Lateral ligament* (4): *stress testing for complete lateral ligament tears* (3): If tilting of the talus in the ankle mortice is demonstrated, repeat the examination on the other side and compare the films.

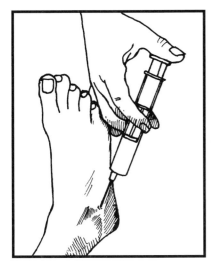

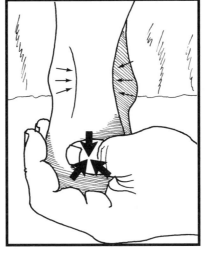

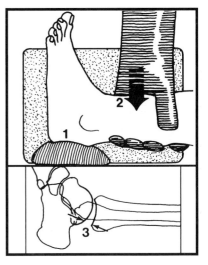

10. *Lateral ligament* (5): *stress testing for complete lateral ligament tears* (4): If the injury is fresh and painful, the examination may be more readily permitted after the injection of 15–20 ml of 0.5% lignocaine widely in the region of the lateral ligament.

11. *Lateral ligament* (6): *stress testing of the anterior talo-fibular component of the lateral ligament:* Instability may sometimes follow tears of the anterior talo-fibular portion only of the lateral ligament. With the patient prone, press downwards on the heel, looking for anterior displacement of the talus, which is often accompanied by dimpling of the skin on either side of the tendo calcaneus.

12. *Lateral ligament* (7): *stress testing of the anterior tibio-fibular ligament* (2): anterior displacement may be confirmed by radiographs taken in the prone position; alternatively, with the patient supine (and preferably with local anaesthesia), support the heel on a sandbag (1) and press firmly downwards on the tibia (2) for 30 seconds up to exposure. A gap between the talus and tibia of > 6 mm is regarded as pathological (3).

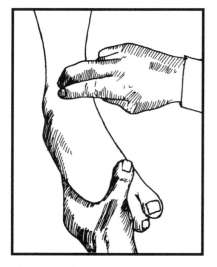

13. *Inferior tibio-fibular ligament* (1): In tears of this ligament (which has anterior and posterior components) tenderness is present over the ligament just above the line of the ankle joint.

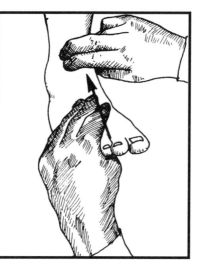

14. *Inferior tibio-fibular ligament* (2): In tears of the ligament pain is produced by dorsiflexion of the foot which displaces the fibula laterally.

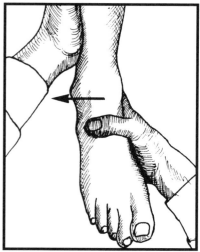

15. *Inferior tibio-fibular ligament* (3): Grasp the heel and try to move the talus directly laterally in the ankle mortice. Lateral displacement indicates a tear of the ligament.

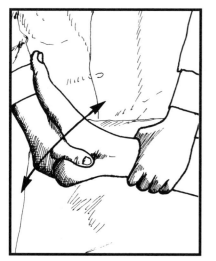

16. *Movements* (1): First confirm that the ankle is mobile, and that any apparent movement is not arising in the mid-tarsal or more distal joints. Firmly grasp the foot proximal to the mid-tarsal joint; try to produce dorsiflexion and plantar flexion.

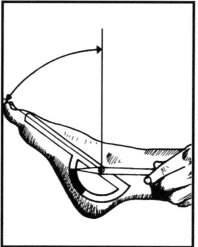

17. *Ankle joint movements* (2): Measure *plantar flexion* from the zero position. This reference lies at right angles to the line of the leg. *Normal range: 55°.*

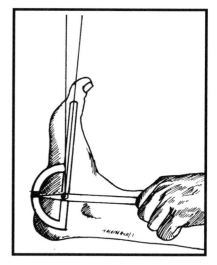

18. *Ankle joint movements* (3): Measure the range of *dorsiflexion*. Always compare the sides. *Normal range: 15°.*

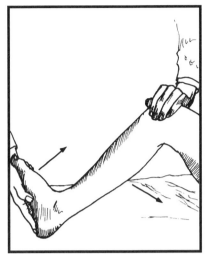

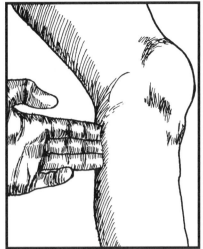

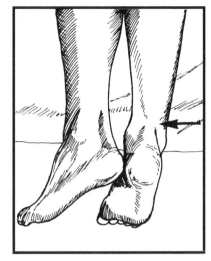

19. *Ankle joint movements* (4): If dorsiflexion is restricted, bend the knee. If this restores a normal range, the Achilles tendon is tight. If it makes no difference, joint pathology (such as osteoarthritis, rheumatoid arthritis or infection) is the likely cause.

20. *Ankle joint movements* (5): If there is loss of active dorsiflexion (drop foot) a full neurological examination is required. The commonest causes are stroke, old poliomyelitis, prolapsed lumbar intervertebral discs and local lesions of the common peroneal (lateral popliteal) nerve.

21. *Tendo calcaneus (Achilles tendon)* (1): The patient should be prone, with the feet over the edge of the couch. Defects in the contour of the tendon may be obvious. Note any enlargement of the bursae related to the tendon.

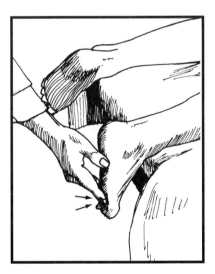

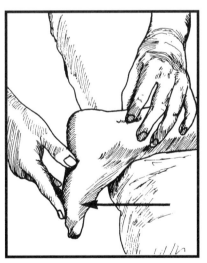

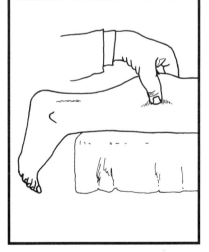

22. *Tendo calcaneus* (2): Test the power of plantar flexion by asking the patient to press the foot against your hand. Compare one side with the other, and note the shape of each contracting calf and the prominence of each tendon.

23. *Tendo calcaneus* (3): Palpate the tendon while the patient continues resisted plantar flexion. Compare the sides. Any gap in the tendon (ruptured tendo calcaneus) should be obvious. The integrity of the tendon may also be tested by inserting a needle vertically into the middle of the calf. Normally the needle should tilt when the ankle is passively dorsiflexed and plantar flexed.

24. *Tendo calcaneus* (4): *Thomson test:* Normally when the calf is squeezed the foot moves as the ankle plantar flexes. Loss of this movement is pathognomonic of an acute rupture of the tendo calcaneus.

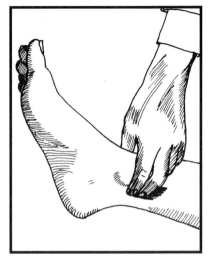

25. *Tenosynovitis* (1): *medial* (1): Look for tenderness along the line of the long flexor tendons. Tenderness is usually diffuse and linear in pattern. Note the site and extent of any local thickening.

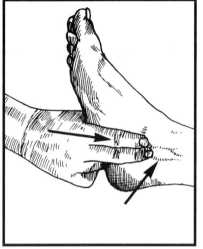

26. *Tenosynovitis* (2): *medial* (2): Look for synovitis in relation to the flexor tendons. There may be obvious swelling. Demonstrate the presence of any excess synovial fluid by milking the tendon sheaths in a proximal direction.

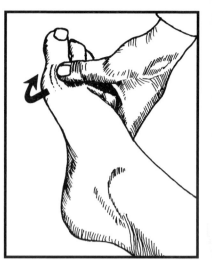

27. *Tenosynovitis* (3): *medial* (3): Plantar flex and evert the foot. This may produce pain where tenosynovitis involves the tendon of tibialis posterior.

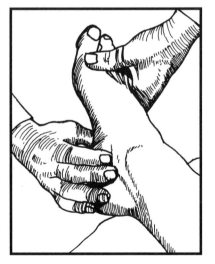

28. *Tenosynovitis* (4): *medial* (4): With the foot held in the plantar flexed and everted position, look for tenderness or gaps (spontaneous rupture) in the line of the tendon of tibialis posterior. Spontaneous rupture is seen most frequently in flat foot and rheumatoid arthritis.

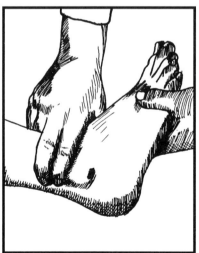

29. *Tenosynovitis* (5): *lateral* (1): Examine the peroneal tendons for tenderness and the presence of excess synovial fluid in their sheaths.

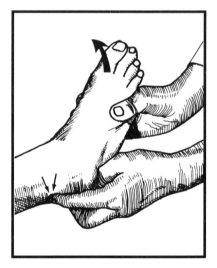

30. *Tenosynovitis* (6): *lateral* (2): Force the foot into plantar flexion and inversion. This will give rise to pain and increase tenderness along the line of the peroneal tendons if tenosynovitis of the peroneal tendons is present.

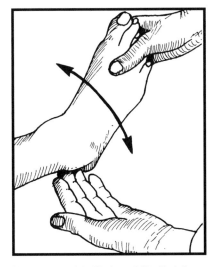

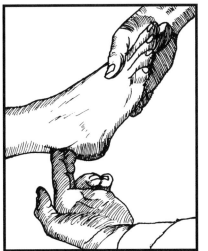

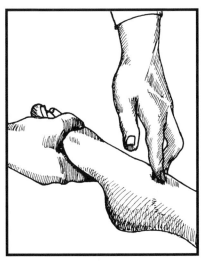

31. *Tenosynovitis* (7): *lateral* (3): Feel for crepitus along the line of the tendon sheaths behind both malleoli as the foot is swung backwards and forwards between inversion and eversion. Confirm by auscultation.

32. *Peroneal tendons:* Lightly palpate the peroneal tendons with the fingers; look and feel for displacement of the tendons as the patient everts the foot against light resistance. Displacement occurs in the condition known as 'snapping peroneal tendons'.

33. *Articular surfaces* (1): Forcibly plantar flex the foot to allow palpation of the anterior part of the superior articular surface of the talus. Tenderness occurs in arthritic conditions and in osteochondritis of the talus. A tender exostosis may be palpable in cases of footballer's ankle.

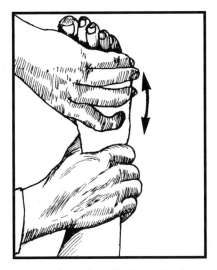

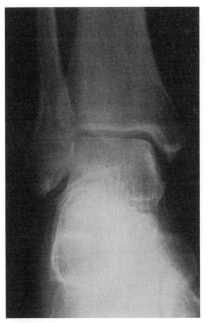

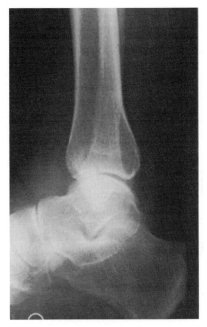

34. *Articular surfaces* (2): Place a hand across the front of the ankle and passively dorsiflex and plantar flex the foot. Crepitus, which may be confirmed by auscultation, suggests articular surface damage.

35. *Radiographs* (1): Normal antero-posterior radiograph of the ankle.

36. *Radiographs* (2): Normal lateral radiograph of the ankle.

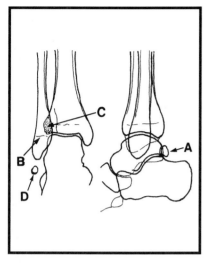

37. *Radiographs* (3): In the standard AP and lateral projections do not mistake (A) the common os trigonum accessory bone and (B) the epiphyseal line of the fibula for fracture. The amount of tibio-fibular overlap (C) is dependent on positioning and any diastasis. The os fibulare (D) is thought to represent an avulsion of the anterior talo-fibular ligament, and may be associated with instability.

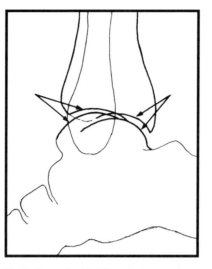

38. *Radiographs* (4): The articular margins of tibia and talus should appear as two congruent circular arcs. If there is some difficulty in positioning which cannot be improved upon, four arcs will be seen. Two pairs should be congruent as shown. If not, there is a subluxation.

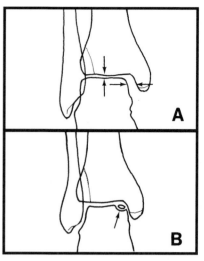

39. *Radiographs* (5): Note any widening of the gap (A) between talus and medial malleolus: this is suggestive of diastasis (compare its size with the one between the upper surfaces of the talus and tibia — both should normally be equal). (B) Note the presence of any defects in the articular surface of the talus, suggestive of osteochondritis tali. A CAT scan may help in the doubtful case.

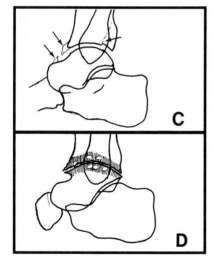

40. *Radiographs* (6): Note any irregularity in the joint surfaces which may suggest previous fracture, e.g. of the posterior malleolus (C). Examine the articular margins for exostoses: these are a feature of footballer's ankle (where there may be corresponding changes in the talus) and of osteoarthritis (D), where there may be other signs such as joint space narrowing and cystic change.

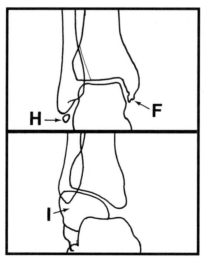

41. *Radiographs* (7): Look at the malleoli, where deformity (F) or rounded shadows (H) suggest previous avulsion injuries. Distortion of the talus occurs in association with talipes deformities (I) and after injuries which have resulted in avascular necrosis where there may be increases in bone density.

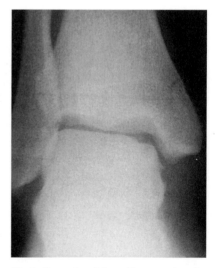

42. *Radiographs of the ankle: examples of pathology* (1): The upper articular surface of the talus is distorted on its medial side. The appearances are typical of osteochondritis dissecans. More complete assessment of the defect may be obtained by a CAT scan.

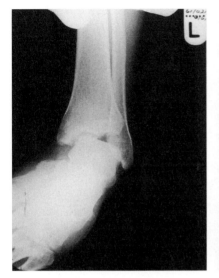

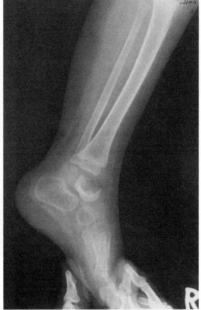

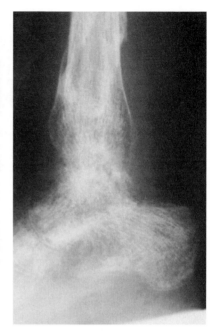

43. *Pathology* (2): This inversion film shows tilting of the talus in the ankle mortice. There was no tilting elicited in comparison films of the other side, indicating a unilateral complete tear of the lateral ligament.

44. *Pathology* (3): There is a large defect in the talus which also shows increased density inferiorly: the diagnosis is tuberculosis of the talus.

45. *Pathology* (4): There is gross decalcification of the ankle as a result of Sudeck's atrophy (post-traumatic osteodystrophy); this followed a minor fracture in the foot, and was associated with marked swelling, stiffness and pain in the joint.

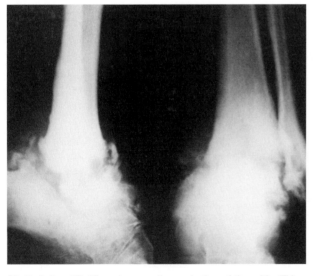

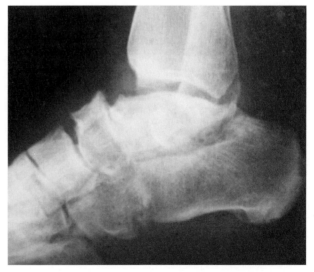

46. *Pathology* (5): There is gross disorganisation of the ankle. This is a syphilitic neuropathic joint (Charcot's disease).

47. *Pathology* (6): The upper articular surface of the talus is flattened. The bony collapse follows a dislocation of the talus, which although successfully reduced, has been complicated by avascular necrosis. The secondary osteoarthritic changes are associated with pain, swelling and stiffness.

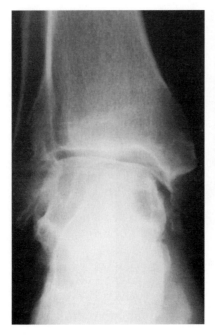

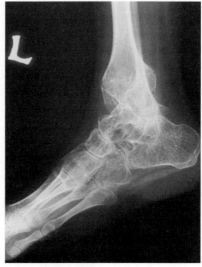

49. *Pathology* (8): Bony ankylosis of the ankle following a chronic infection (TB).

48. *Pathology* (7): Osteoarthritis of the ankle joint. Note the narrowing of the joint space and the rounding of the upper articular surface of the talus (the so-called 'ball and socket' ankle joint of osteoarthritis in the foot).

14. The foot

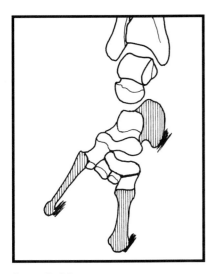

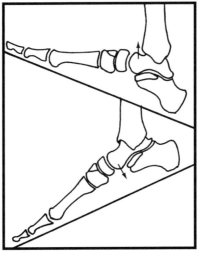

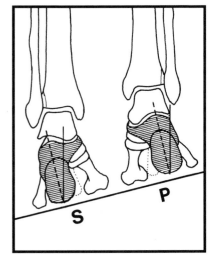

Anatomical features
Fig. 14.A *Tripod action of the foot:* To maintain perfect ground contact, each foot acts as a tripod, with the legs of the tripod being represented by the calcaneus and the heads of the first and fifth metatarsals. To maintain balance, the centre of gravity (in front of S2) must fall within the area covered by one or both feet, and to make this possible each foot must be capable of movement in two planes.

Fig. 14.B *Planes of movement (1): In the X-axis,* nearly all of the movement occurs in the *ankle,* and this allows balance to be maintained when going up and down slopes. (Some very slight movement in the same plane occurs in the mid-tarsal and tarso-metatarsal joints, and minimally in the subtalar joint.)

Fig. 14.C *Planes of movement (2): In the Z-axis,* supination (S) occurs when the soles of the feet are turned inwards to face one another; pronation (P) involves movement in the opposite direction. This allows the feet to adapt to a surface sloping at right angles to the direction of travel. The major part of this movement involves the subtalar joint (but the mid-tarsal and tarso-metatarsal joints are also involved).

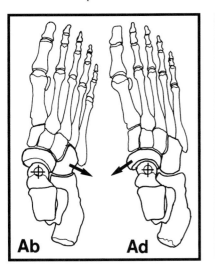

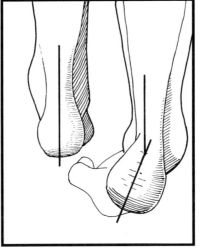

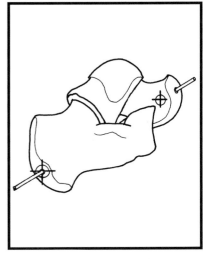

Fig. 14.D *Planes of movement (3): In the Y-axis,* at right angles to the others, a very limited range of abduction and adduction of the forefoot may occur. Most of this occurs in the mid-tarsal joint, but some takes place in the tarso-metatarsal joints and in the ankle. This is of relatively little importance, although a fixed metatarsus adductus is a well-known, self-limiting deformity generally of childhood.

Fig. 14.E *Inversion: Inversion of the heel* occurs when the calcaneus tilts into *varus.* This movement occurs in the subtalar joint. As the heel tilts, it carries the rest of the foot with it (the foot is directly connected to the calcaneus through the calcaneo-cuboid joint), and this results in supination of the foot. (*Valgus* tilting of the heel (eversion) results in *pronation* of the foot.)

Fig. 14.F *Subtalar movements (1):* Movements in the subtalar joint, which involves two pairs of articular surfaces, are highly complex, the only joints which they resemble being those between the radius and ulna. There is, however, a relatively fixed axis of movement which passes through the centre of the head of the talus in front, and through the postero-lateral tubercle of the calcaneus behind.

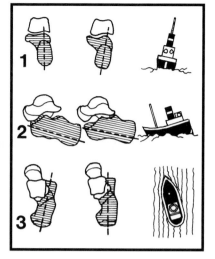

Fig. 14.G *Subtalar movements* (2): The complex pattern of calcaneal movements which occur in inversion are sometimes compared with the three-plane movements of ships or aircraft: the calcaneus rolls (1), pitches (2) and yaws (turns) (3) under the talus.

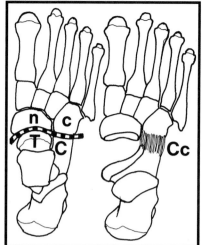

Fig. 14.H *The mid-tarsal joint* (1): This links the hind foot with the mid foot. It is formed by the head of the talus (T) and the navicular (n) on the medial side, and on the lateral by the calcaneus (C) and the cuboid (c). The latter joint (Cc), which permits only a limited range of movements, ensures that when the heel moves, the rest of the foot follows.

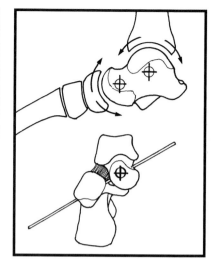

Fig. 14.I *The mid-tarsal joint* (2): The joint has in effect two axes of movement. Firstly, it acts as a hinge allowing slight dorsiflexion and plantar flexion (like the ankle). The axis of this hinge passes through the centre of the head of the talus, so that this movement is coordinated with subtalar movement (which passes through the same point). The plane of this axis is tilted at 45° relative to the horizontal.

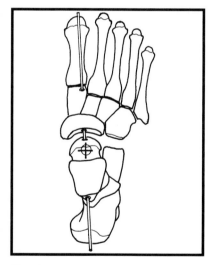

Fig. 14.J *The mid-tarsal joint* (3): In addition to movements in (roughly) the X-axis, a limited amount of pronation and supination (Z-axis) is possible; the navicular slides and rotates round the head of the talus, and the cuboid slides on the calcaneus. This axis of rotation also passes through the centre of the head of the talus.

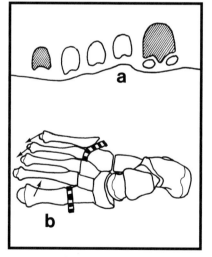

Fig. 14.K *Tarso-metatarsal movements:* (a) While the heads of the first and fifth metatarsals form the anterior limbs of each foot tripod, the other metatarsal heads can adapt to any irregularity in the surface of the ground. (b) Elevation of the first metatarsal head and depression of the others can contribute an appreciable amount to overall supination of the foot (e.g. first tarso-metatarsal movement amounts to 15°).

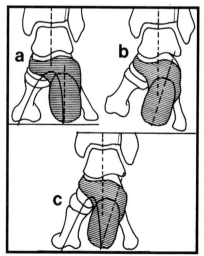

Fig. 14.L *Heel posture* (1): Normally, in the weight-bearing foot the axis of the heel is in alignment with the tibia (a). If the heel posture is abnormal, and tilts into varus, then under normal circumstances the foot would supinate and the first metatarsal head would not contact the ground (b). To correct this, the foot distal to the subtalar joint must pronate, and this leads to accentuation of the medial longitudinal arch (c).

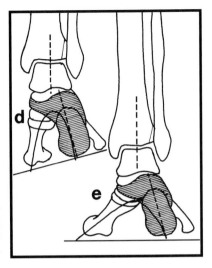

Fig. 14.M *Heel posture* (2): If, on the other hand, the heel posture is one of valgus (d), then to allow all the metatarsal heads to contact the ground the foot distal to the subtalar joint must supinate, leading to flattening of the medial arch (e). The important practical points to note are that *valgus heels are associated with flat foot, and varus heels with pes cavus.*

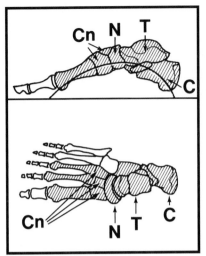

Fig. 14.N *The arches* (1): These are well-known features of the foot. The medial longitudinal arch is the most important, and the one *primarily* affected in pes planus and pes cavus. It is formed by the calcaneus (C), talus (T), navicular (N), cuneiforms (Cn), and medial three metatarsals. Flattening of the arch is common, and is assessed clinically, although weight-bearing lateral radiographs may be helpful.

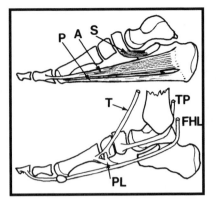

Fig. 14.O *The arches* (2): *The medial arch is supported by the spring ligament (S),* which shoulders the head of the talus; the plantar fascia (P), which acts as a tie; abductor hallucis (A) and flexor digitorum brevis, which act as spring ties; tibialis anterior (T), which lifts the centre of the arch (and with peroneus longus (PL) forms a stirrup-like support for it); tibialis posterior (TP), which adducts the mid-tarsal joint and reinforces the action of the spring ligament; and flexor hallucis longus (FHL), which acts as a long spring tie and helps support the head of the talus.

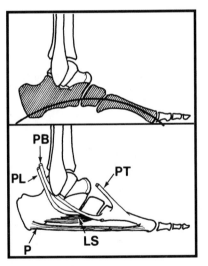

Fig. 14.P *The arches* (3): *The lateral longitudinal arch* is formed by the calcaneus, cuboid, and fourth and fifth metatarsals; it is very shallow, and generally flattens out on weight-bearing. It is supported by the long and short plantar ligaments (LS), the plantar fascia (P), flexor digitorum brevis, flexor and abductor digiti minimi (not shown), peroneus tertius (PT), peroneus brevis (PB) and peroneus longus (PL).

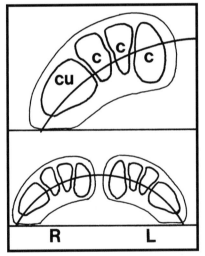

Fig. 14.Q *The arches* (4): *The transverse arch* is formed by the cuneiforms (c) and cuboid (cu). It stretches across the sole in the coronal plane. It is in fact a half-arch: the whole arch is completed with the other foot. It is of no particular clinical significance as its presence and size are precisely related to those of the medial longitudinal arch. The shape of the cuneiforms (likened to voussoirs) helps maintain the arch.

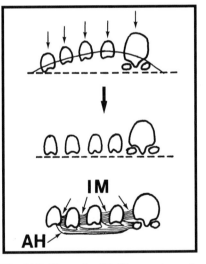

Fig. 14.R *The arches* (5): *The anterior arch* lies in the coronal plane; its bony components constitute the metatarsal heads. It is not a feature of the weight-bearing foot as under load the metatarsal heads flatten out. The metatarsal heads are prevented from spreading out (splaying) by the intermetatarsal ligaments (IM) and the intrinsic muscles, especially the transverse head of adductor hallucis (AH).

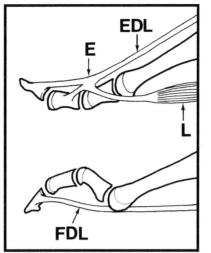

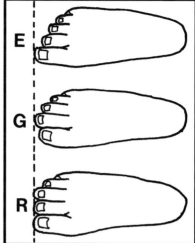

Fig. 14.S *The toes* (1): Extensor digitorum longus (EDL) extends the MP and both IP joints of each toe. The interosseous and lumbrical muscles (L), through their attachment to the extensor expansions (E), extend the toes at the proximal and distal interphalangeal joints, and flex the MP joints; if they become weak or fail, the unchecked pull of flexor digitorum longus (FDL) results in clawing of the toes.

Fig. 14.T *The toes* (2): The relative length of the toes is subject to variation, many of which are regarded as normal. The commonest arrangement is the *Egyptian foot* (E) when the great toe is longest, and the succeeding toes progressively shorter. In the so-called *Greek foot* (G), the second is the longest. In the *rectangular or intermediate foot* (R), the great and second toes (and often the third) are of equal length.

Conditions commencing or seen first in childhood

Talipes equino varus. This is the commonest of the major congenital abnormalities affecting the foot, and all newly born children should be examined to exclude this condition. The deformity is a complex one; characteristically there is a varus deformity of the heel and adduction of the forefoot accompanied by some degree of plantar flexion and supination. Treatment in the form of corrective stretching of the foot and splintage must be started immediately if a good result is to be achieved. In some cases, especially when there is a delay in starting treatment or where there is a failure to respond, simple measures may not be enough. More radical treatments include (a) serial corrective plasters; (b) surgery to release contracted soft tissues (e.g. lengthening of the Achilles tendon and division of the plantar fascia at the heel); (c) procedures which stretch soft tissues and influence bone growth, especially those using the Ilizarov method (this involves the insertion of wires through bony elements in the leg and foot, connecting them with a frame, and repeatedly adjusting their spacing and orientation). In untreated cases the primary anomaly which affects the soft tissues is followed by alteration in tarsal bone growth. In such cases, wedge excision of bone and fusion of the mid-tarsal and subtalar joints is required to obtain a plantigrade foot (Dunn's arthrodesis, triple fusion).

When an incomplete correction has been obtained, the commonest residual deformities seen in the older child and adult are persistent adduction of the forefoot, shortening of the Achilles tendon and some stunting in overall growth of the foot.

Talipes calcaneus. This is a much less common congenital abnormality in which the dorsum of the child's foot lies against the shin. There are frequently associated deformities of the subtalar and mid-tarsal joints, with the heel lying in the varus or valgus position (talipes calcaneo-varus, talipes calcaneo-valgus). This condition is also treated by stretching and splintage as soon as the diagnosis has been made.

Intoeing. After walking has commenced, parents may seek advice because the child is walking with the feet turned inwards (intoeing, hen-toed gait). The feet may be internally rotated to such an extent that the child is constantly tripping and falling. Sometimes this may be due to torsional deformity of the tibiae (which must always be excluded), but more often it is the result of a postural deformity of the hips (internal rotation) or excessive anteversion of the femoral neck. The condition generally corrects spontaneously by the age of 6. Continued observation is advised until correction occurs, but active treatment is seldom required.

Flat foot. The arches of the foot do not start to form until a child starts walking, and they are not fully formed until about the age of 10; *the young child's foot is normally flat*. Nothing is known to speed up the process of arch formation; orthopaedic shoes, heel cups and plastic moulded insoles have all been shown to be valueless. Failure of establishment of the arches is quite rare, but if this occurs it can lead to awkwardness of gait, rapid, uneven wear and distortion of the shoes, but seldom pain or other symptoms. Persistent flat foot may be associated with valgus deformities of the heel, knock knees, torsional deformities of the tibiae, and shortening of the Achilles tendon. Rarely it may result from an abnormal talus (vertical talus), or neuromuscular disorders of the limb (e.g. poliomyelitis, muscular dystrophies). In the older child, gross deformities with a clear organic basis may require surgery, the nature of which is dependent on the pathology (e.g. calcaneal osteotomy for severe valgus heels).

Pes cavus. Abnormally high longitudinal arches are produced by muscle imbalance which disturbs the forces controlling the formation and maintenance of the arches. In many cases there is a varus deformity of the heel and a first metatarsal drop (an increase in the angle between the first metatarsal and the tarsus). Two distinct groups are seen: those in which subtalar mobility is maintained, and those in which subtalar movements are decreased or absent. A neurological abnormality should always be sought, and sometimes this may be obvious (e.g. spastic diplegia or old poliomyelitis). Many cases are associated with spina bifida occulta, which may be confirmed by clinical and radiological examination. Rarely fibrosis of the muscles of the posterior compartment of the leg from ischaemia may be the cause. In the more severe cases there is weakness of the intrinsic muscles of the foot, with clawing of the toes; the abnormal distribution of weight in the foot leads to excessive callus formation under the metatarsal heads and the heel.

When the deformity is marked, surgery is indicated to relieve symptoms and lessen the chances of ultimate skin breakdown under the metatarsal heads. Where there is a varus deformity of the heel, correction of this defect alone may give good results; in some cases a wedge osteotomy of the distal tarsus or metatarsal bases is required to flatten the highly curved arch and improve the weight distribution in the foot. Where clawing of the toes is the most striking finding, proximal interphalangeal joint fusions of the toes or transplanting the flexor into the extensor tendons may be helpful.

Köhler's disease. This is an osteochondritis of the navicular occurring in children between the ages of 3 and 10. Pain of a mild character is centred over the medial side of the foot. Symptoms settle spontaneously over a few months and are not influenced by treatment.

Sever's disease. Chronic pain in the heel in children in the 6–12 age group generally arises from the calcaneal epiphysis which radiologically often shows increased density and fragmentation. The condition is usually referred to as Sever's disease, which although originally considered to be an osteochondritis, is now believed to be due to a traction injury of the Achilles tendon insertion. Symptoms settle spontaneously without treatment.

Conditions affecting the adolescent foot

Hallux valgus. In adolescence, and particularly in girls where there is competition between the rapidly growing foot, tight stockings and often small, high-heeled, unsuitable shoes, valgus deformity of the great toe first appears. In some cases a hereditary short and varus first metatarsal may contribute to the problem. As the deformity progresses, the drifting proximal phalanx of the great toe uncovers the metatarsal head, which presses against the shoe and leads to the formation of a protective bursa (bunion), often associated with recurrent episodes of inflammation (bursitis). The great toe may pronate, and further lateral drift results in crowding of the other toes; the great toe may pass over the second toe or more commonly the second toe may ride over it. The second toe may press against the toe cap of the shoe where there is little room for it, and develop painful calluses. Later it may dislocate at the metatarso-phalangeal joint. The sesamoid bones under the first metatarsal head may sublux laterally, leading to sharply localised pain under the first metatarso-phalangeal joint. In the late stages of the condition, arthritic changes may develop in the metatarso-phalangeal joint. More commonly, there is associated disturbance of the mechanics of the forefoot, leading to anterior metatarsalgia.

A number of surgical procedures are available to correct hallux valgus deformity. The most popular are: (a) fusion of the metatarso-phalangeal joint in a corrected position; (b) Keller's arthroplasty (excision of the prominent part of the metatarsal head and removal of the basal portion of the proximal phalanx); (c) osteotomy of the first metatarsal neck (Mitchell operation); and (d) in early cases, simple excision of the prominent part of the metatarsal head, which may give relief. Silicone replacement of the metatarso-phalangeal joint is not advocated, as it has been found that a silicone granuloma almost invariably develops in the region within 4 years of surgery.

Peroneal (spastic) flat foot. In adolescents (boys in particular), painful flat foot may be found in association with apparent spasm of the peroneal muscles. The foot is held in a fixed, everted position. Inversion of the foot is not permitted, and there is often marked disturbance of gait. The condition is frequently associated with ossification in a congenital cartilaginous bar bridging the calcaneus and navicular (tarsal coalition). This anomaly may be demonstrated radiologically. Surgery, in the form of excision of the bar, is now the normal treatment for this condition.

Exostoses. Apart from the exposure and prominence of the medial side of the first metatarsal head commonly seen in association with hallux valgus (and referred to as a first metatarsal head exostosis), several exostoses may give rise to trouble in adolescence:

1. *Calcaneal exostosis.* Prominence of the calcaneus above and to the sides of the Achilles tendon insertion may cause problems with friction against the counter of the shoe (blisters, calluses, difficulty in shoe-fitting).
2. *Cuneiform exostosis.* An exostosis formed on the dorsum of the foot by arthritic lipping at the margins of the joint between the first metatarsal and medial cuneiform may cause similar difficulties.
3. *Fifth metatarsal head.* Prominence of the fifth metatarsal head may occur and is often associated with a varus deformity of the fifth toe (quinti varus).

All the above conditions are treated by local excision of the prominence.

4. *Fifth metatarsal base.* The base of the fifth metatarsal is sometimes enlarged and unduly prominent, especially in the narrow foot; it may sometimes cause pressure against the shoe, but surgical treatment is seldom required.

Conditions affecting the adult foot

Hallux rigidus. Primary osteoarthritis of the metatarso-phalangeal (MP) joint of the great toe often commences in adolescence and gives rise ultimately to pain and stiffness in this joint. It is commoner in males, and is not associated with hallux valgus. Sometimes the toe is held in a flexed position (hallux flexus), and the proximal phalanx and metatarsal head are thickened following joint narrowing and circumferential exostosis formation. Treatment is usually by fusion or Keller's arthroplasty.

Adult flat foot. Gradual flattening of the medial longitudinal arch (incipient flat foot) may occur in those who spend much of the day on their feet. This is often associated with increase in body weight and the degenerative changes of ageing in the supporting structures of the arch. When these changes are rapid, they give rise to pain ('medial foot strain'). Secondary (tarsal) arthritic changes may also give rise to pain in long-standing flat foot and are associated with loss of movement in the foot (rigid flat foot). Nevertheless, in two-thirds of cases of flat foot, mobility is preserved in the ankle and subtalar joints (flexible or mobile flat foot) and there is no cause for clinical concern, or significant potential for disability. (Ballet dancers and many professional footballers have grotesquely flat feet which do not interfere with their activities.)

In the early stages, incipient flat foot may be helped by weight reduction, physiotherapy and arch supports. In the later stages, surgical shoes with moulded insoles may be the most helpful measure.

Splay foot. Widening of the foot at the level of the metatarsal heads is known as splay foot. This may occur as a variation in the normal pattern of foot growth, causing no difficulty apart from that of obtaining suitable footwear. Splay foot may also be seen in association with metatarsus primus varus, hallux valgus and pes cavus.

Anterior metatarsalgia. In anterior metatarsalgia there is complaint of pain under the metatarsal heads. The condition is particularly common in the middle-aged woman and is also often associated with some splaying of the forefoot. Symptoms may be triggered off by periods of excessive standing or increase in weight, and there is often a concurrent flattening of the medial longitudinal arch. Weakness of the intrinsic muscles is usually present, so that there is a tendency to clawing of the toes; hyperextension of the toes at the MP joints leads to exposure of the plantar surfaces of the metatarsal heads, which give high spots of pressure against the underlying skin. In turn this produces pain and callus formation in the sole.

This pathological process is by far the commonest cause of forefoot pain, but in every case March fracture, Freiberg's disease, plantar digital neuroma and verruca pedis should be excluded.

The majority of cases of anterior metatarsalgia respond to skilled chiropodial measures, which may include trimming of calluses and provision of supports — these distribute the weight-bearing loads more evenly on the metatarsal heads. Where there is much splaying of the forefoot and associated toe deformities, surgical shoes may be required. Where there is a marked hallux valgus deformity, an MP joint fusion may improve the mechanics of the forefoot with relief of pain.

March fracture. This occurs in young adults and involves the second or less commonly the third or fourth metatarsals. The fracture usually follows a period of unaccustomed activity (there is no history of injury) and pain settles after 5–6 weeks when the fracture unites.

Freiberg's disease. This is an osteochondritis of the second metatarsal head associated with palpable deformity and pain. Pain may persist for 1–2 years and in severe cases excision of the metatarsal head may become necessary. Excellent results have also been claimed for a dorsiflexion osteotomy of metatarsal neck.

Plantar (digital) neuroma (Morton's metatarsalgia). A neuroma situated on one of the plantar digital nerves just prior to its bifurcation at one of the toe clefts may give rise to piercing pain in the foot. It most commonly affects the plantar nerve running between the third and fourth metatarsal heads to the third web space, but any of the digital nerves may be affected. It most commonly occurs in women, particularly in the 25–45 age group, and is treated by excision of the affected nerve.

Verruca pedis (plantar wart). Verrucae, thought to be viral in origin, are common in the metatarsal region, the great toe and the heel. They must be differentiated from calluses, and are most frequently treated by the careful application of caustic preparations such as salicylic acid, acetic acid and carbon dioxide snow.

Plantar fasciitis. Pain in the heel is a common complaint in the middle-aged and may be due to tearing of the calcaneal attachment of the plantar fascia following degenerative changes in its structure. Treatment is by the use of Sorbo-rubber pads in the heel of the shoe, physiotherapy in the form of ultrasound, or by the local infiltration of hydrocortisone.

Mallet toe, hammer toe, claw toe, curly toe. In a *mallet* toe, there is a fixed flexion deformity of the distal interphalangeal joint of the toe. In a *hammer* toe there is a fixed flexion deformity of the proximal interphalangeal joint of a toe: the distal IP and MP joints are extended. In a *claw* toe both interphalangeal joints are flexed, and the MP joint extended. In a *curly* toe, all three joints are flexed. All may develop corns where the deformed toe presses against the footwear. Treatment may be conservative, by local chiropodial measures, or surgical, by means of interphalangeal joint fusions or occasionally in the case of mallet toe, by amputation. Simultaneous correction of an accompanying hallux valgus deformity may be required if a straightened second hammer toe is prevented from lying correctly because of the position of the hallux. Multiple clawed toes seen in association with pes cavus may be treated by IP joint fusions and flexor/extensor tendon transfers.

The nail of the great toe. Ingrowing of the great toe nail gives rise to pain and a tendency to recurrent infection at the nail fold. If infection is not a problem, skilled chiropody treatment (e.g. by nail training using a prosthetic device) is usually successful.

Where infection is marked, avulsion of the nail to permit drainage and healing is often required. In chronic cases, ablation of the nail bed (e.g. by phenolisation) may give a permanent cure.

Gross thickening and deformity of the nail (onychogryphosis) may also be treated by ablation of the nail bed or by regular chiropody.

Subungual exostosis, often a source of great pain, is treated by surgical removal of the exostosis.

Deformities of the nails may result from mycelial infections and are very resistant to treatment.

Irregularity of nail growth is a common feature of psoriasis and is usually associated with skin lesions elsewhere. There may be an accompanying psoriatic arthritis.

Rheumatoid arthritis. The foot is commonly involved in rheumatoid arthritis and the deformities are often multiple and severe. They frequently include pes planus, splay foot, hallux valgus, clawing of the toes and subluxation of the toes at the MP joints. Anterior metatarsalgia is often marked. Sometimes a single deformity, such as a hammer toe, may be the main source of the patient's symptoms and may be amenable to a simple local surgical procedure. Where there are many deformities, the prescription of surgical shoes with moulded insoles may be the best treatment. Where there is gross crippling deformity, Fowler's operation, which is an arthroplasty of all the metatarso-phalangeal joints combined with a plastic reconstruction of the metatarsal weight-bearing pad, is often helpful in the older patient; the best results may be obtained when the procedure is combined with fusion of the first MP joint.

Gout. Gout classically affects the MP joint of the great toe, but in severe cases the other MP joints and even the tarsal joints are involved in the arthritic process. The treatment is mainly medical but surgical footwear may be required.

Tarsal tunnel syndrome. The posterior tibial nerve may become compressed as it passes beneath the flexor retinaculum into the sole of the foot, giving rise to paraesthesia and burning pain in the sole of the foot and in the toes. The condition is uncommon, but is relieved by division of the flexor retinaculum. The superficial peroneal nerve may also be compressed as it runs under the extensor retinaculum on the dorsum of the foot, giving paraesthesia in the area of its distribution.

Diagnosis of foot complaints

The following table lists the commonest disorders and relates them to the age groups in which they have the highest incidence.

Table 14.1

	Heel pain	*Pain on dorsal and medial side of foot*	*Great toe pain*	*Forefoot pain*
Children	Sever's disease	Köhler's disease	Tight shoes and stockings; Ingrowing toe nail;	Verruca pedis
Adolescents	Calcaneal exostosis; Bursitis	Cuneiform exostosis; Peroneal flat foot	Early hallux rigidus; Bunion	March fracture; Freiberg's disease
			Hallux valgus, nail problems	Pes cavus; Verruca pedis
Adults	Plantar fasciitis	Flat foot	Hallux valgus and bunion	Anterior metatarsalgia; Plantar neuroma
		Osteoarthritis		
		Rheumatoid arthritis	Hallux rigidus	Pes cavus
			Gout, nail problems	Rheumatoid arthritis; Gout; Verruca pedis; Tarsal tunnel syndrome

In assessing flat foot and pes cavus, the following table may be helpful:

Table 14.2

	Factors in flat foot	*Factors in pes cavus*
Infants	'Normal foot'	In all age groups, this is due to muscle imbalance often from a neurological disorder, e.g. spastic diplegia, poliomyelitis, Friedreich's ataxia, peroneal muscle atrophy, spina bifida (usually occulta). Many cases are associated with varus heels
	Vertical talus	
Children	Knock knees	
	Valgus heels	
	Neurological disturbance	
	Torsional deformities of the tibia	
Adolescents	Continuation of childhood factors	
	Peroneal flat foot	
Adults	Continuation of childhood factors	
	Overweight, excessive standing	
	Degenerative processes	

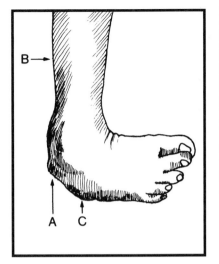

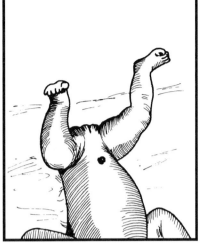

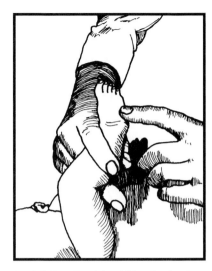

1. *Club foot* (1): *talipes equino varus:* In the untreated case there is (A) persisting varus of the heel; (B) atrophy of the calf muscles; (C) callus where the child walks on the lateral border of the foot. It is commoner in males, may be bilateral, and may be associated with other anomalies.

2. *Club foot* (2): The newborn child often holds the foot in plantar flexion and inversion (giving a false impression of deformity). First observe the child as it kicks to see if this position is maintained.

3. *Club foot* (3): If the child maintains the foot in the inverted position, support the leg and lightly scratch the side of the foot.

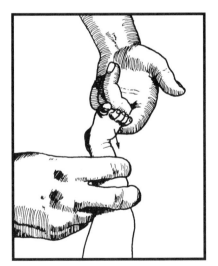

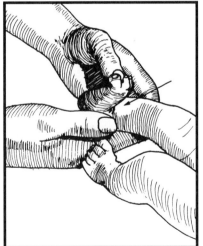

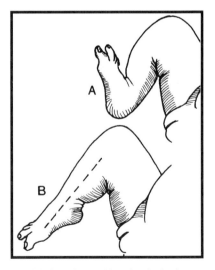

4. *Club foot* (4): In the normal foot the child will respond by dorsiflexion of the foot, eversion, and fanning of the toes. This reaction does not take place if the child has a talipes deformity.

5. *Club foot* (5): If the child does not respond in a normal fashion, gently dorsiflex the foot. In the normal child, the foot can be brought into contact or close to the tibia without effort.

6. *Club foot* (6): (A) Note that in the less common talipes calcaneus deformity, the foot is held in a position of dorsiflexion. (B) Note that in the normal infant the foot can be plantar-flexed to such a degree that the foot and tibia are in line.

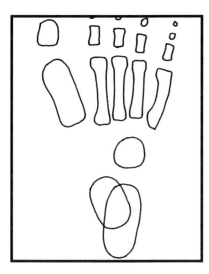

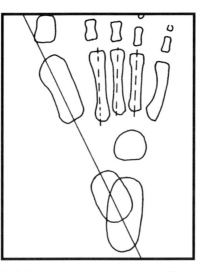

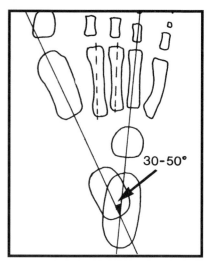

7. *Radiographs: antero-posterior view* (1):
Interpretation is difficult due to the
incompleteness of ossification. Centres for
the talus, calcaneus, metatarsals, phalanges
and often the cuboid are present at birth.
Begin by drawing a line through the long
axis of the talus.

8. *Radiographs: antero-posteror view* (2):
This line normally passes through the first
metatarsal, or lies along its medial edge.
Note also that the axes of the middle three
metatarsals are roughly parallel. Now draw a
second line through the long axis of the
calcaneus.

9. *Radiographs: antero-posterior view* (3):
Note (A) the axial line of the calcaneus
passes through or close to the fourth
metatarsal. (B) The axes of the talus and
calcaneus subtend at an angle of 30–50°
(see 14, 114 for radiographic appearance of
vertical talus).

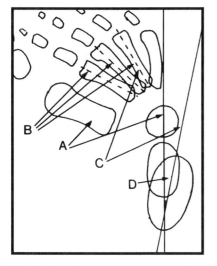

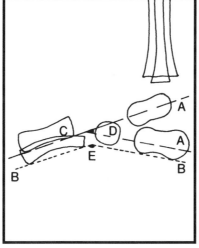

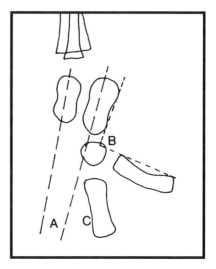

10. *Radiographs: antero-posterior view* (4):
In club foot, the previously described
relations are altered due to forefoot
adduction. Note (A) the talar axis does not
cut the first metatarsal; (B) the middle three
metatarsal axes are not parallel; (C) the
calcaneal axis does not strike the fourth
metatarsal; (D) the angle between the talus
and calcaneus is reduced.

11. *Radiographs: lateral* (1): Draw (A) axes
through talus and calcaneus, and (B)
tangents to the calcaneus and fifth
metatarsal. Note (C) the talar axis passes
below the first metatarsal (at birth); (D) the
interaxial angle is 25–50°; (E) the angle
between the tangents is 150–175°.

12. *Radiographs: lateral* (2): In club foot,
note (A) the talar and calcaneal axes are
nearly parallel; (B) the angle of the tangents
is less obtuse; (C) the talar axis does not
pass below the first metatarsal. Geometric
analysis of the type discussed on this page
may be of help in the doubtful case and in
assessing progress.

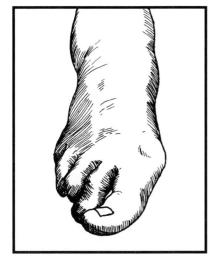

13. *Appearance:* Note the shape of the foot, and the presence of any obvious deformities, abnormal callus formation etc.

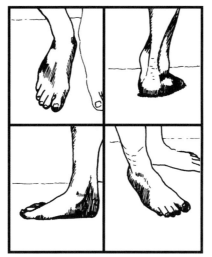

14. *Weight-bearing posture:* Examine the weight-bearing foot, from above, from behind and from the sides.

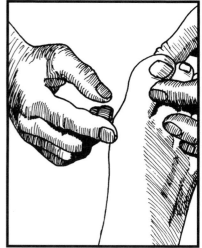

15. *Palpation:* Look for tenderness. Note any joint crepitus. Note any increase or decrease in skin temperature.

The mature foot — summary of key stages in examination (13–18)

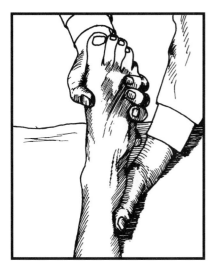

16. *Movements:* Examine the mobility of the toes, foot and ankle.

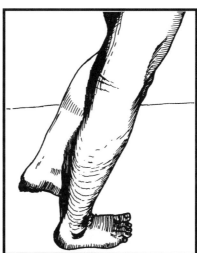

17. *Gait:* Examine the gait, with and without shoes. If indicated, screen the ankles, knees, hips, spine, central nervous system and the circulation. Note the footprint and examine the shoes.

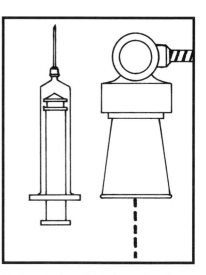

18. *Investigations:* Study the results of special investigations, e.g. radiographs, serum uric acid, sedimentation rate, rheumatoid factor etc.

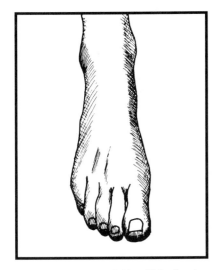

19. *Inspection: general:* Note if the foot is normally proportioned. If not, look at the hands and assess the rest of the skeleton. The feet, for example, are long and thin in Marfan's syndrome (arachnodactyly, spider bones).

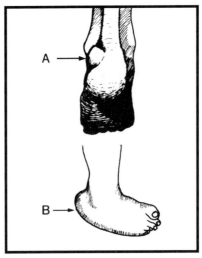

20. *Inspection: heel:* Is there (A) a calcaneal prominence ('calcaneal exostosis') with overlying callus or bursitis? Is there deformity of the heel suggesting old fracture or (B) talipes deformity?

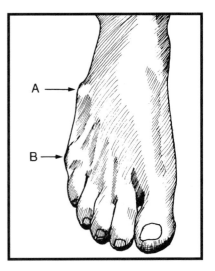

21. *Inspection: dorsum* (1): Is there (A) prominence of the fifth metatarsal base? (B) An 'exostosis' from prominence of the fifth metatarsal head? (Both are sources of local pressure symptoms.)

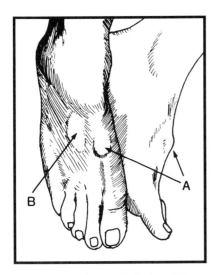

22. *Inspection: dorsum* (2): Is there (A) a cuneiform exostosis? (B) A dorsal ganglion?

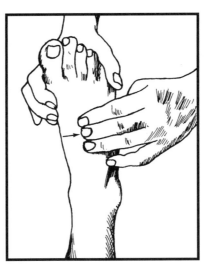

23. *Inspection: dorsum* (3): Note the general state of the skin and nails. If there is any evidence of ischaemia, a full examination is required. In all cases, the presence of the dorsalis pedis pulse should be sought routinely.

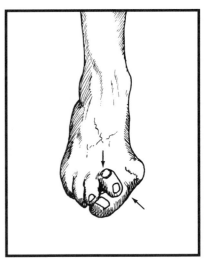

24. *Inspection: great toe* (1): Note any hallux valgus deformity. If the deformity is severe, the great toe may under- or override the second, and it may pronate. The second toe may sublux at the MP joint. Always re-assess any valgus deformity with the foot weight-bearing.

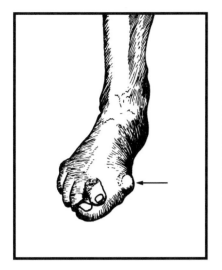

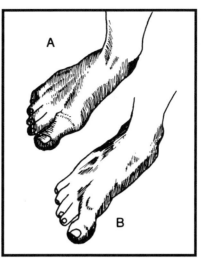

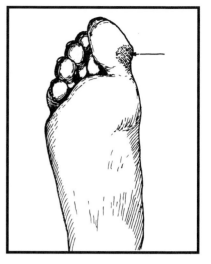

25. *Inspection: great toe* (2): Note the presence of any bursa over the MP joint (bunion) and whether active inflammatory changes are present (from friction or infection). Discoloration of the joint with acute tenderness is suggestive of gout.

26. *Inspection: great toe* (3): Note if (A) the great toe is thickened at the MP joint, suggesting hallux rigidus (osteoarthritis of the first metatarso-phalangeal joint), or (B) held in a flexed position (hallux flexus), again generally due to osteoarthritis.

27. *Inspection: great toe* (4): Note the presence of excess callus under the great toe. This is suggestive of hallux rigidus.

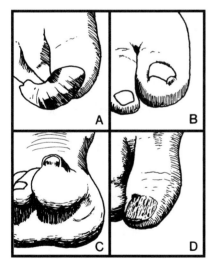

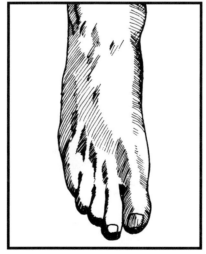

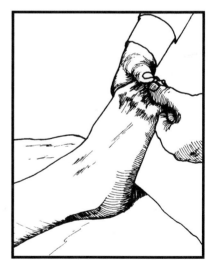

28. *Inspection: great toe nail:* Note if the great toe nail is (A) deformed (onychogryphosis); (B) ingrowing, possibly with accompanying inflammation; (C) elevated (suggesting subungual exostosis); (D) of uneven texture and growth (suggesting fungal infection or psoriasis).

29. *Inspection: toes* (1): Note the relative lengths of the toes. A second toe longer than the first may occasionally become clawed or throw additional stresses on its MP joint.

30. *Inspection: toes* (2): Flex the toes and note the relative lengths of the metatarsals. Abnormally short first or fifth metatarsals are a potential cause of forefoot imbalance and pain. When both are short, there is often painful callus under the second metatarsal.

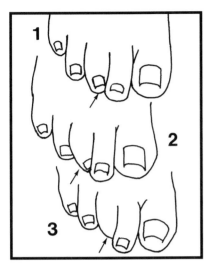

31. *Inspection: toes* (3): *curly toe:* In this deformity a degree of fixed flexion develops in both IP joints and the MP joint. It is generally caused by interosseous muscle weakness. In *grade 1*, the toe is mildly flexed, with or without some adduction; in *grade 2*, there is a degree of under- or overriding; and in *grade 3*, the nail is not visible from the dorsum.

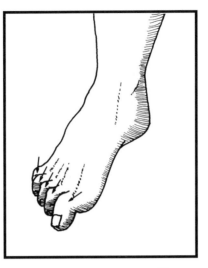

32. *Inspection: toes* (4): *claw toes:* The toes are said to be clawed when they are extended at the metatarso-phalangeal joints and flexed at the interphalangeal joints. If all the toes are involved, this suggests that there may be an associated pes cavus, or some other cause of intrinsic muscle insufficiency (the lumbricals and interossei flex the MP joints and extend the IP joints).

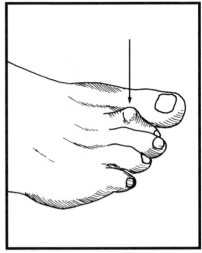

33. *Inspection: toes* (5): Is there a *hammer toe* deformity, where the toe is flexed at the proximal interphalangeal joint and extended at the MP and distal IP joint? The second toe is most commonly affected, often due to an associated hallux valgus deformity. There is usually callus over the prominent interphalangeal joint from shoe pressure.

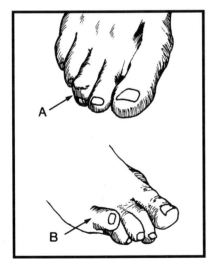

34. *Inspection: toes* (6): Note the presence of (A) a mallet toe deformity (flexion deformity of the distal interphalangeal joint). There is usually callus under the tip of the toe or deformity of the nail; (B) an overlapping fifth toe or quinti varus deformity (often congenital).

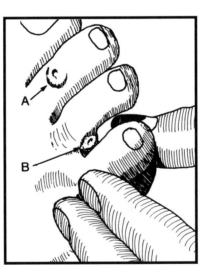

35. *Inspection: toes* (7): Note the presence of (A) *hard corns*. These are areas of hyperkeratosis which occur over bony prominences, and are generally caused by pressure against the shoes. (B) *Soft corns* are macerated hyperkeratotic lesions occurring between the toes and are not associated with pressure or friction.

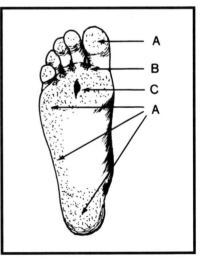

36. *Inspection: sole* (1): Note (A) hyperidrosis; (B) evidence of fungal infection or athlete's foot; (C) ulceration of sole suggesting pes cavus or neurological disturbance.

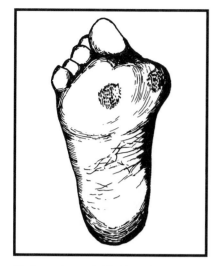

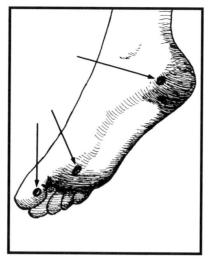

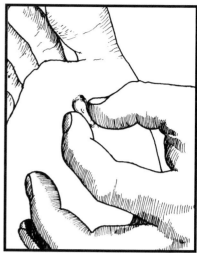

37. *Inspection: sole* (2): Note the presence of callus, indicating uneven or restricted areas of weight-bearing. Be careful to distinguish between abnormal, local thickening, and diffuse, moderate thickening at the heel and under the metatarsal heads (which is normal).

38. *Inspection: sole* (3): Note the presence of a verruca (plantar wart). Note the three classical sites at the heel, under the great toe, and in the forefoot in the region of the metatarsal heads. In the sole they are situated *between* the metatarsal heads; unlike calluses, they *do not occur in pressure areas.*

39. *Inspection: sole* (4): *verruca ctd.* A verruca is exquisitely sensitive to side-to-side pressure. Calluses are much less sensitive, and only to direct pressure. A magnifying lens may be used to confirm the central papillomatous structure of the verruca if there is any remaining doubt.

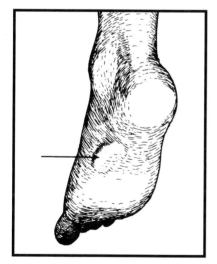

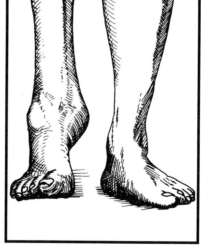

40. *Inspection: sole* (5): Note any localised fibrous tissue masses in the sole typical of Dupuytren's contracture of the feet. These tissue thickenings arise from the plantar fascia, and are attached to the skin. Always inspect the hands, as both upper and lower limbs are often involved together in this process.

41. *Posture* (1): Examine the patient standing. Are both the heel and forefoot squarely on the floor (plantigrade foot)? If the heel does not touch the ground, examine for shortening of the leg (see 10, 5) or shortening of the tendo calcaneus (see 13, 19).

42. *Posture* (2): *intoeing:* If this deformity is present, examine for (A) torsional deformity of the tibia (see 12, 6), (B) increased internal rotation of the hips (see 10, 45), or (C) adduction of the forefoot. Most cases of intoeing in children resolve spontaneously by age 6.

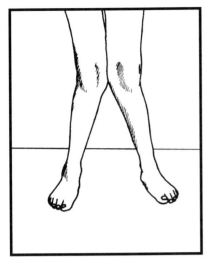

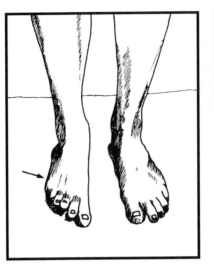

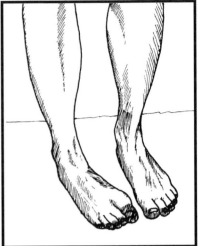

43. *Posture* (3): *genu valgum:* Note the presence of genu valgum, which is frequently associated with valgus flat foot (see 11, 41). Genu valgum in turn is most commonly seen as a result of a growth disturbance about the knee, or as a complication of rheumatoid arthritis.

44. *Posture* (4): *eversion:* If the foot is everted, this suggest (A) peroneal spastic flat foot, (B) a painful lesion on the lateral side of the foot, or (C) if less marked, pes planus.

45. *Posture* (5): *inversion:* If the foot is inverted, this suggests (A) muscle imbalance from stroke or other neurological disorder, (B) hallux flexus or rigidus, (C) pes cavus, (D) residual talipes deformity, or (E) painful condition of the forefoot.

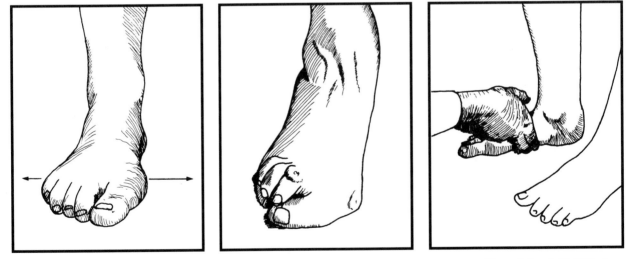

46. *Posture* (6): *splaying:* Note if there is broadening of the forefoot. This is often the result of intrinsic muscle weakness, and may be associated with pes cavus, callus under the metatarsal heads, hallux valgus, anterior metatarsalgia and trouble with shoe-fitting.

47. *Posture* (7): *the toes:* Re-assess the toes for curling, clawing, mallet toes and hammer toes. Re-assess the great toe, particularly for the degree of hallux valgus and overriding of adjacent toe(s).

48. *Posture* (8): *medial arch* (1): With the patient weight-bearing, look at the medial longitudinal arch and try to assess its height. Try to slip the fingers under the navicular. In pes cavus, the fingers may penetrate a distance of 2 cm or more from a vertical line dropped from the medial edge of the foot.

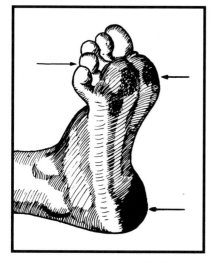

49. *Posture (9): medial arch (2):* If the arch appears high and accentuated, this suggests a degree of pes cavus. Look for confirmatory clawing of the toes, callus or ulceration under the metatarsal heads, and alteration of the footprint.

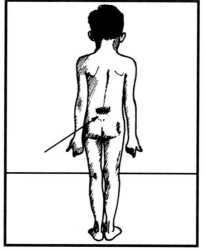

50. *Posture (10): medial arch (3):* If *pes cavus* is present, carry out a full neurological examination. Look at the lumbar spine for dimpling of the skin, a hairy patch or pigmentation suggesting spina bifida or neurofibromatosis. Radiography of the lumbar spine is desirable.

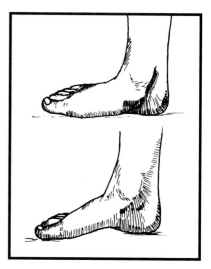

51. *Posture (11): medial arch (4):* In *pes planus*, the medial arch is obliterated. The navicular is often prominent, and the fingers cannot be inserted under it. Ask the patient to attempt to arch the foot. In mobile flat foot the arch can often be restored voluntarily.

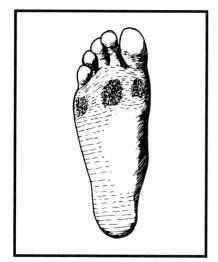

52. *Posture (12): medial arch (5):* If pes planus is suspected, re-examine the sole for confirmatory evidence of callus under the metatarsal heads, and an increase in the area of the sole involved in weight-bearing (i.e. extension of the narrow lateral strip). The footprint will be abnormal in these circumstances. Note also the presence of any knock-knee deformity.

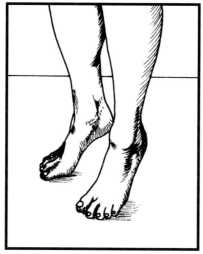

53. *Posture (13): medial arch (6):* In pes planus, assess the mobility of the foot first by asking the patient to stand on the toes, while at the same time examining the alteration in the shape of the foot by sight and feel. Later in the examination carefully note the range of inversion and eversion.

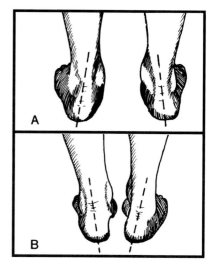

54. *Posture (14): heel (1):* Look at the foot from behind, paying particular attention to the slope of the heels. Note (A) valgus heels are associated with pes planus; (B) varus heels are associated with pes cavus.

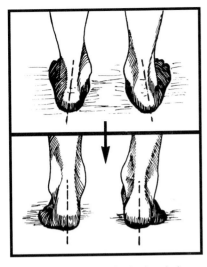

55. *Posture* (15): *heel* (2): Again ask the patient to stand on the toes, observing the heels. If the heel posture corrects, this indicates a mobile subtalar joint. Where the heel is valgus it may suggest shortening of the tendo calcaneus.

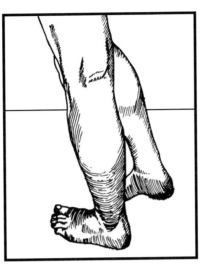

56. *Gait:* Watch the patient walking, first bare-footed and then in shoes, to assess the gait. Examine from behind, from in front and from the side. A child should also be made to run. A reluctant child can usually be coaxed to walk holding its mother's hand. Highly technical, specialised methods are available using force plates, videoanalysis etc.

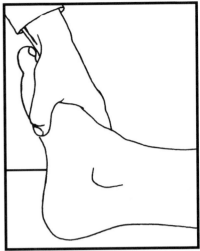

57. *Skin temperature:* Grasp the foot and assess the skin temperature, comparing one side with other. Take into account the effects of local bandaging and the ambient temperature. A warm foot is particularly suggestive of rheumatoid arthritis or gout.

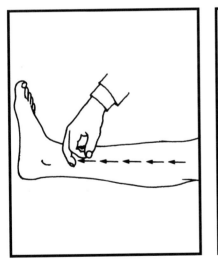

58. *Circulation* (1): If the foot is cold, note the skin temperature gradient along the length of the limb. You should have already observed any trophic changes or discoloration of the skin suggestive of ischaemia.

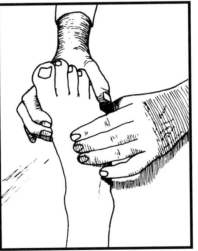

59. *Circulation* (2): Attempt to palpate the dorsalis pedis artery. The vessel lies just lateral to the tendon of extensor hallucis longus and its pulsation should be felt against the middle cuneiform. A good pulse is against any significant degree of ischaemia.

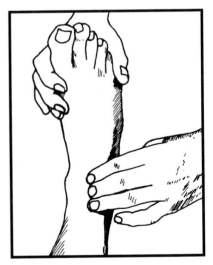

60. *Circulation* (3): Now try to feel the anterior tibial pulse near the midline of the ankle just above the joint line, where the vessel crosses the distal end of the tibia.

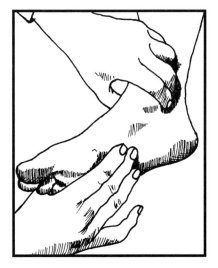

61. *Circulation* (4): The posterior tibial artery is often difficult to find, and it is helpful to invert the foot while palpating behind the medial malleolus.

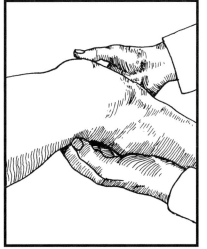

62. *Circulation* (5): Next seek the popliteal artery. When the patient is supine it can only be felt by applying strong pressure in an anterior direction, with the knee flexed, to force the vessel against the femoral condyles. Alternatively, it may be sought with the patient prone.

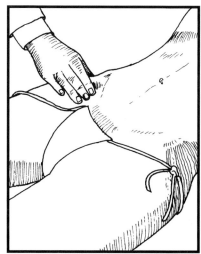

63. *Circulation* (6): The femoral pulse may be felt a little to the medial side of the midpoint of the groin, when the artery can be compressed against the superior pubic ramus.

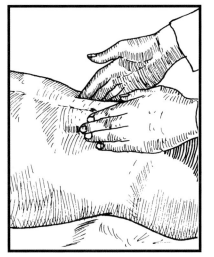

64. *Circulation* (7): Examine the abdomen, palpating the abdominal aorta. Note the presence of pulsation as it is compressed against the lumbar spine, and note any evidence of aneurysmal dilatation.

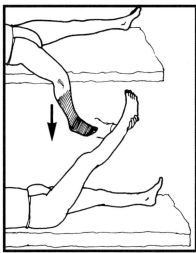

65. *Circulation* (8): Note any cyanosis of the foot when dependent and blanching on elevation suggestive of marked arterial insufficiency.

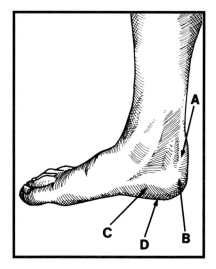

66. *Tenderness* (1): *heel:* Tenderness round the heel is present in (A) Sever's disease; (B) superior calcaneal exostosis and tendo calcaneus bursitis; (C) plantar fasciitis and inferior calcaneal exostosis; (D) pes cavus.

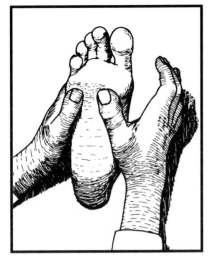

67. *Tenderness* (2): *forefoot* (1): Diffuse tenderness under all the metatarsal heads is common in (A) anterior metatarsalgia; (B) pes cavus and pes planus; (C) gout and rheumatoid arthritis.

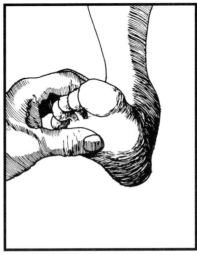

68. *Tenderness* (3): *forefoot* (2): Tenderness *under* the second metatarsal head and *over* the second metatarso-phalangeal joint is found when the second toe subluxes as a sequel to hallux valgus or rheumatoid arthritis.

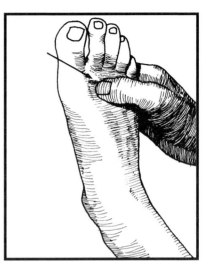

69. *Tenderness* (4): *forefoot* (3): Puffy, localised swelling on the dorsum of the foot, palpable thickening of the second metatarso-phalangeal joint, pain on plantar flexion of the toe, and joint tenderness are diagnostic of *Freiberg's disease.*

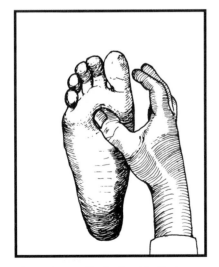

70. *Tenderness* (5): *forefoot* (4): Tenderness on *both* plantar and dorsal surfaces of the second or third metatarsal necks or shafts occurs in March fracture.

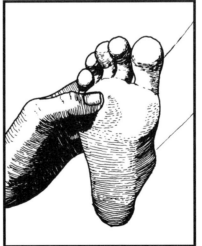

71. *Tenderness* (6): *forefoot* (5): *plantar neuroma* (1): Sharply defined tenderness between the metatarsal heads (most commonly between the third and fourth) is found in *plantar digital neuroma.*

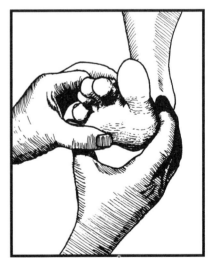

72. *Plantar neuroma* (2): *Morton's metatarsalgia:* Occasionally the neuroma may be felt to move by compressing the metatarsal heads with one hand while simultaneously pressing from the sole towards the dorsal surface and back.

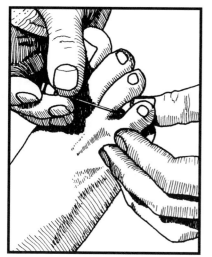

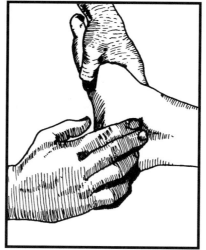

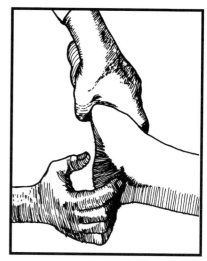

73. *Plantar neuroma* (3): Sometimes the patient complains of paraesthesia in the toes, and sensory impairment should be sought on both sides of the web space involved.

74. *Tenderness* (7): *tarsal tunnel syndrome* (1): Tenderness may occur over the posterior tibial nerve in the tarsal tunnel syndrome.

75. *Tarsal tunnel syndrome* (2): *Tinel's sign:* In the tarsal tunnel syndrome, tapping over the posterior tibial nerve may give rise to paraesthesia in the sole of the foot.

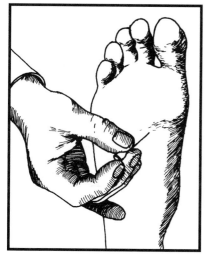

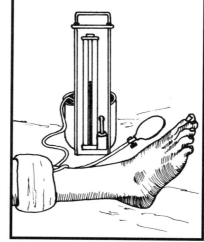

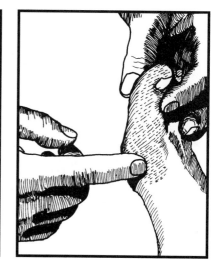

76. *Tarsal tunnel syndrome* (3): Test sensation over the whole of the sole of the foot and the toes in the area of supply of the medial and lateral plantar nerves (the two terminal divisions of the posterior tibial nerve). Compare the feet. Sensory loss is in fact rather uncommon in tarsal tunnel syndrome.

77. *Tarsal tunnel syndrome* (4): In doubtful cases, apply a tourniquet to the calf and inflate to just above the systolic blood pressure. If this brings on the patient's symptoms in 1–2 minutes, the diagnosis is confirmed. Pain and paraesthesia on the *dorsum* of the foot may be encountered in the much rarer *superficial peroneal nerve compression syndrome*.

78. *Tenderness* (8): *great toe* (1): *In gout,* tenderness is often most acute, but is diffusely spread round the whole metatarso-phalangeal joint and often the entire toe. There is often a reddish blue discoloration of the skin round the toe.

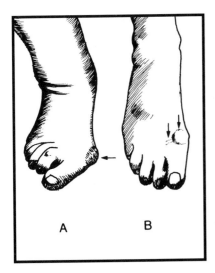

79. *Tenderness* (9): *great toe* (2): (A) *In hallux valgus* tenderness is often absent, or confined to the bunion. (B) *In hallux rigidus* there is usually tenderness over the exostoses which form on the metatarsal head and proximal phalanx, often on the dorsal surface of the joint as well as the lateral side.

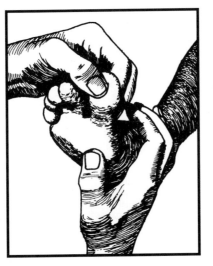

80. *Tenderness* (10): *In sesamoiditis*, there is tenderness over the sesamoid bones which are situated under the first metatarsal head. Pain is produced if the toe is dorsiflexed while pressure is maintained on the sesamoid bones.

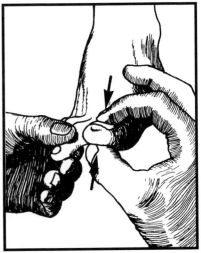

81. *Tenderness* (11): *great toe nail:* In *subungual exostosis*, pain is produced by squeezing the toe in the vertical plane. In *ingrowing toe nail*, pain is produced by side-to-side pressure.

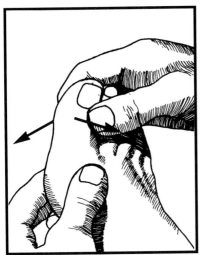

82. *Crepitus:* Move the great toe in an up-and-down direction while palpating the metatarso-phalangeal joint. Repeat with the interphalangeal joint. Crepitus, indicating osteoarthritic change, is constant in the metatarso-phalangeal joint in hallux rigidus. Interphalangeal joint crepitus is considered a contra-indication for MP joint fusion.

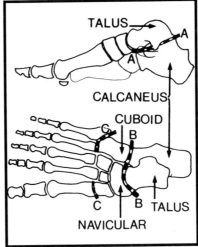

83. *Movements* (1): In assessing foot movements, remember that the total range of supination and pronation in the foot is made up of movements which occur in the subtalar joint (A–A), the mid-tarsal joint (B–B), and the tarso-metatarsal joints (C–C). In the latter, the main movements occur in the joints at the bases of the first, fourth and fifth metatarsals.

84. *Movements* (2): *supination:* Ask the patient to turn the soles of the feet towards one another. The patellae should be vertical. The resulting angle may be measured. If the legs are squarely placed on the couch, its end may be used as a guide. *Normal range: 35° approximately.* Note that this is a summation of movements occurring at the three levels previously described.

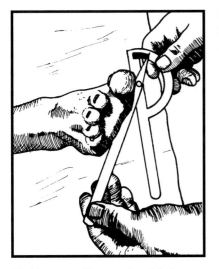

85. *Movements* (3): *pronation:* Ask the patient to turn the feet outwards. The range of movements may be measured in a similar fashion. *Normal range: 20° approximately.*

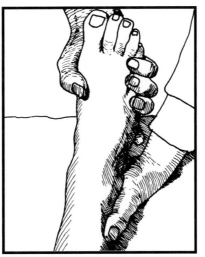

86. *Movements* (4): If supination and pronation are restricted, fix the heel with one hand and with the other assist the patient to repeat these movements. No reduction in the range means a stiff subtalar joint. Presence of some movement shows that the mid-tarsal and tarso-metatarsal joints preserve some mobility.

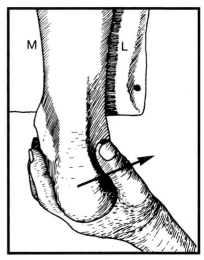

87. *Movements* (5): Turn the patient face down with the feet over the edge of the examination couch. Evert the heel and note the presence of movement in the subtalar joint by the position of the heel. The normal range of eversion of the heel is about 10°.

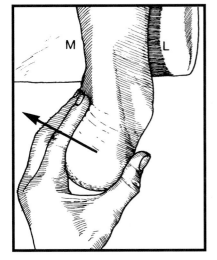

88. *Movements* (6): Repeat, forcing the heel into inversion. The normal range of inversion measurable at the heel is about 20°. Loss of movement indicates a stiff subtalar joint (e.g. old calcaneal fracture, rheumatoid or osteoarthritis, spastic flat foot).

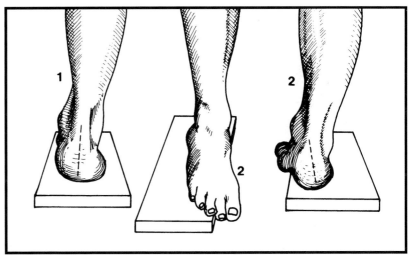

89. *Movements* (7): In idiopathic pes cavus, and pes cavus secondary to neuromuscular disease, the subtalar joint is generally mobile; in pes cavus secondary to congenital talipes equino varus the subtalar joint is often stiff. As a further guide to the differentiation of these cases, mark the axis of the heel with a skin pencil, and note its position with the patient standing on a 2 cm block of wood — first squarely (1), and then with the forefoot over the medial edge (2). A change in the axis (3) indicates a mobile subtalar joint.

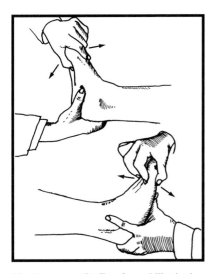

90. *Movements* (8): Test for mobility in the first, fourth and fifth tarso-metatarsal joints by steadying the heel with one hand and attempting to move the metatarsal heads individually in a dorsal and plantar direction.

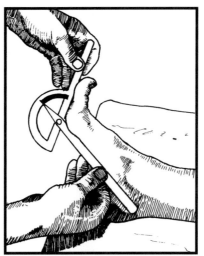

91. *Movements* (9): *great toe* (1): Note the range of extension in the great toe at the metatarso-phalangeal joint. *Normal range: 65°.*

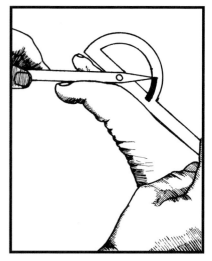

92. *Movements* (10): *great toe* (2): Note the range of flexion at the metatarso-phalangeal joint. *Normal range: 40°.* Metatarso-phalangeal movements are severely restricted and painful in hallux rigidus. There is often little impairment in hallux valgus unless secondary arthritic changes are quite severe.

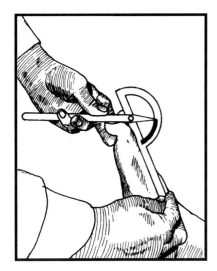

93. *Movements* (11): *great toe* (3): Note the range in the interphalangeal joint. *Normal flexion: 60°. Extension: 0°.* Restriction is common after fractures of the terminal phalanx, and is generally regarded as being a contra-indication to metacarpo-phalangeal joint fusion.

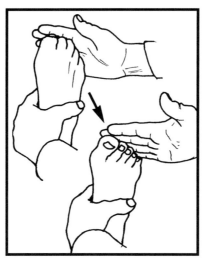

94. *Movements* (12): *toes:* Overall mobility may be roughly assessed by alternately curling and straightening the toes. Accurate measurement of individual ranges is seldom needed. Restriction is often seen in gout, rheumatoid arthritis, Sudeck's atrophy and ischaemic conditions of the foot and leg.

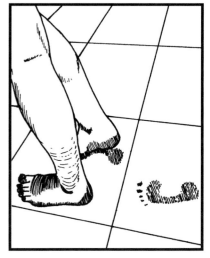

95. *Footprint* (1): It is sometimes helpful to see the pattern of weight distribution in the foot: note the imprint of the sweaty foot on a vinyl floor, or (A) apply olive oil to the sole and dust the imprint with talc, or (B) use ink on paper (or 'fix' on an X-ray plate and develop it). A pedoscope may also be used for this purpose.

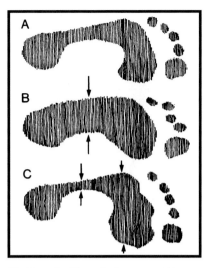

96. *Footprint* (2): *typical patterns:* (A) Normal foot; (B) pes planus: note the increase in area of the central part of sole taking part in weight-bearing; (C) pes cavus: note the decrease in area of contact in the mid-sole and the splaying of the anterior part of the foot. In extreme cases the lateral weight-bearing strip may disappear.

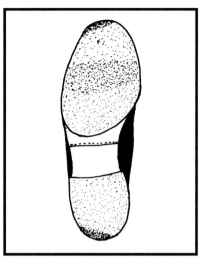

97. *Shoes* (1): The patient's only complaint may be shoe wear. Inspection is expected and may be helpful. In the normal sole wear is fairly even, being maximal across the tread and at the tip (to the lateral side). At the back of the heel, maximum wear is also to the lateral side.

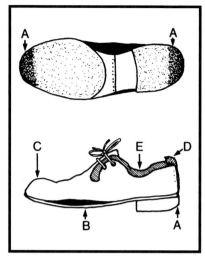

98. *Shoes* (2): *the too-short shoe:* Note (A) excessive wear of the toe and heel. (B) Gap may appear above sole. (C) Toe cap may bulge and inside of shoe may be marked by toes. (D) The heel may give at seam. There may be blistering of the heel, and sock wear. (E) Gap may appear at ankle.

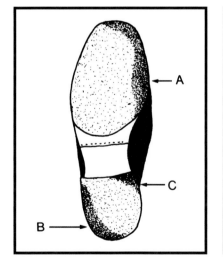

99. *Shoes* (3): *pes planus* (1): (A) Wear on medial side of sole extending to the tip. (B) Wear on outer side of heel. (C) In severe cases, wear on diagonal corner of heel.

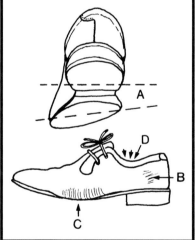

100. *Shoes* (4): *pes planus* (2): (A) Shoe twisted when viewed from behind (heel and sole on different planes). (B) Scuff marks on medial side. (C) The upper bulges over the sole on the medial side. (D) The quarter bulges away from the foot.

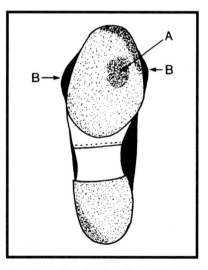

101. *Shoes* (5): *splay foot:* Note (A) Excess wear in the region of the first or second metatarsal heads. (B) The upper bulges over the sole anteriorly.

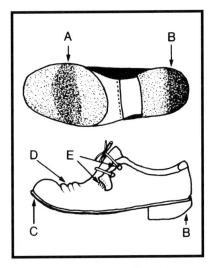

102. *Shoes* (6): *pes cavus:* Note (A) Excessive wear under the metatarsal head region. (B) Excessive wear at back of heel. (C) Raising of toe. (D) Creases. (E) Giving-way of lacings.

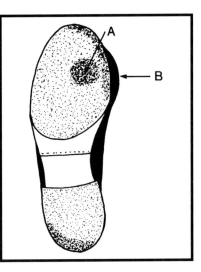

103. *Shoes* (7): *hallux valgus:* There is often (A) excess wear as in splay foot under the area of the first and second metatarsal heads; (B) bulging of upper to accommodate the prominent first metatarsal head.

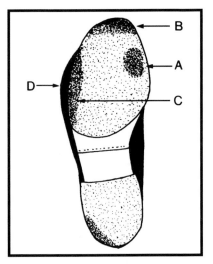

104. *Shoes* (8): *hallux rigidus:* Note (A) excessive wear under the first metatarsal head and (B) at the tip of the sole; (C) excess wear on the lateral side (through walking on the side of the foot); (D) lateral overhang. The toe of the shoe may be up-turned.

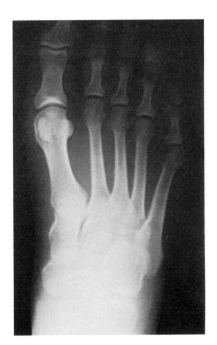

105. *Radiographs* (1): Normal antero-posterior radiograph of the foot.

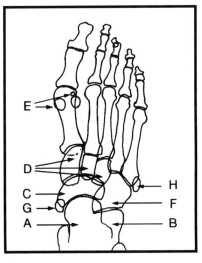

106. *Radiographs* (2): An antero-posterior view is routine, with a lateral or oblique. (A) talus; (B) calcaneus; (C) navicular; (D) cuneiforms; (E) sesamoids (often bi- or tripartite); (F) cuboid. Inconstant accessory bones may be mistaken for fracture or loose bodies, e.g. (G) os tibiale externum; (H) os vesalianum.

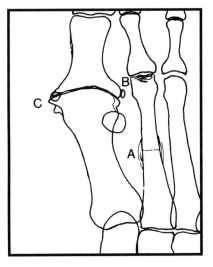

107. *Radiographs* (3): In the antero-posterior view, note bone texture and typical anomalies such as (A) March fracture (periosteal reaction occurs in healing stages); (B) Freiberg's disease; (C) osteoarthritic changes with exostosis formation (hallux rigidus).

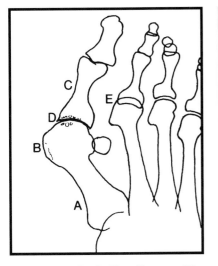

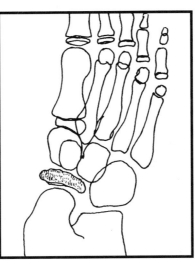

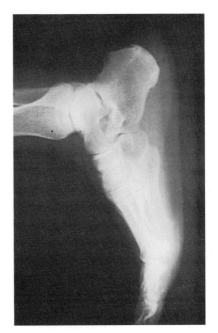

108. *Radiographs* (4): Note, if present, (A) metatarsus primus varus; (B) first metatarsal 'exostosis'; (C) hallux valgus; (D) joint narrowing or cyst formation, suggestive of osteoarthritis, rheumatoid arthritis or gout; (E) metatarso-phalangeal joint subluxation secondary to hallux valgus or to rheumatoid arthritis.

109. *Radiographs* (5): In the child note any increased density of the navicular, suggestive of Köhler's disease. The bone may appear reduced in size.

110. *Radiographs* (6): Normal lateral radiograph of the foot.

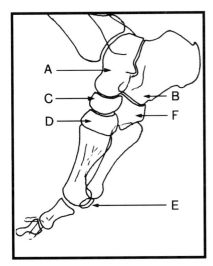

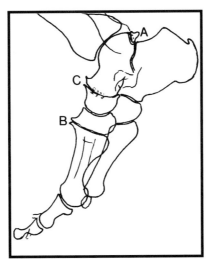

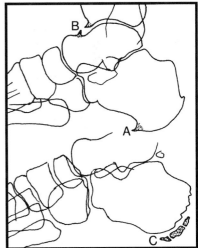

111. *Radiographs* (7): In the lateral radiographs, it is often difficult to trace the outline of individual metatarsals due to superimposition, although the first and fifth are usually quite clear. (A) Talus; (B) calcaneus; (C) navicular; (D) medial cuneiform; (E) sesamoid; (F) cuboid.

112. *Radiographs* (8): Note if present (A) the accessory os trigonum (often mistaken for a fracture); (B) cuneiform exostosis; (C) narrowing of the mid-tarsal joint and other changes suggestive of mid-tarsal rheumatoid or osteoarthritis.

113. *Radiographs* (9): Note if present in the adult (A) calcaneal spur, sometimes associated with plantar fasciitis; (B) footballer's ankle; (C) in the child, increased density and fragmentation of the calcaneal epiphysis, seen in Sever's disease.

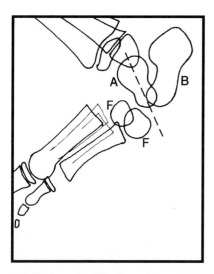

114. *Radiographs* (10): Congenital vertical talus, which is associated with dislocation of the talo-navicular joint, has a classical radiographic appearance. Note the direction of the long axis of the talus. (A) Talus; (B) calcaneus; (F) both centres of ossification in the cuboid.

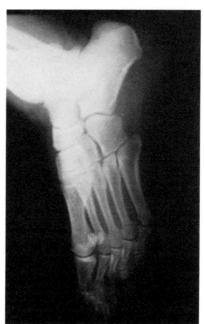

115. *Radiographs* (11): Normal oblique radiograph of the foot.

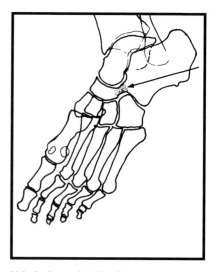

116. *Radiographs* (12): Calcaneo-navicular bar or synostosis (and the commonest of the tarsal coalitions) is best seen in oblique projections of the foot, and is found in association with spastic flat foot.

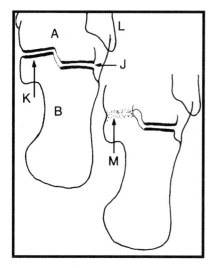

117. *Radiographs* (13): An axial or tangential projection of the heel shows (A) talus, (B) calcaneus, (J) posterior talo-calcaneal joint, (K) sustentaculum tali, (L) base of fifth metatarsal. A talo-calcaneal synostosis, sometimes found in spastic flat foot, may be demonstrated by this view (M).

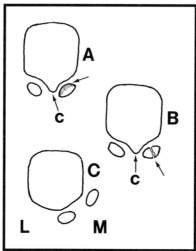

118. *Radiographs* (14): A tangential projection may be used when the sesamoid bones are suspect, showing for example (A) osteochondritic changes, (B) stress fracture, (C) dislocation and loss of the crista (c), seen most commonly in association with advanced hallux valgus.

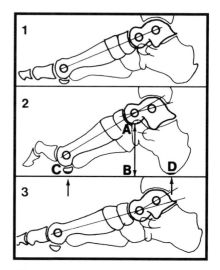

119. *Radiographs* (15): A weight-bearing lateral projection is of value in assessing deformities involving the longitudinal arches and toe. The axes of the talus and first metatarsal normally coincide, and the height of the arch may be assessed by noting the ratio AB/CD. (1) Normal; (2) pes cavus; (3) pes planus.

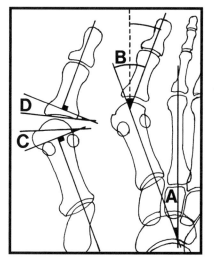

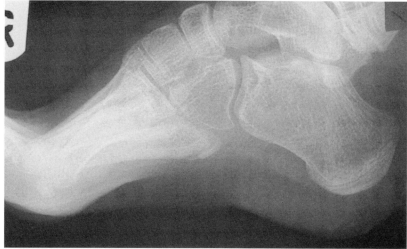

120. *Radiographs* (16): In assessing hallux valgus, note (A) the *intermetatarsal angle* is normally 9° or less — more suggests metatarsus primus varus; (B) the so-called *hallux valgus angle* is normally 16° or less. (*True* valgus of the hallux is B–A.) The normal *distal metatarsal articular* and *proximal phalangeal articular angles* (C & D) are respectively 15° and 5° (or less).

121. *Radiographs of the foot: examples of pathology* (1): Note the accentuation of both the medial and lateral longitudinal arches of the foot typical of pes cavus.

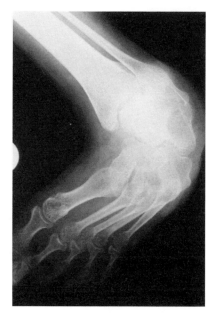

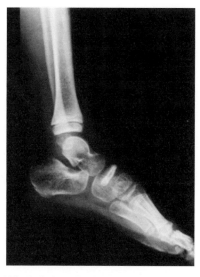

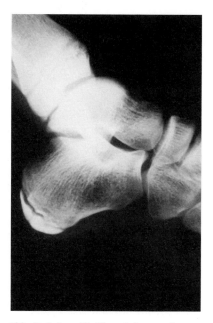

123. *Pathology* (3): There is increased density of the navicular due to Köhler's disease.

122. *Pathology* (2): There is gross deformity of the tarsus as a result of an untreated club foot.

124. *Pathology* (4): There is increased density and fragmentation of the calcaneal epiphysis typical of Sever's disease.

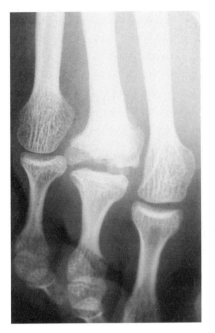

125. *Pathology* (5): There is marked destruction of the second metatarsal head typical of advanced Freiberg's disease.

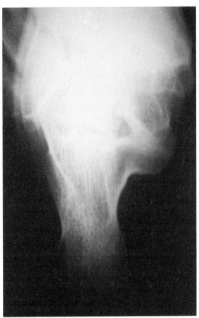

126. *Pathology* (6): This axial (tangential) view of the calcaneus shows a talo-calcaneal synostosis (coalition) in the region of the sustentaculum tali. This was associated clinically with a rigid flat foot.

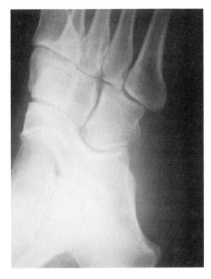

127. *Pathology* (7): This oblique radiograph shows a complete calcaneo-navicular synostosis; this was associated clinically with a spastic flat foot.

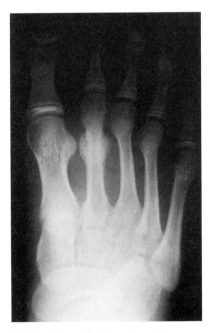

128. *Pathology* (8): There is new bone formation in the second metatarsal shaft typical of a healing March fracture.

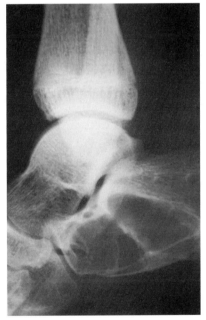

129. *Pathology* (9): There is distortion of the normal architecture of the calcaneus due to the presence of a simple, multilocular bone cyst.

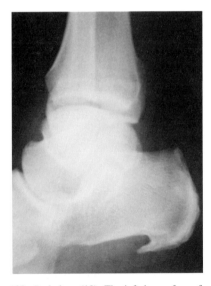

130. *Pathology* (10): The inferior surface of the calcaneus is elongated to form a calcaneal spur. This was found in a case of plantar fasciitis.

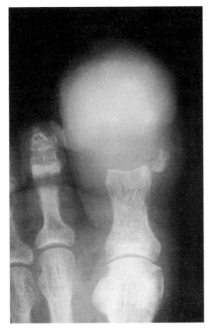

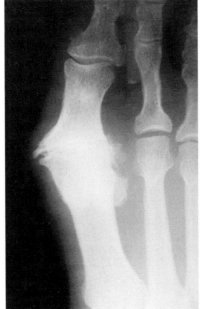

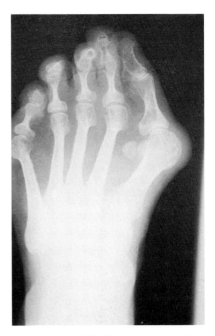

131. *Pathology* (11): The terminal phalanx has virtually disappeared, and there is gross soft tissue swelling of the toe due to a severe nail infection which has spread locally, leading to a destructive osteitis.

132. *Pathology* (12): The metatarso-phalangeal joint of the great toe is narrowed, and there is marked osteoarthritic lipping typical of an advanced hallux rigidus.

133. *Pathology* (13): The first metatarsal is short and medially inclined (metatarsus primus varus). The forefoot is splayed. There is a marked hallux valgus deformity, with pronation of the phalanges.

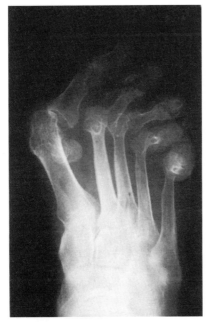

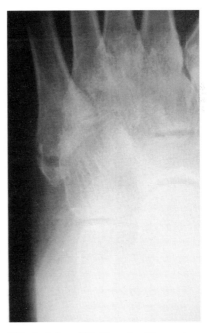

134. *Pathology* (14): As a result of rheumatoid arthritis, there are multiple deformities which include valgus angulations of all the toes. The lesser toes are dislocated at the MP joints.

135. *Pathology* (15): There is widespread decalcification and disturbance of bone texture typical of Sudeck's atrophy (post-traumatic osteodystrophy). This has followed an avulsion fracture (produced by peroneus brevis) of the base of the fifth metatarsal.

Biochemical values

	Serum calcium	Serum phosphate	Alkaline phosphatase	Total acid phosphatase	Remarks
Normal range	2.12–2.62 mmol/litre 8.5–10.5 mg/100 cc	Adults: 0.8–1.4 mmol/litre 2.5–4.3 mg/100 cc Children: 1.3–2.0 mmol/litre 4–6.2 mg/100 cc	Adults: 21–106 IU/litre Children: 21–142 IU/litre Infants: 21–210 IU/litre	2.0–5.5 IU/litre	
Laboratory accuracy	±2%	±2%	±10%	±10%	
Hyperparathyroidism	Raised	Lowered	Raised if bone involved	Normal	
Hypoparathyroidism	Lowered	Raised	Normal	Normal	
Pseudo hypo-parathyroidism	Lowered	Raised	Normal	Normal	
Osteoporosis	Normal	Normal	Normal	Normal	

Osteomalacia	Normal to low	Low	Slight increase	Normal	Ca × PO₄ < 2.25 SI units or 28.0 mg/100 cc units

Condition					
Osteomalacia	Normal to low	Low	Slight increase	Normal	$Ca \times PO_4 < 2.25$ SI units or 28.0 mg/100 cc units
Rickets	Normal to low	Low	Slight increase	Normal	
Paget's disease	Normal, raised in immobilisation	Normal	Raised	Raised	
Uraemic osteodystrophy	Low or normal	Raised	Raised	Normal	
Myelomatosis	Often raised	Normal	Normal	Normal	High ESR
Bone metastases	Normal or raised	Normal or low	Raised	Normal or raised	ESR raised
Sarcoidosis	Often raised	Usually normal	Normal	Normal	ESR raised
Prostatic neoplasm	Normal or raised	Normal or low	Normal or high	Normal or high, raised in 15% of cases without and in 65% with metastases	Prostatic acid phosphatase fraction of total acid phosphatase affected but not in highly malignant undifferentiated tumours

	SI units	*mg/100 cc or μg/100 cc*
Total serum protein	60–80 g/litre	6.0–8.0 mg/100 cc
Albumin	33–50 g/litre	3.3–5.0 mg/100 cc
Globulin	20–35 g/litre	2.0–3.5 mg/100 cc
Bilirubin	5–20 μmol/litre	0.29–1.17 mg/100 cc
Urea	2.5–7.5 mmol/litre	15–45 mg/100 cc
Serum urate	Males:	
	0.13–0.45 mmol/litre	2.2–7.6 mg/100 cc
	Females:	
	0.13–0.35 mmol/litre	2.2–5.9 mg/100 cc
Serum iron	Males:	
	14–32 μmol/litre	78–180 μg/100 cc
	Females:	
	10–30 μmol/litre	56–168 μg/100 cc
Total iron binding capacity (TIBC)	45–70 μmol/litre	250–390 μg/100 cc
Fasting blood glucose	3.3–5.6 mmol/litre	60–100 mg/100 cc
Serum cholesterol	3.6–8.5 mmol/llitre	140–330 mg/100 cc

Index